Percutaneous Vertebroplasty and Kyphoplasty

Second Edition

Percutaneous Vertebroplasty and Kyphoplasty

Second Edition

John M. Mathis, MD, MSc
Professor and Chairman, Department of Radiology, Virginia College of Osteopathic Medicine, Blacksburg, Virginia; Medical Director, Centers for Advanced Imaging, Roanoke, Virginia

Hervé Deramond, MD
Service d'imagerie médicale, Centre Hospitalier Universitaire de Fort de France, Hopital Pierre Zobda-Quitman, Fort de France, France

Stephen M. Belkoff, PhD
Associate Professor, Director, Biomechanical Instrumentation Laboratory, Department of Orthopedic Surgery, Johns Hopkins University, Baltimore, Maryland

Editors

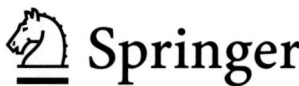

John M. Mathis, MD, MSc
Professor and Chairman
Department of Radiology
Virginia College of Osteopathic
  Medicine
Blacksburg, VA
and
Medical Director
Centers for Advanced Imaging
Roanoke, VA
USA

Hervé Deramond, MD
Service d'imagerie médicale
Centre Hospitalier
  Universitaire de Fort de
  France
Hopital Pierre Zobda-Quitman
Fort de France
France

Stephen M. Belkoff, PhD
Associate Professor
Director
Biomechanical Instrumentation
  Laboratory
Department of Orthopedic
  Surgery
Johns Hopkins University
Baltimore, MD
USA

Library of Congress Control Number: 2005932543

ISBN-10: 0-387-29078-8
ISBN-13: 978-0387-29078-2

Printed on acid-free paper.

© 2006, 2002 Springer Science+Business Media, Inc.
All rights reserved. This work may not be translated or copied in whole or in part without the written permission of the publisher (Springer Science+Business Media, Inc., 233 Spring Street, New York, NY 10013, USA), except for brief excerpts in connection with reviews or scholarly analysis. Use in connection with any form of information storage and retrieval, electronic adaptation, computer software, or by similar or dissimilar methodology now known or hereafter developed is forbidden.
The use in this publication of trade names, trademarks, service marks, and similar terms, even if they are not identified as such, is not to be taken as an expression of opinion as to whether or not they are subject to proprietary rights.
While the advice and information in this book are believed to be true and accurate at the date of going to press, neither the authors nor the editors nor the publisher can accept any legal responsibility for any errors or omissions that may be made. The publisher makes no warranty, express or implied, with respect to the material contained herein.

Printed in China.   (BS/EVB)

9 8 7 6 5 4 3 2 1

springer.com

Preface

Since the first edition of this book was published in 2002, there have been many advances in our knowledge of percutaneous vertoplasty (PV), particularly about how to perform the procedure more safely and how to approach more complex case situations. Additionally, materials that were initially used "off label" or that simply were not FDA approved have completed their governmental review and have received FDA approval. This has increased the legitimacy of the procedure from the legal and reimbursement perspective.

Controversy over height restoration and device selection has become a progressively bigger issue over time. Kyphoplasty (balloon assisted vertebroplasty) has received tremendous emphasis. This book compares and contrasts data and claims that differentiate kyphoplasty from percutaneous vertebroplasty. We also look at other methods that potentially can be used for height restoration.

New procedures that deal with bone augmentation in other anatomic regions have evolved (i.e., sacroplasty) and are discussed. As this revolution in image-guided percutaneous bone augmentation has developed, multiple medical specialties have embraced these procedures in their training programs for both residents and practicing physicians.

All these factors have contributed to the need for an updated edition of the book that encompasses new developments in the field of percutaneous bone augmentation and compares and contrasts the various procedures that are in use world wide. It presents recommendations by national societies that have published "Standards of Practice." Complications, that have become more apparent since the procedures inception, are discussed in detail along with methods for their avoidance. Finally, this edition presents cases that the student or practitioner may likely face and describes the methods used to analyze and treat these various problems.

It has been our pleasure and honor to be associated with the development, dissemination, and investigation of these various procedures and the materials that are used to accomplish the numerous types of image-guided bone augmentations discussed.

John M. Mathis, MD, MSc
Hervé Dermond, MD
Stephen M. Belkoff, PhD

Contents

Preface v
Contributors xi

Section I Basic Science and Techniques

Chapter 1   History and Early Development of Percutaneous
            Vertebroplasty 3
            *John M. Mathis, Stephen M. Belkoff,
            and Hervé Deramond*

Chapter 2   Spine Anatomy 8
            John M. Mathis

Chapter 3   The Medical Management of Bone Health
            and Osteoporosis 33
            Michele F. Bellantoni

Chapter 4   Surgical Options for Vertebral Compression
            Fractures 51
            Aleksandar Curcin and Richard Henrys

Chapter 5   Patient Evaluation and Selection 60
            M.J.B. Stallmeyer and Gregg H. Zoarski

Chapter 6   Biomechanical Considerations 89
            Stephen M. Belkoff

Chapter 7   Percutaneous Vertebroplasty: Procedure
            Technique 112
            John M. Mathis

Chapter 8   Balloon Kyphoplasty and Lordoplasty 134
            Paul F. Heini, René Orler, and Bronek Boszczyk

Chapter 9	Vertebroplasty Versus Kyphoplasty: A Comparison and Contrast *John M. Mathis, A. Orlando Ortiz, and Gregg H. Zoarski*	145
Chapter 10	Tumors *Hervé Deramond, Jacques Chiras, and Anne Cotten*	157
Chapter 11	Extreme Vertebroplasty: Techniques for Treating Difficult Lesions *John D. Barr and John M. Mathis*	185
Chapter 12	Sacroplasty *Keith Kortman, John M. Mathis, and A. Orlando Ortiz*	197
Chapter 13	Complications Associated with Vertebroplasty and Kyphoplasty *John M. Mathis and Hervé Deramond*	210
Chapter 14	Standards for the Performance of Percutaneous Vertebroplasty: American College of Radiology and Society of Interventional Radiology Guidelines	223

Section II Case Studies

Case 1	Single-Level Vertebroplasty and Biopsy *John M. Mathis*	249
Case 2	Multilevel Vertebroplasty *James Ball and John M. Mathis*	255
Case 3	Vertebra with a Cleft or Cavity *John M. Mathis*	259
Case 4	The Mobile Vertebra: Height Restoration *John M. Mathis*	263
Case 5	Extreme Vertebral Collapse *John M. Mathis*	267
Case 6	Anterior Cervical Approach *John D. Barr and John M. Mathis*	272
Case 7	Vertebral Refracture After Percutaneous Vertebroplasty *Jon Kim and John M. Mathis*	277

Case 8	Percutaneous Sacroplasty .... *John M. Mathis*	281
Case 9	Percutaneous Pelvic Augmentation: Supra-Acetabular Region .... *John M. Mathis*	285
Case 10	Kyphoplasty in Osteoporotic Compression Fractures .... *A. Orlando Ortiz and John M. Mathis*	289
Case 11	Femoral Neck Augmentation .... *Paul F. Heini and Torsten Franz*	295
Index	....	299

Contributors

James Ball, MD, Chief of Neuroradiology, Department of Diagnostic Radiology, Florida Hospital Medical Center, Orlando, FL, USA.

John D. Barr, MD, Chief, Interventional Neuroradiology, Department of Radiology, Baptist Memorial Hospital, Memphis, TN, USA.

Stephen M. Belkoff, PhD, Associate Professor, Director, Biomechanical Instrumentation Laboratory, Department of Orthopedic Surgery, Johns Hopkins University, Baltimore, MD, USA.

Michele F. Bellantoni, MD, Associate Professor of Medicine, Division of Geriatric Medicine and Gerontology, Department of Medicine, Johns Hopkins University School of Medicine, Baltimore, MD, USA.

Bronek Boszczyck, MD, Attending, Department of Orthopedic Surgery, University of Bern, Bern, Switzerland.

Jacques Chiras, MD, Professor, Department of Neuroradiology, Groupe Hospitalier Pitie-Salpetriere, Paris, France.

Anne Cotten, MD, Service de Radiologie Osteo-articulaire, Hôpital Roger Salengro, Centre Hospitalier Universitaire de Lille, Lille, France.

Aleksandar Curcin, MD, MBA, Spine Fellowship Director, Department of Orthopedic Surgery, Sinai Hospital of Baltimore, Baltimore, MD, USA.

Hervé Deramond, MD, Service d'imagerie médicale, Centre Hospitalier Universitaire de Fort de France, Hopital Pierre Zobda-Quitman, Fort de France, France.

Torsten Franz, MD, Attending, Department of Orthopedic Surgery, University of Bern, Bern, Switzerland.

Paul F. Heini, PhD, MD, Head, Spine Surgery, Department of Orthopedic Surgery, University of Bern, Bern, Switzerland.

Richard Henrys, MD, Spine Fellow, Department of Orthopedic Surgery, Sinai Hospital of Baltimore, Baltimore, MD, USA.

Jon Kim, MS, Third Year Medical Student, Virginia College of Osteopathic Medicine, Blacksburg, VA, USA.

Keith Kortman, MD, Neuroradiologist, Chief, Department of Radiology, Sharp Memorial Hospital, San Diego, CA, USA.

John M. Mathis, MD, MSc, Professor and Chairman, Department of Radiology, Virginia College of Osteopathic Medicine, Blacksburg, VA; Medical Director, Centers for Advanced Imaging, Roanoke, VA, USA

René Orler, MD, Orthopädische Chirurgie, Universitätsspital Bern, Bern, Switzerland.

A. Orlando Ortiz, MD, MBA, Chairman, Department of Radiology, Winthrop-University Hospital; Professor, Department of Clinical Radiology, Stony Brook University School of Medicine, Mineola, NY, USA.

M.J.B. Stallmeyer, MD, PhD, Assistant Professor, Department of Radiology, University of Maryland School of Medicine, Baltimore, MD, USA.

Gregg H. Zoarski, MD, Director, Diagnostic and Interventional Neuroradiology, Associate Professor, Department of Radiology, University of Maryland School of Medicine, Baltimore, MD, USA.

Section I

Basic Science and Techniques

1
History and Early Development of Percutaneous Vertebroplasty

John M. Mathis, Stephen M. Belkoff, and Hervé Deramond

For several decades, vertebroplasty has been performed as an open procedure to augment the purchase of pedicle screws for spinal instrumentation (1) and to fill voids resulting from tumor resection (2–5). The procedure introduces bone graft or acrylic cement into vertebral bodies to mechanically augment their structural integrity (2–4,6–12). In some cases, however, the risk of an open procedure is not indicated. It was one such case that served as the impetus for the development of percutaneous vertebroplasty (PV). Percutaneous vertebroplasty achieves the benefits of surgical vertebroplasty without the morbidity associated with an open procedure. Vertebral augmentation is accomplished by injecting polymethylmethacrylate (PMMA) cement into a vertebral body via a percutaneously placed cannula.

The procedure was first performed in 1984 by Galibert and Deramond in the Department of Radiology of the University Hospital of Amiens, France (13), on a woman, aged 54, who had complained of severe cervical pain for several years. In 1979, plain radiographs of her cervical spine indicated normal findings, but in 1984, when she presented with unbearable pain associated with a severe radiculopathy localized to the C2 nerve root, plain radiographs showed a large vertebral hemangioma (VH) involving the entire C2 vertebra. An axial computed tomography (CT) scan confirmed epidural extension of the disease. A C2 laminectomy was first performed, and the epidural component was excised. To obtain structural reinforcement of the C2 vertebral body, it was decided that cement would be injected percutaneously. A 15-gauge needle was inserted into the C2 vertebral body via an anterolateral approach (Figure 1.1A). The amount of PMMA injected was estimated to be 3 mL (Figure 1.1B). The patient experienced complete pain relief. The results of the procedure were so impressive that the procedure was subsequently used for six other patients. A report describing the outcomes was published in 1987 (13).

The experience gained from these patients, and from some experimental work conducted on fresh cadaveric vertebral bodies, helped establish the main technical points of the procedure (13–15). These technical points include the use of large-bore (10–13 gauge) needles in the

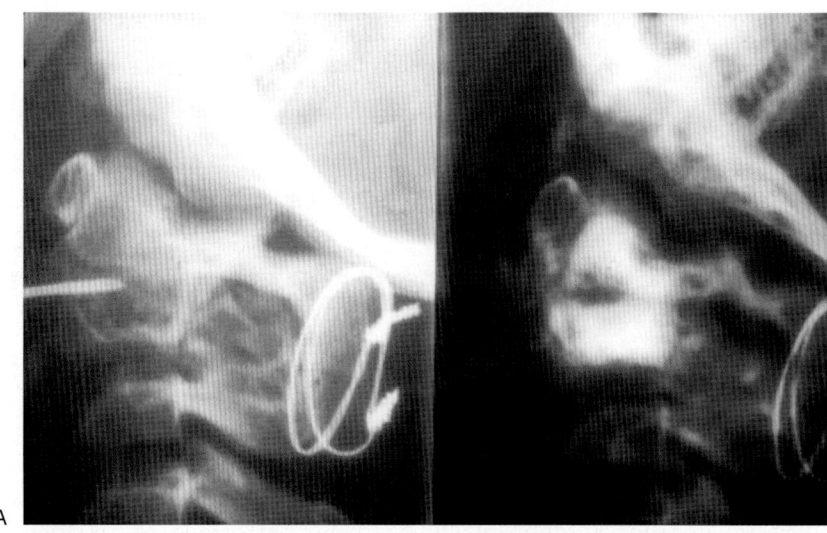

Figure 1.1. The first PV case. **(A)** Lateral view of C2 with a cannula in place in the VH cavity. **(B)** Lateral view of C2 after PMMA injection (white arrows). This resulted in complete pain resolution for this patient. (From JM Mathis, H Deramond, SM Belkoff [eds], Percutaneous Vertebroplasty. New York: Springer, 2002, with permission.)

thoracic and lumbar spine and smaller bore (13–15 gauge) needles in the cervical spine. An opacification agent was added to the PMMA cement to facilitate fluoroscopic visualization of the distribution of the cement during injection. Early in the clinical experience, a posterolateral approach for the needles was used in the thoracic spine, but after cement leakage along the track of the needle induced a case of intercostal radiculopathy, a transpedicular needle approach was developed. With the transpedicular approach, the needle passes through the pedicle into the vertebral body, resulting in a lower risk of cement discharging posteriorly along the needle track.

Inspired by the success of the initial PV cases, clinicians from the neuroradiologic and neurosurgical teams of the University Hospital in Lyons (France) (16,17) used a slightly modified technique (18-gauge needles) to inject PMMA into the weakened vertebral bodies of seven patients: four with osteoporotic vertebral compression fracture (VCFs), two with VHs, and one with spinal metastasis. These clinicians reported good (one patient) to excellent (six patients) pain relief in these seven initial patients (16).

In the early 1990s, PV (performed with Deramond's technique) was introduced into clinical practice in the United States at the University of Virginia (18). Since that time, PV has become a more commonly used method for treating painful vertebral lesions. The European experience has predominantly focused on treating pain related to tumor involvement (both benign and malignant) (13,19–22), whereas the U.S. experience focused on treating painful osteoporotic VCFs. This distinction has become blurred as clinicians on both continents have responded to changing patient demographics (e.g., increased longevity, increased incidence of osteoporosis, and increased numbers of patients surviving cancer—all of whom have higher risks of VCFs). Severe pain associated with VCF is a very common medical problem; it affects between 700,000 and 1,000,000 patients every year in the United States alone (23–25). The disease demographics are similar in Europe. Most of these fractures are the result of bone mineral loss due to primary osteoporosis (occurring progressively with age). However, an increasing number of fractures also result from secondary osteoporosis caused by therapeutic drugs such as catabolic steroids, anticonvulsants, cancer chemotherapy, and heparin (26).

Until the introduction of PV, there were few treatment options other than bed rest and pain management for osteoporotic VCFs. The immediate and lasting pain relief attained with PV is quickly making the procedure an accepted treatment for osteoporotic VCFs and is challenging the standard medical treatment of bed rest and analgesics. Similarly, because patients with metastatic lesions are surviving longer, there is an increased demand to improve their quality of life and provide mobility during the end stages of their disease. In cases of spinal metastases, PV reportedly relieves pain and structurally augments vertebral bodies compromised by osteolytic lesions, providing some palliation and allowing the patient to continue with weight-bearing activities of daily living.

Since the first edition of this book was published, substantial progress has been made in our understanding of the requirements for providing an adequate percutaneous augmentation of a vertebra following VCF. Numerous companies are producing devices and materials to aid in the performance of PV. Bone cements for percutaneous vertebroplasty and kyphoplasty now have Food and Drug Administration approval (in the United States) or have obtained the Conformitè Europèene mark (in Europe). In the United States, reimbursement for PV is available through Medicare and numerous independent insurance carriers. This coverage is now being expanded to allow the procedure to be performed in outpatient offices.

The second edition of this book contains the most current information available on both patient selection and the techniques of the procedures used for percutaneous augmentation of the vertebra and other areas of the skeleton. The book also contains new information on the materials used in the procedures. We have added a section with case reports to show the reader interesting clinical problems and the methods used to solve them. These cases provide practical information to enhance the core didactic chapters, and the result is a complete body of information on how to perform each of these procedures with maximal effectiveness and safety.

References

1. Kostuik JP, Errico TJ, Gleason TF. Techniques of internal fixation for degenerative conditions of the lumbar spine. Clin Orthop 1986; 203:219–231.
2. Cybulski GR. Methods of surgical stabilization for metastatic disease of the spine. Neurosurgery 1989; 25(2):240–252.

3. Alleyne CH, Jr., Rodts GE, Jr., Haid RW. Corpectomy and stabilization with methylmethacrylate in patients with metastatic disease of the spine: a technical note. J Spinal Disord 1995; 8(6):439–443.
4. Sundaresan N, Galicich JH, Lane JM, et al. Treatment of neoplastic epidural cord compression by vertebral body resection and stabilization. J Neurosurg 1985; 63(5):676–684.
5. Scoville WB, Palmer AH, Samra K, et al. The use of acrylic plastic for vertebral replacement or fixation in metastatic disease of the spine. Technical note. J Neurosurg 1967; 27(3):274–279.
6. Cortet B, Cotten A, Deprez X, et al. [Value of vertebroplasty combined with surgical decompression in the treatment of aggressive spinal angioma. Apropos of 3 cases]. Rev Rhum Ed Fr 1994; 61(1):16–22.
7. Harrington KD. Anterior decompression and stabilization of the spine as a treatment for vertebral collapse and spinal cord compression from metastatic malignancy. Clin Orthop 1988; 233:177–197.
8. Harrington KD, Sim FH, Enis JE, et al. Methylmethacrylate as an adjunct in internal fixation of pathological fractures. Experience with three hundred and seventy-five cases. J Bone Joint Surg 1976; 58A(8):1047–1055.
9. Mavian GZ, Okulski CJ. Double fixation of metastatic lesions of the lumbar and cervical vertebral bodies utilizing methylmethacrylate compound: report of a case and review of a series of cases. J Am Osteopath Assoc 1986; 86(3):153–157.
10. O'Donnell RJ, Springfield DS, Motwani HK, et al. Recurrence of giant-cell tumors of the long bones after curettage and packing with cement. J Bone Joint Surg 1994; 76A(12):1827–1833.
11. Persson BM, Ekelund L, Lovdahl R, et al. Favourable results of acrylic cementation for giant cell tumors. Acta Orthop Scand 1984; 55(2):209–214.
12. Knight G. Paraspinal acrylic inlays in the treatment of cervical and lumbar spondylosis and other conditions. Lancet 1959; (ii):147–149.
13. Galibert P, Deramond H, Rosat P, et al. [Preliminary note on the treatment of vertebral angioma by percutaneous acrylic vertebroplasty]. Neurochirurgie 1987; 33(2):166–168.
14. Deramond H, Darrason R, Galibert P. [Percutaneous vertebroplasty with acrylic cement in the treatment of aggressive spinal angiomas]. Rachis 1989; 1(2):143–153.
15. Darrason R. Place de la vertebroplastie percutanee acrylique dans le traitement des hemangiomes vertebraux agressifs. Doctoral Thesis (Medicine). Universite de Picardie, October 26, 1988.
16. Lapras C, Mottolese C, Deruty R, et al. [Percutaneous injection of methylmethacrylate in osteoporosis and severe vertebral osteolysis (Galibert's technic)]. Ann Chir 1989; 43(5):371–376.
17. Bascoulergue Y, Duquesnel J, Leclercq R, et al. Percutaneous injection of methyl methacrylate in the vertebral body for the treatment of various diseases: percutaneous vertebroplasty [abstr]. Radiology 1988; 169P:372.
18. Jensen ME, Evans AJ, Mathis JM, et al. Percutaneous polymethylmethacrylate vertebroplasty in the treatment of osteoporotic vertebral body compression fractures: technical aspects. Am J Neuroradiol 1997; 18(10): 1897–1904.
19. Cotten A, Dewatre F, Cortet B, et al. Percutaneous vertebroplasty for osteolytic metastases and myeloma: effects of the percentage of lesion filling and the leakage of methyl methacrylate at clinical follow-up. Radiology 1996; 200(2):525–530.
20. Kaemmerlen P, Thiesse P, Jonas P, et al. Percutaneous injection of orthopedic cement in metastatic vertebral lesions [letter]. N Engl J Med 1989; 321(2):121.

21. Kaemmerlen P, Thiesse P, Bouvard H, et al. [Percutaneous vertebroplasty in the treatment of metastases. Technic and results]. J Radiol 1989; 70(10): 557–562.
22. Weill A, Chiras J, Simon JM, et al. Spinal metastases: indications for and results of percutaneous injection of acrylic surgical cement. Radiology 1996; 199(1):241–247.
23. Melton LJ, III. Epidemiology of spinal osteoporosis. Spine 1997; 22(24 Suppl):2S–11S.
24. Melton LJ, Kan SH, Wahner HW, et al. Lifetime fracture risk: an approach to hip fracture risk assessment based on bone mineral density and age. J Clin Epidemiol 1988; 41(10):985–994.
25. Kanis JA, Johnell O. The burden of osteoporosis. J Endocrinol Invest 1999; 22(8):583–588.
26. Miller KK, Klibanski A. Clinical review 106: amenorrheic bone loss. J Clin Endocrinol Metab 1999; 84(6):1775–1783.

2
Spine Anatomy

John M. Mathis

Percutaneous vertebroplasty (PV), kyphoplasty (KP), and percutaneous sacroplasty (PS) require accurate localization of the bone region to be treated and careful identification of the trajectory that must be followed for safe device insertion. The normal anatomic structures and pathologic factors that affect the spine must be understood to accomplish this goal. This chapter describes the pertinent anatomy of the spine for these image-guided procedures and discusses how special variations or situations can affect the choice of devices and appropriate needle trajectories.

General Spine Anatomy

The spine is made up of 33 bones: 24 vertebrae consisting of 7 cervical, 12 thoracic, and 5 lumbar elements. The sacrum and coccyx provide unique variations. The sacrum is composed of 5 segments that are fused. The coccyx has 4 segments that are variably fused (1).

The multiple spine segments are joined by intervening discs and structurally augmented by connecting ligaments and muscles. The entire spine is depicted in Figure 2.1A, demonstrating the natural curvature that changes from segment to segment. Viewed from the lateral projection, there is normally lordosis in the cervical and lumbar segments and mild kyphosis in the thoracic and sacral regions. These variations in curvature are important as they affect the orientation of the individual vertebra and critical vertebral components like the pedicles that are commonly used for device access to the vertebral body in PV and KP (Figure 2.1B).

The vertebrae progressively enlarge from the cervical through the lumbar region. There is also variability in vertebra size at any particular level based on the individual's size. For instance, an upper thoracic vertebra in a small woman may have a diameter of only 2–2.5 cm (similar to a U.S. quarter). A large male may have a vertebra at the same level that is one to two times larger. These variations in size affect the initial volume of each vertebra, which will ultimately affect the amount

Chapter 2 Spine Anatomy 9

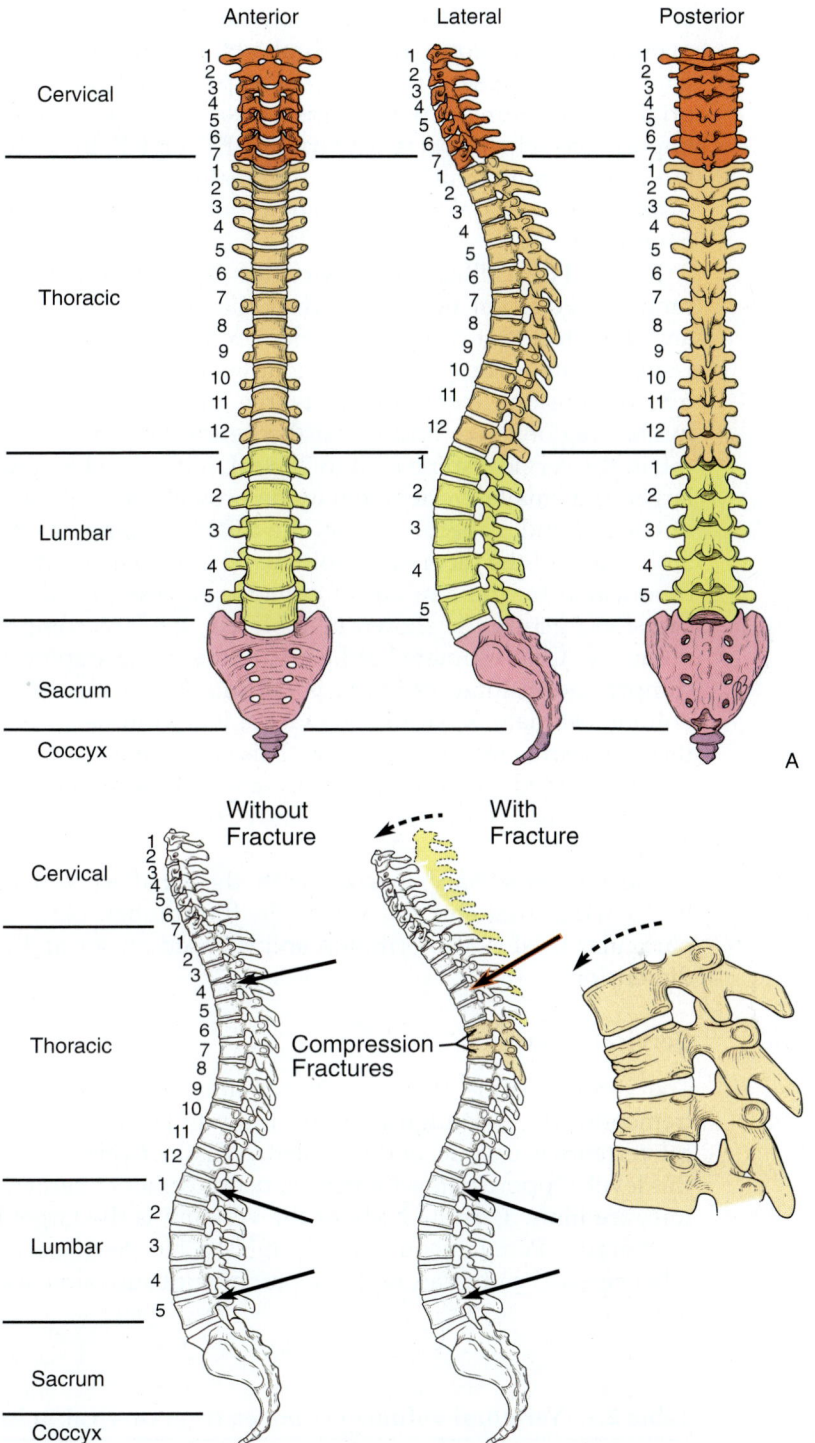

Figure 2.1. (A) AP, lateral and posterior depictions of the entire spine. The lateral view shows the normal lordotic curve found in the cervical and lumbar regions. A kyphotic curve is normal in thoracic and sacral regions. These curves can be modified or accentuated in disease. **(B)** Drawing to show how the usual transpedicular needle entry angle (black arrows) changes as vertebrae experience compression deformity and kyphosis increases in the thoracic spine. Increasing kyphosis occurs with compression fractures of the thoracic spine (dashed arrow).

of cement that can be used safely to augment a fracture without overfilling. Variations in vertebral volume are also affected by the amount of collapse a vertebra has experienced during fracture. The original and ultimate (postcollapse) sizes of the vertebra are of extreme importance when one is performing PV or KP. In both procedures, the most common side effects are created by cement leaks (2). This results from natural and pathologic holes in the vertebra as well as overfilling.

To avoid overfilling it is important to appreciate the general volume range of vertebral bodies between the cervical and lumbar regions and the effect that compression has on the initial volumes (Table 2.1). Using volumes computed for a hollow cylinder (and with representative dimensions taken for vertebrae in the cervical, thoracic, and lumbar regions), we find initial theoretical volumes ranging from 7.2 mL in the cervical spine (C5) to 22.4 mL in the lumbar spine (L3). Both larger and smaller vertebrae may be present. Because of the thickness of cortical and trabecular bone, the fillable volume is on the order of 50% or less of the theoretical volume. The fillable volume will again be diminished by the amount of collapse experienced during the compression fracture. As shown in Table 2.1, the 50% compressed, *fillable* volume of C5 is estimated at 1.8 mL. In the thoracic spine at T9 the 50% compressed volume estimate is 3.8 mL. At L3 the 50% compressed volume estimate is 5.6 mL. Actual cement volumes used to augment these vertebrae may be even less. This shows that quite small volumes will be needed to biomechanically augment a vertebra after fracture and that larger volumes will simply lead to overfilling and cement leak.

The vertebrae vary in size, with the smallest vertebra found in the cervical area and the largest in the lumbar. Size variation at a particular level is also common and is based on sex and general body dimensions.

Cervical Spine

The cervical spine (Figure 2.2) contains seven segments that vary tremendously in configuration from top to bottom (3). The first cervical vertebra is unique, and little actual distinct vertebral body exists at this level. Opportunities for percutaneous cement augmentation, therefore, are limited, as the body of the vertebra is the target for this type of therapy. Percutaneous vertebroplasty has been performed in all other cervical vertebrae, with the pathologic cause almost always being

Table 2.1. Vertebral volume estimates from cervical to lumbar spine.

Vertebral Level	Theoretical Volume (mL)	Fillable Volume (mL)	50% Compressed Volume (mL)
C5	7.2	3.6	1.8
T9	15.3	7.65	3.8
L3	22.4	11.2	5.6

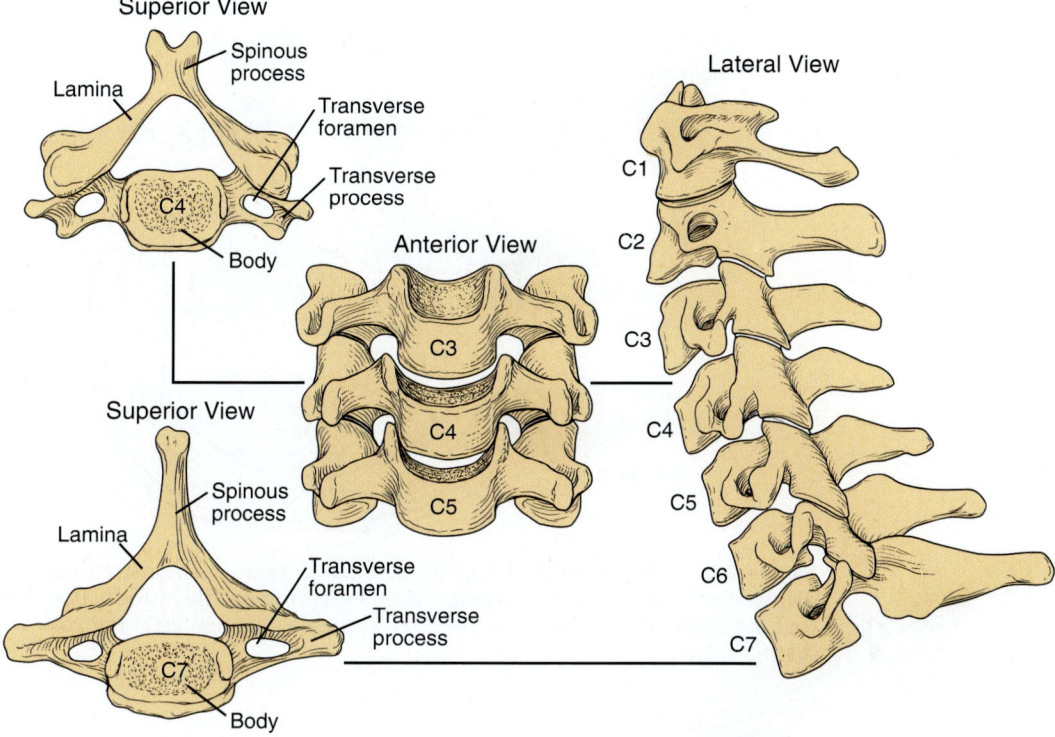

Figure 2.2. The cervical spine and vertebrae.

some form of neoplastic destruction with a subsequent compression fracture. Osteoporotic fractures are rare in the cervical spine.

The most common approach to the cervical spine for percutaneous bone augmentation has been via the anterolateral approach. This usually requires an accompanying manual maneuver that transiently displaces the carotid–jugular complex out of the way while a guide or primary needle is inserted into the margin of the vertebral body (Figure 2.3). The right side is chosen to avoid the needle transiting the esophagus (which lies behind or to the left of the trachea). The angle of the mandible can make access to high cervical vertebra, particularly C2, difficult. An occasional procedure has been performed via a trans-oral approach (4). The angle in this situation is improved by going through the mouth, but one cannot eliminate the added risk of trans-oral contamination of bacteria. For this reason, this route must not be considered optimum at C2. The lateral approach has also been used and is not optimum because of the potential for injury to the vertebral artery, which is fixed along the lateral aspect of the vertebral body (Figure 2.4). At C2–C6 the vertebral artery courses through the foramen transversarium and cannot be displaced as can the carotid–jugular complex during needle insertion. Regardless of the needle approach, computed

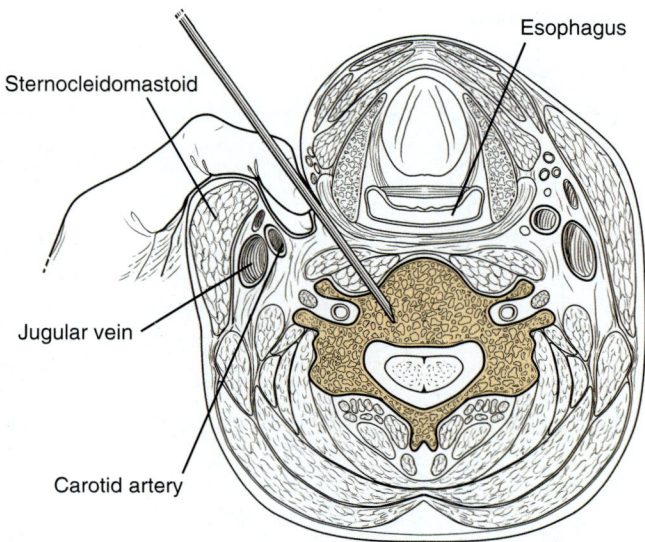

Figure 2.3. Anterior cervical approach. Axial drawing demonstrates manual displacement of the carotid–jugular complex during needle introduction. Note that the right side is chosen to best avoid the esophagus (as is the case with discography).

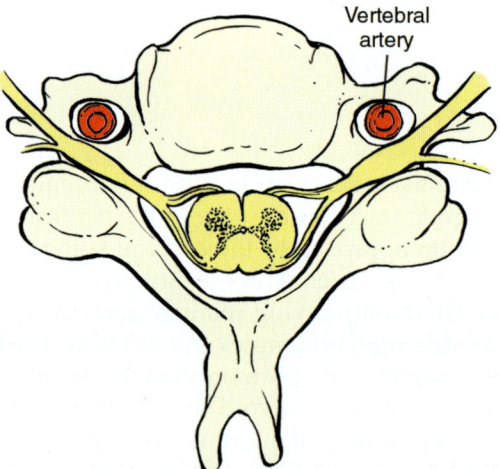

Figure 2.4. Drawing of a cervical vertebral body shows the position of the vertebral artery along the lateral aspect of the vertebral body in the foramina transversarium. A lateral needle approach would put the vertebral artery at risk. (From Mathis [2], with permission).

tomography (CT) offers an accurate method of visualizing structure that must be avoided during needle introduction.

Thoracic Spine

The thoracic spine is made up of 12 thoracic vertebra aligned with a gentle kyphosis in the normal, healthy spine. There is less variation in vertebral shape from top to bottom here than in the cervical region. Size variation is considerable and amounts to approximately a factor of 2 from T1 to T12. All thoracic vertebrae have a junction with a rib on each side, with ligaments attaching the rib head to the vertebral body and the adjacent rib to the vertebral transverse process (Figure 2.5). Just as there is substantial variation in the size of the thoracic vertebrae from top to bottom, there is considerable variation in the size and orientation of the pedicles as well (5). Pedicles at the lower aspect of the thoracic spine are relatively large and oriented in almost a direct anteroposterior (AP) direction (Figure 2.6A). Ascending toward the upper thoracic spine there is a progressive decrease in the size of the pedicles. Orientation remains AP until the most superior thoracic vertebrae (T1 and T2). The uppermost thoracic vertebrae have a more obliquely oriented pedicle (Figure 2.6B).

The vertebrae have a convex anterior margin and concave posterior margin when viewed from above (Figure 2.6). This is important, as

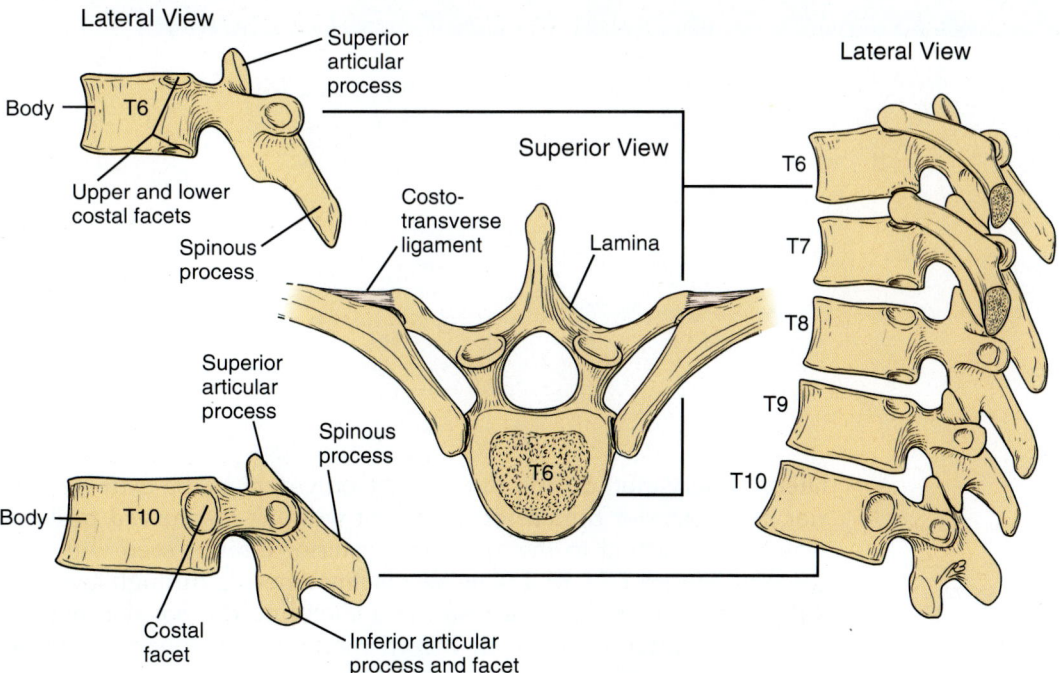

Figure 2.5. Artist's depiction of the thoracic vertebrae. There is considerable change in vertebral size from T1 to T12.

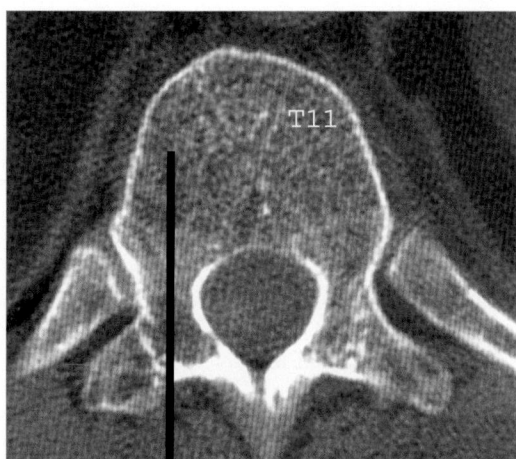
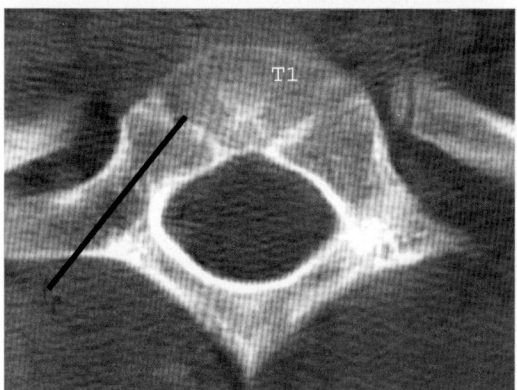
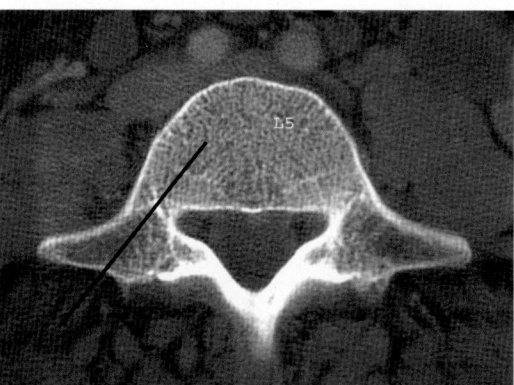

Figure 2.6. (A) The T11 vertebra is shown. The transpedicular angle is essentially straight in the anterior to posterior direction. The black line shows the angle and the needle direction that a transpedicular approach will take. All vertebrae from about T3 to L3 have a similar transpedicular angle. **(B)** This is the T1 level. Note the large change in the transpedicular angle compared with T11 (above). A transpedicular approach will have a much more lateral to medial approach (black line). **(C)** This level is L5. The high thoracic and lowest lumbar vertebrae show the most extreme transpedicular angles (away from AP).

lateral observation during fluoroscopy only depicts the extreme anterior and posterior dimensions. Cement will exit the curved posterior wall before getting to the apparent posterior limit as seen with fluoroscopy (Figure 2.7A,B). Likewise, placing a needle through a straight AP pedicle orientation will result in a lateral needle position that can breech the anterolateral wall before reaching the apparent anterior limit, as shown in the lateral projection (Figure 2.7C).

The needle approach to the T3–T12 thoracic spine is either transpedicular (through the pedicle) or parapedicular (transcostovertebral)

Figure 2.7. (A) A lateral radiograph after PV demonstrates the apparent anterior and posterior vertebral margins (black arrowheads). Cement in the back of the vertebra (white arrow) appears to stop before reaching the posterior vertebral margin. **(B)** Computed tomography scan of the same vertebra as in A. Note the concave posterior margin of the vertebra and the small cement leak (white arrow). The actual vertebral margin ends before the apparent margin as seen on the lateral radiograph. Cement injection should be stopped when cement enters the posterior quarter of the vertebra. **(C)** An axial CT scan of a thoracic vertebra demonstrates its very convex anterior margin. The black line depicts a straight transpedicular approach. Note that this approach would breach the anterior cortex long before the needle reaches the apparent anterior margin when seen in the lateral projection.

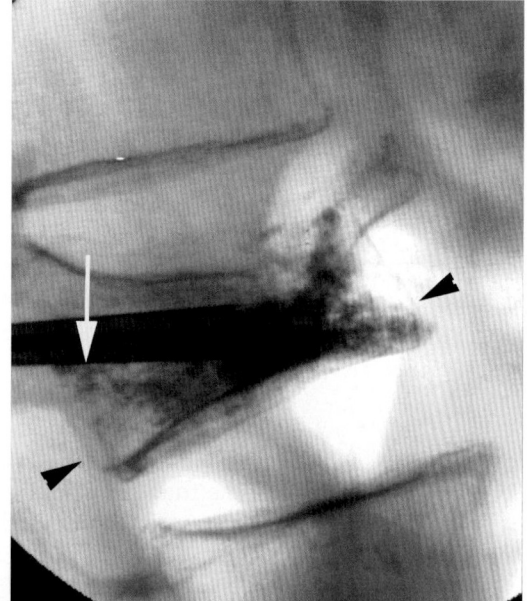

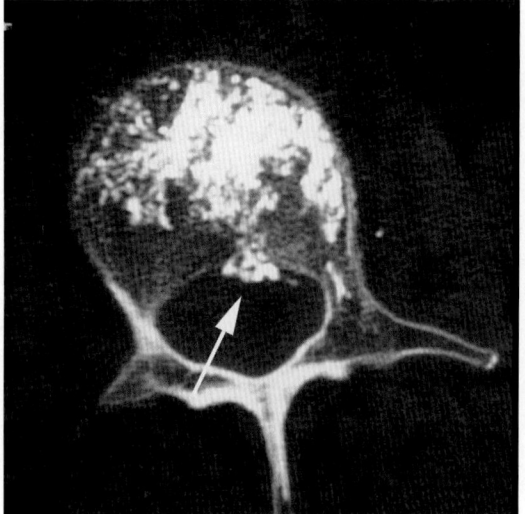

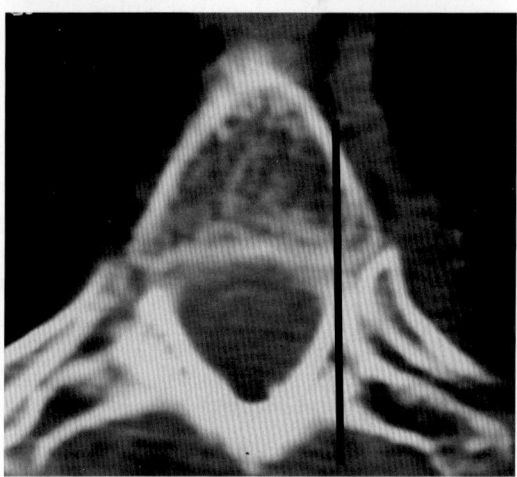

(6,7,8) through the junction of the rib and transverse process. The transpedicular approach (Figure 2.8A) is the most commonly used and safest, but small pedicle size may make it difficult to use large-bore needles (10–11 gauge). Reducing needle size to 13 gauge will eliminate this problem in adults regardless of thoracic level. The parapedicular approach (Figure 2.8B,C) allows placement of a needle above the transverse process and lateral to the pedicle. This has been found useful for larger instruments (commonly used in KP) or when the pedicle is destroyed or not adequately visualized because of severe osteoporosis. It is not recommended as the primary access method because of its higher potential complication rate related to either pneumothorax or hemorrhage.

The upper thoracic spine (T1–T2) can also be approached via the anterolateral method described for the cervical region (9,10,11). This transitional region has similarities of both the cervical and thoracic spine that allows these options. Pedicle orientation differences at these levels must be considered if a transpedicular approach is used (see Figure 2.6B).

Lumbar Spine

There are five lumbar vertebrae that make up the largest of the vertebrae found in the spine (Figure 2.9). These vertebrae have mild size variations from L1 to L5 (8). Pedicle orientation is quite different from L1 to L5. The pedicles of the upper lumbar region are similar to the lower thoracic with a nearly straight AP orientation. This gradually becomes a more oblique angle toward the lower lumbar spine and is maximal at L5 (see Figure 2.6C).

The approach to the lumbar spine for PV or KP is almost always transpedicular (see Figure 2.8A). The pedicles of the lumbar spine are large and allow access in most adults with 10–11 gauge needles without difficulty. The parapedicular (Figure 2.8B,C) approach remains a viable option but is much less needed because of the generous pedicle size in this region. The posterolateral approach is of historical value only (a low approach below the transverse process that places the exiting nerve root at risk of injury) and used only by manufactures' of instruments that are large and not required for the standard, minimally invasive procedure of PV or KP.

Sacrum

The sacrum (and coccyx) forms the terminal end of the lower spine. It is composed of five segments that are fused (Figure 2.10A). The lower lumbar spine joins the sacrum from above through the L5–S1 disc, making an articulation similar to other intervertebral junctions. The sacrum is joined to the pelvis via the sacroiliac (SI) joints. It is shaped like a "keystone," tapering to a narrower transverse width along its inferior margin (Figure 2.10B). This aids weight transfer to the pelvis without allowing slippage between the sacrum and pelvis through the SI joints. However, this anatomic shape and junction at the SI joints

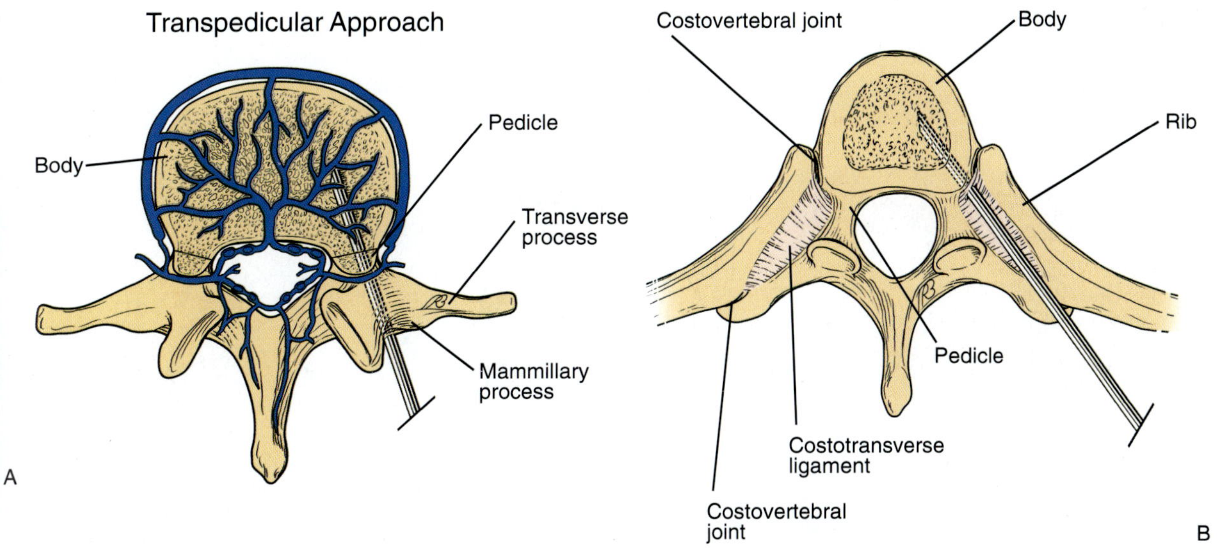

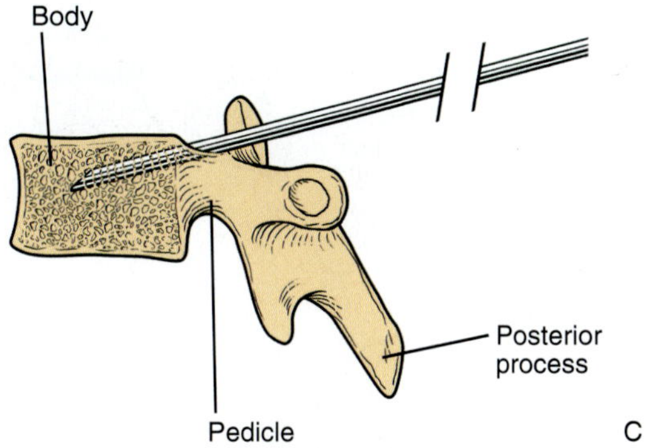

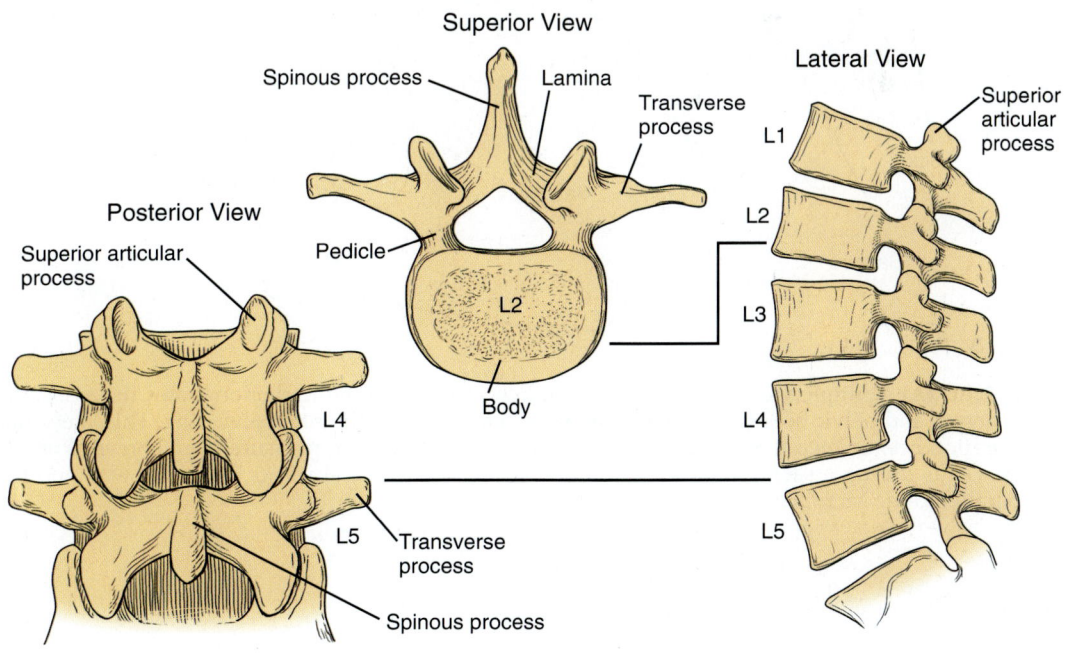

Figure 2.8. (A) Artist's concept of a transpedicular needle approach. Note that the angle is slightly away from the lateral margin and places the needle in the anterior half of the vertebral body. (B) Axial drawing of a thoracic vertebra with a needle entering via the parapedicular (transcostovertebral) approach. The entry site is along the lateral vertebral margin (lateral to the pedicle). (C) A lateral vertebral drawing shows the parapedicular approach. The needle enters above the transverse process. To enter below the pedicle would put the exiting nerve root at risk of damage.

Figure 2.9. The lumbar vertebrae.

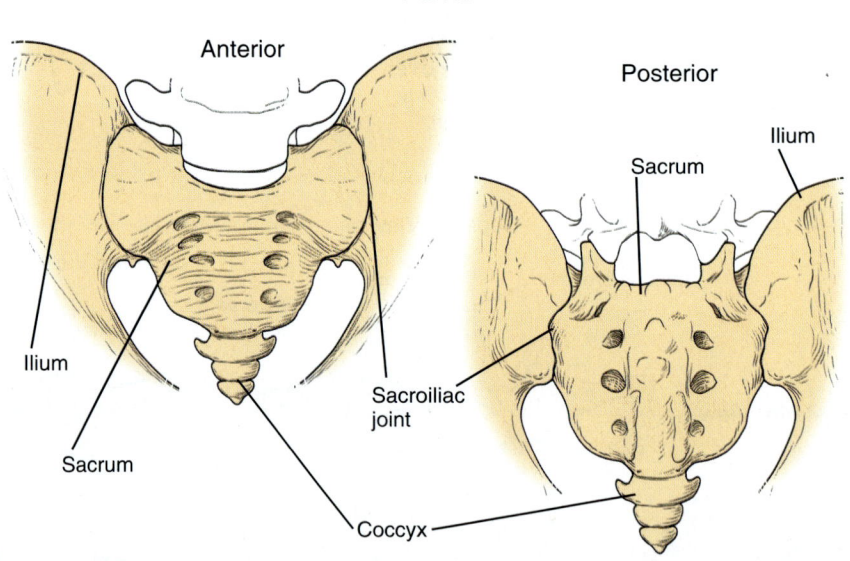

Figure 2.10. **(A)** Multiple views of the sacrum and coccyx. **(B)** Drawing demonstrates the association of the sacrum and pelvic bones. The sacrum forms a "keystone" within the pelvic ring. This "keystone" configuration acts to keep the sacrum from slipping downward with pressure from above. When the sacrum yields during a sacral insufficiency fracture, the lateral sacral wings (ala) give way and fracture parallel to the sacroiliac joints.

does create the unique fractures seen in the sacrum due to osteoporosis and trauma (see below).

Sacral insufficiency fractures may be percutaneously augmented to relieve pain such as compressed vertebrae. However, needle access is different because of the unique anatomic structure of the sacrum (compared with the vertebrae) and the different configuration of the fractures. Access to the sacral wings is usually from a posterior-oblique approach (Figure 2.11). This will require two needles if there is a bilateral sacral wing fracture. If the fracture extends into the central body of the sacrum, a needle approach through the SI joint or between the spinal canal and foramina may be necessary.

The size of the sacrum is large compared with a single vertebra, and therefore cement augmentation usually requires considerably more cement for similar filling of the fracture region.

Vascular Anatomy

The arterial supply to the vertebral bodies comes from arterial branches that leave the aorta and run along the lateral margins of the vertebrae supplying the vertebral body, the epidural space, and exiting nerve roots (Figure 2.12) (2,9). Communications between these branches exist up and down the paraspinous region. Supply to the spinal cord is intermittent and not dependably found at any one level.

Three interconnecting, valveless venous systems (interosseous, epidural, and paravertebral) make up the vertebral venous supply (1).

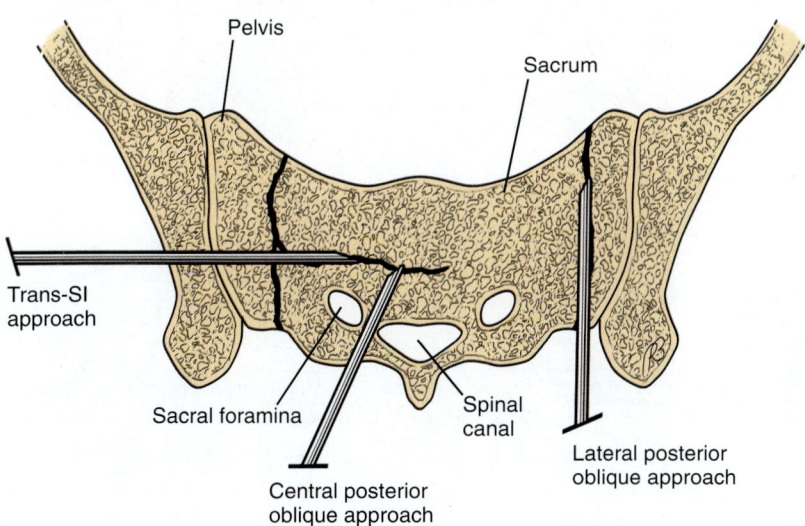

Figure 2.11. This drawing demonstrates the various needle angles that can be used to access the fractures of a sacral insufficiency fracture. The most common is the posterolateral that parallels the sacroiliac joint.

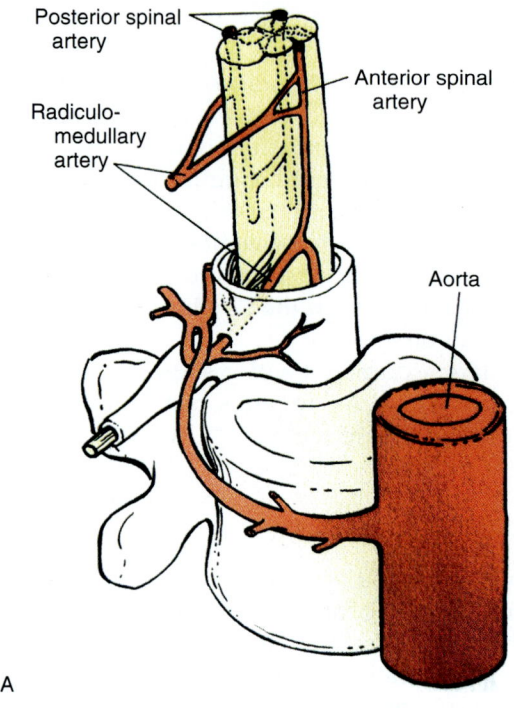

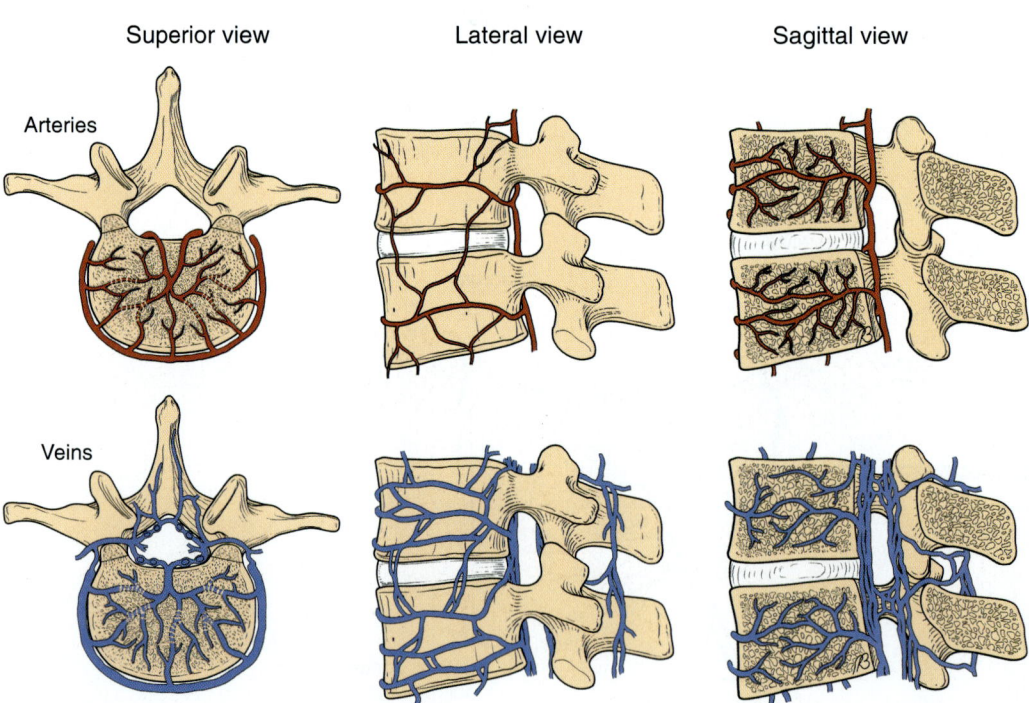

Figure 2.12. (**A**) Drawing of the aortic arterial branch that supplies the vertebral body and gives branches into the foramina and ultimately to the spinal cord. The cord supply is variable at each segment. The branches are found bilaterally. (**B**) Multiple projections of the arterial and venous supply to the vertebral bodies and epidural space. The venous elements are more numerous at all levels compared with the arteries. (A, from Mathis [2], with permission).

Through these systems there is intimate communication with the intraosseous, intertrabecular space (Figure 2.12B). Blood products and marrow fat are harbored in this space and commingled with flowing blood at venous pressure. This space in the axial skeleton becomes a primary source of blood-forming elements in the older adult. It is this space into which the cement is injected during PV or KP. Communication of the intertrabecular space via connecting venous systems can allow potential posterior, lateral, or anterior cement leaks to occur. Posterior communication is via the basivertebral venous system (Figure 2.13A–C), which usually forms the largest draining veins from the vertebrae. These veins connect directly to the epidural venous system that surrounds the exiting nerve roots and the thecal sac.

Lateral drainage from the vertebrae communicates to the paravertebral veins. Paravertebral veins form a system along the lateral aspect of the vertebrae running in both vertical and horizontal directions and that interconnect the posterior epidural and anterior central venous elements (Figure 2.13D,E). The central venous elements are large central channels composed of the azygos and caval veins that ultimately return venous blood to the lungs.

Direct entry of cement into the exiting vascular channels is minimized by needle placement away from the majority of these vessels. This risk is highest in the posterior aspect of the vertebra. Lateral and anterior communications are generally much smaller than to the basivertebral plexus (Figure 2.13A). The cement distribution is controlled by least resistance flow. Injecting away from the large (low pressure) channels forces intertrabecular distribution of cement preferentially. Large channels can be encountered accidentally, and continuous observation for this type of cement filling and distribution will limit leaks and prevent serious consequences.

Percutaneous Needle Approaches (Additional Considerations)

Individual needle approaches were generally described above with each segment of the spine for which they are applicable. The transpedicular approach is the most commonly used and provides the safest method of accessing the vertebral body (see Figure 2.8A). This occurs because the pedicle provides a discreet target that is visualized during image-guided needle placement. There are no structures within the pedicle that can be damaged during accurate transpedicular needle insertion. Percutaneous vertebroplasty can be accomplished in 85%–95% of cases using this route, as most compression fractures occur from T6 to L5 and the pedicle structure is adequate for needle insertion throughout this region. Complications that can occur with alternate routes (pneumothorax and bleeding with parapedicular; damage to vascular structures with anterolateral) are avoided with the transpedicular route. It should be the mainstay for needle placement with alternate routes reserved for relatively rare situations.

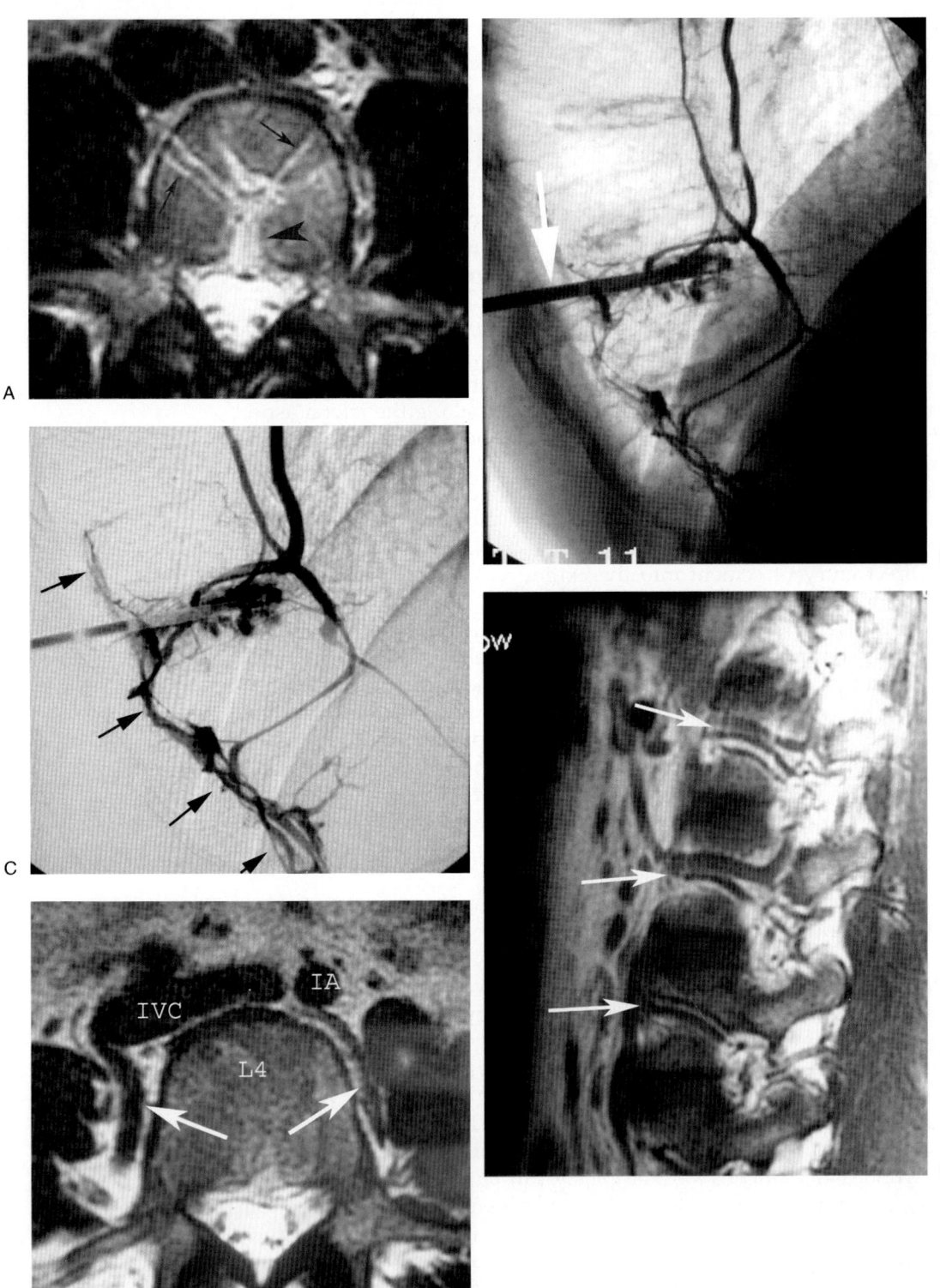

The parapedicular route may be used when the pedicle is absent (due to tumor), not seen because of severe osteoporosis, or too small (see Figure 2.8B,C). It does suffer from the potential for pneumothorax or bleeding. Also known as the transcostovertebral needle route, it passes along the rib margin in the thoracic spine. In some patients the lung may bulge beyond the lateral rib margin and put it at risk for pneumothorax. Bleeding may occur to a greater degree than found with the transpedicular approach, as the entry site into bone in the parapedicular approach is along the lateral aspect of the vertebra. Paravertebral arteries and veins run in this location. They can be quite large (Figure 2.13D,E) and are put at risk for puncture or transection with this needle approach. The needle puncture site can be easily compressed with pressure over the stick site in the transpedicular approach. This is not available for the parapedicular region to help limit bleeding, and therefore puncture of the large lateral vertebral vessels may produce more paraspinous bleeding.

The anterolateral approach is not used much as there is relatively little call for cervical or high thoracic PV. Needle placement can be easily accomplished with fluoroscopy in this approach using manual pressure to move the carotid–jugular complex laterally. Confirmation that the needle has missed the vascular structures, however, may be difficult with fluoroscopy alone. For this reason, CT guidance is commonly used for needle placement with this route. As stated above, the trans-oral route is less optimal than the anterolateral approach, as it is impossible to avoid the potential for bacterial contamination going through the mouth.

Fracture Anatomy

Fractures of the vertebrae and sacrum present with typical patterns that are influenced by the biomechanics of each particular spine element. Most compression fractures of the spine result from primary (age-related) or secondary (drug-related) osteoporosis. Relatively minor trauma or vertebra stress may result in compression fracture. These fractures are referred to as *simple* (as opposed to *burst* or *chance* frac-

◄

Figure 2.13. (A) Axial magnetic resonance image (MRI) demonstrates confluence of vessels at the posterior aspect of the vertebral body (black arrowhead). Vascular channels are much smaller, communicating with the paraspinous regions (black arrows). All of the channels give potential avenues for cement leak during injection. (B,C) Lateral intraosseous venograms (C is subtracted) of a lower thoracic vertebra. Posterior epidural vessels communicate over multiple levels (black arrows). There is filling of the lateral (paraspinous) channels and anterior vessels that ultimately communicate with the vena cava and lungs. (D,E) Lateral and axial MRI images show the large vessels that lie along the lateral aspect of the vertebral bodies in the paraspinous region (white arrows). These vessels are always at risk of injury with the parapedicular needle approach. IVC, inferior vena cava; IA, intraaortic.

tures, more common in primary trauma and produced without underlying pathologic weakening of the bone). Because three fourths of the body weight is born in the anterior two thirds of the spine, the paradigm of a simple fracture creates compression of the anterior body with sparing of the posterior vertebral wall and posterior elements. The anterior endplate region is compromised more often than the inferior endplate (Figure 2.14A). At times both endplates are compressed (Figure 2.14B). Single vertebral fractures are more common than multiple fractures at any one presentation. There is a general trend of fractures to cluster about T12–L1 and to a lesser degree around T7–T8 (10). Subsequent fracture risk increases by 5–10 times once the first osteoporotic fracture occurs at any site (11). The amount of vertebral height loss is not related to the amount of clinical pain experienced by the patient or to how long pain will last.

Variations on the simple compression fracture are common. There may be compression of the posterior wall with or without buckling of the wall into the spinal canal (Figure 2.14C). Fortunately, even with considerable posterior buckling there is infrequent symptomatic cord or nerve compression. Percutaneous vertebroplasty and KP procedures should be safe in this situation if there are no clinical symptoms of neurologic compromise.

Compression fractures can create a cavity or cleft in the vertebra that can be fluid- or air-filled (Figure 2.15). These cavities fill preferentially with cement during treatment and demonstrate very good pain relief.

Nonunion of vertebral bodies is recognized to occur due to lack of fracture healing or osteonecrosis. This situation will often present with signs of motion (or change in height) of the vertebra during respiration or change in body position (Figure 2.16). These fractures are known to provide good opportunity for height restoration during either PV or KP, and their treatment with bone cement also results in very good pain relief.

Compression of vertebrae can be extreme, with height loss greater than 70% (Figure 2.17A). These cases present technical challenges for percutaneous cement injection. Very severe compression usually cannot be treated with KP, as the instruments are larger than those used for PV. Percutaneous vertebroplasty can be accomplished in some cases, as lateral sparing of the vertebrae (greater central compression) is commonly found (Figure 2.17B). This will allow the surgeon to place bilateral needles for cement injection into the less compressed lateral segments. However, as the vertebra becomes progressively compressed, technically getting the needle into an adequate position in the anterior part of the vertebra becomes more and more difficult. Extreme collapse will force the endplates to be very close together, and therefore the needle trajectory will have to be essentially parallel to the endplates (Figure 2.17C). A steeper angle of the needle with respect to the endplates, acceptable in less compression, will not achieve an adequately anterior location for safe cement injection in the most severe compressions.

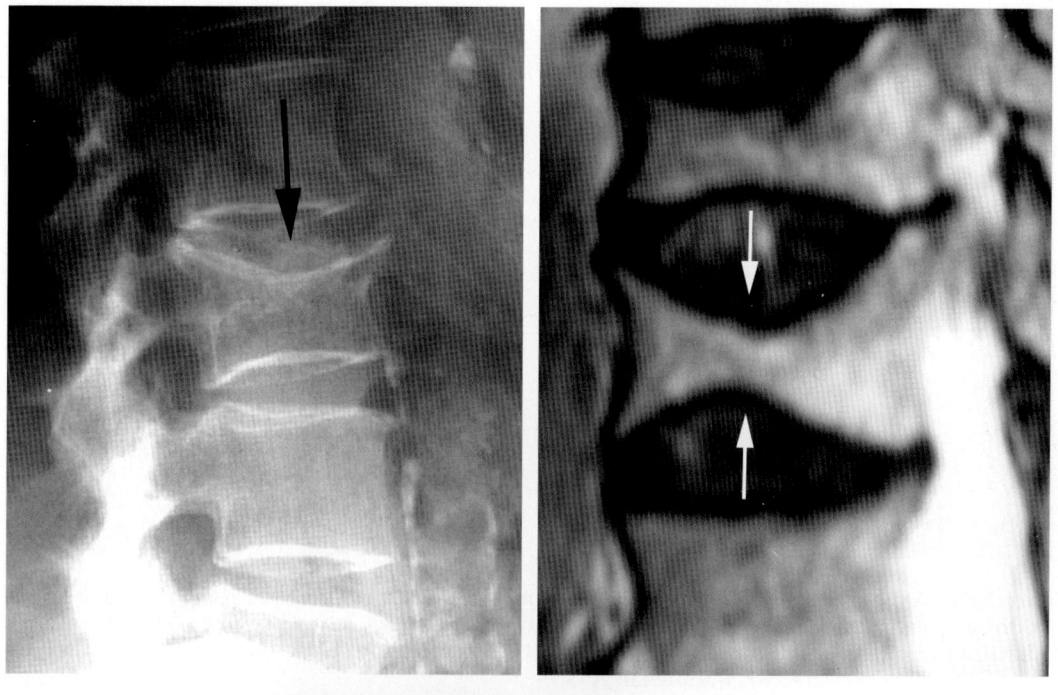
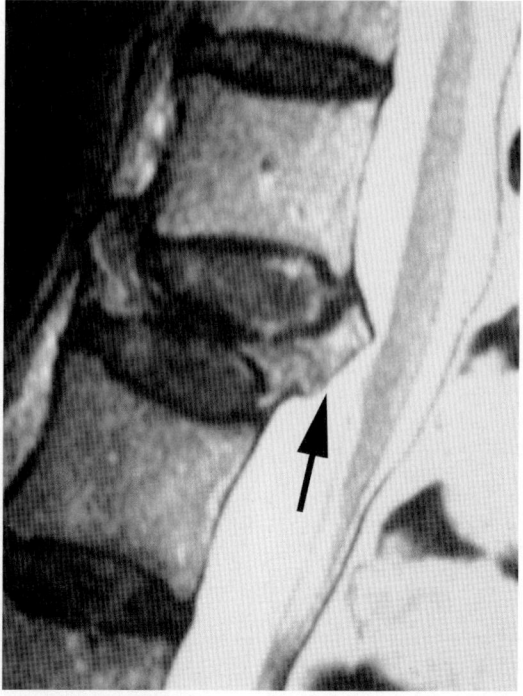

Figure 2.14. **(A)** Radiograph shows a simple compression fracture. The superior endplate is collapsed (black arrow), with most of the height loss in the anterior vertebrae and general sparing of the posterior wall. **(B)** Sagittal MRI shows a compression fracture with both endplate regions affected (white arrows). **(C)** Sagittal MRI shows marked collapse and buckling of the posterior wall (black arrow). There is mild encroachment on the spinal canal. In this patient there were no symptoms of cord compression and no contraindication to PV based on the canal encroachment.

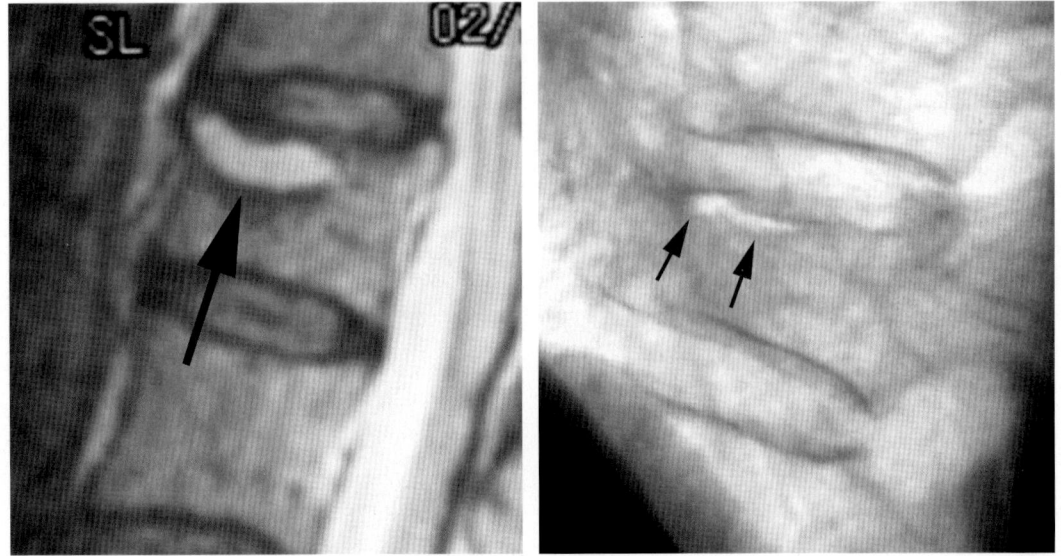

Figure 2.15. **(A)** Sagittal MRI (T2 weighted) demonstrates a localized region of high signal below the superior endplate (black arrow) that represents a cavity that was formed by the compression injury. **(B)** Lateral radiograph that shows a gas-filled cleft (black arrows) below the superior endplate. This finding is equivalent to the MR findings in A.

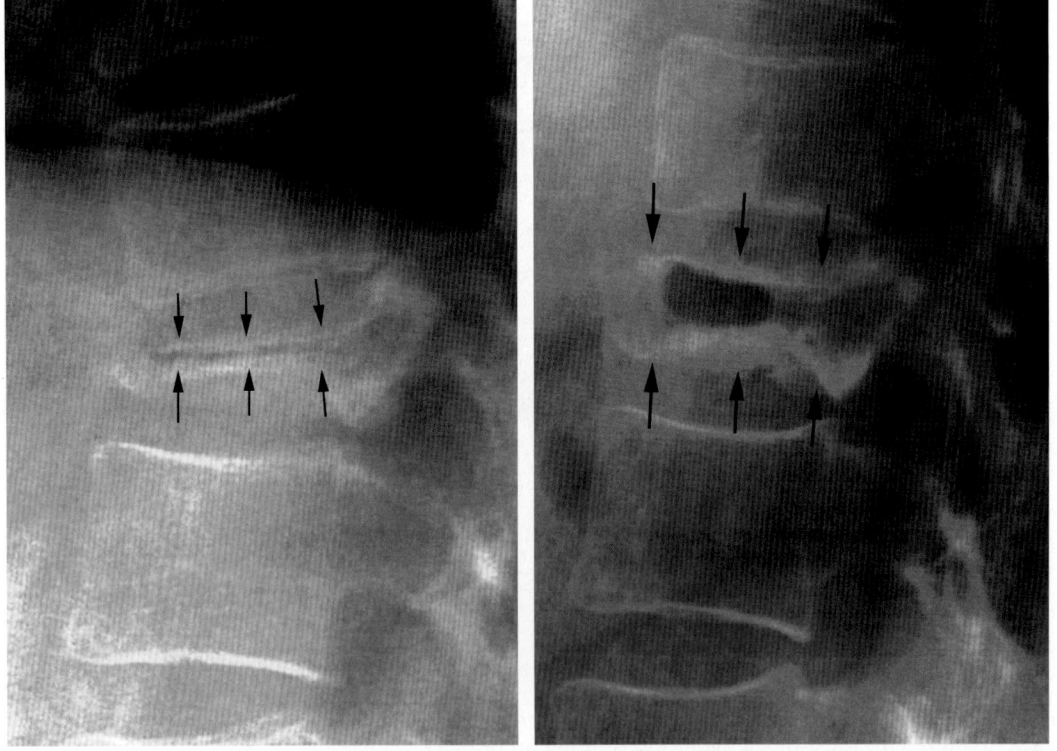

Figure 2.16. **(A)** Lateral radiograph shows a markedly collapsed vertebral body (black arrows). The patient is standing. **(B)** The mobility of the vertebrae (black arrows) is demonstrated with the patient lying prone. This mobility is consistent with vertebral nonunion. Percutaneous vertebroplasty will recapture the height gained during prone positioning.

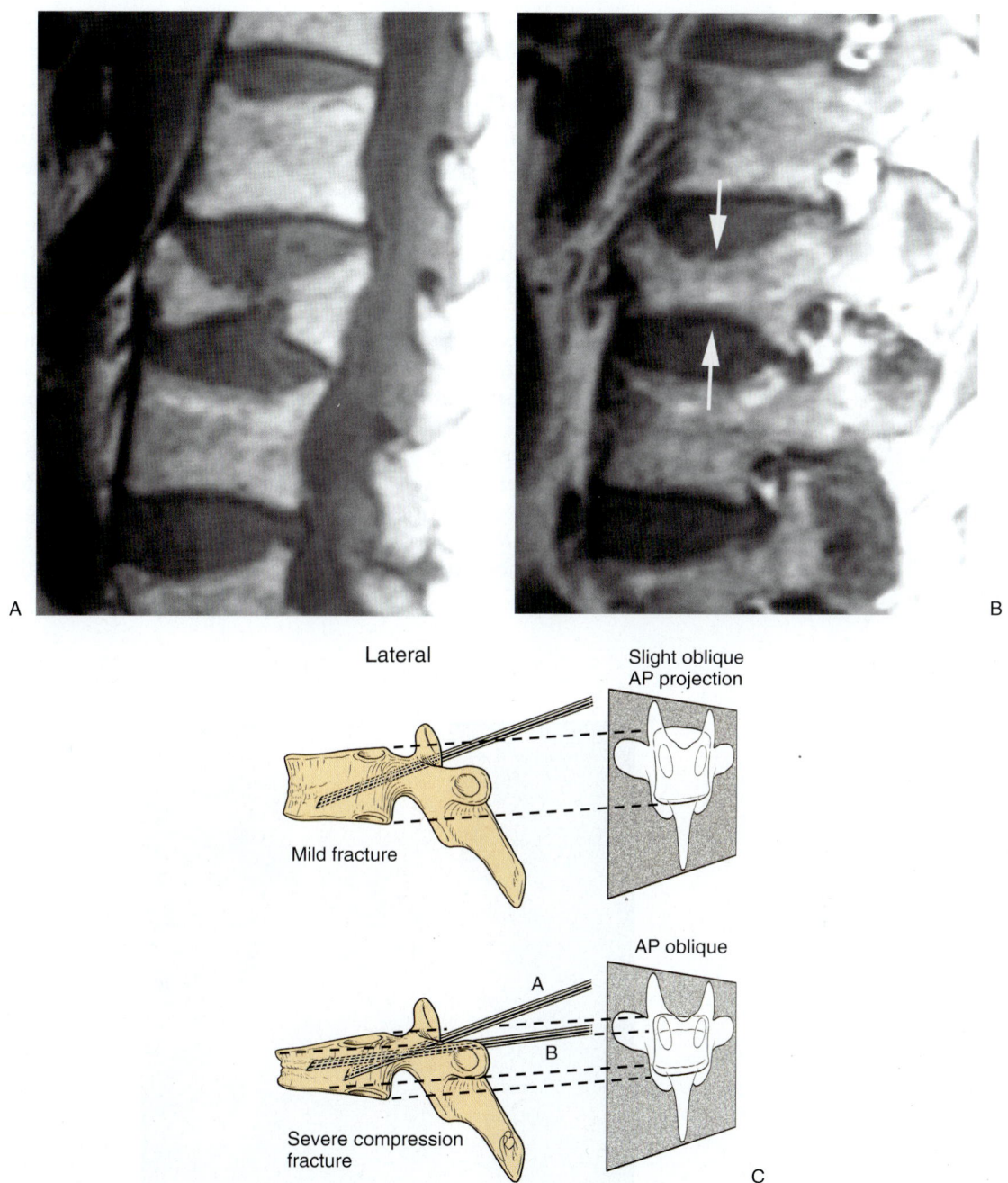

Figure 2.17. **(A)** Sagittal MR image in the midline shows nearly complete collapse of the vertebra centrally. **(B)** A more lateral image of the same patient demonstrates that less compression is present laterally (white arrows). **(C)** With severe compression, a needle angle that is nearly parallel to the endplates **(B)** is required to access the anterior vertebral body. The angle of needle A, acceptable for mild compression, will not work well for extreme compression.

An uncommon presentation is the vertical fractures in which there is literally separation of the anterior and posterior vertebral body (Figure 2.18). These fractures can be treated by "tying" the two halves of the vertebra together with cement. Cement injected in this situation should bridge the fracture site. This is accomplished by achieving an anterior needle location followed by a continuous fill that ties the anterior and posterior portions of the vertebra together.

Although the posterior elements are usually spared with "simple" fractures, there are situations when osteoporotic fractures will involve the posterior elements (Figure 2.19). Cement fixation of the body itself will provide sufficient stabilization in most cases for subsequent healing and pain relief. Injecting cement into fractured pedicles has been described ("pediculoplasty"), but the need for this therapy has not been proved because treatment of the body alone also results in pain relief (12).

Burst and chance fractures are not presently indicated to be appropriate for this procedure, as there are insufficient data to determine whether these fractures can safely be treated with cement injection alone. It has been postulated that first making a cavity (KP) allows a safer method for containing the cement than with

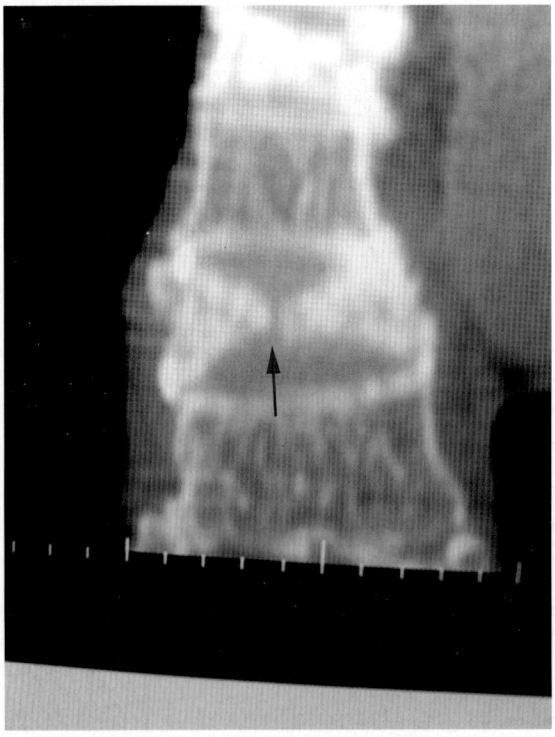

Figure 2.18. A sagittal CT reconstruction demonstrates the vertical fracture that separates the anterior and posterior vertebral body (black arrow).

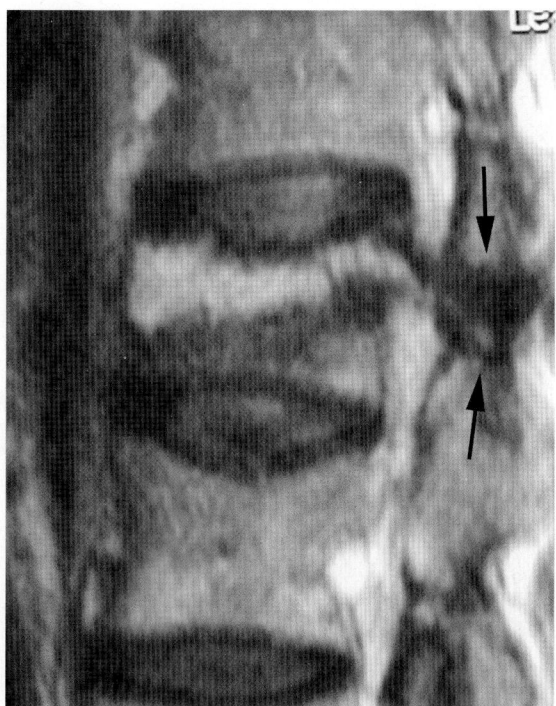

Figure 2.19. A sagittal MR image shows a fracture line extending into the posterior elements of this vertebra (black arrows). This is a common result in ankylosing spondyolitis.

standard PV. Too few cases are available for the technique to be proved at this time.

Sacral insufficiency fractures are sheer fractures rather than the compression injuries, typical of the vertebral bodies. Sacral insufficiency fractures have characteristic anatomic presentations that are seen well with CT, magnetic resonance imaging, and nuclear scanning, but are not well detected with standard radiographs (Figure 2.20). During fracture, the lateral aspect of the sacral ala sheers away from the central sacral body. These fractures may involve one or both sacral wings, with or without involvement of the central sacrum (Figure 2.21). A fracture of a single wing may progress over time to involve both wings and the central body of the sacrum (Figure 2.22).

Sacral insufficiency fractures are complex and often involve the wall of the neural foramina, which can allow direct cement leakage into this space. The complex anatomy of the sacrum makes cement monitoring difficult with fluoroscopy alone.

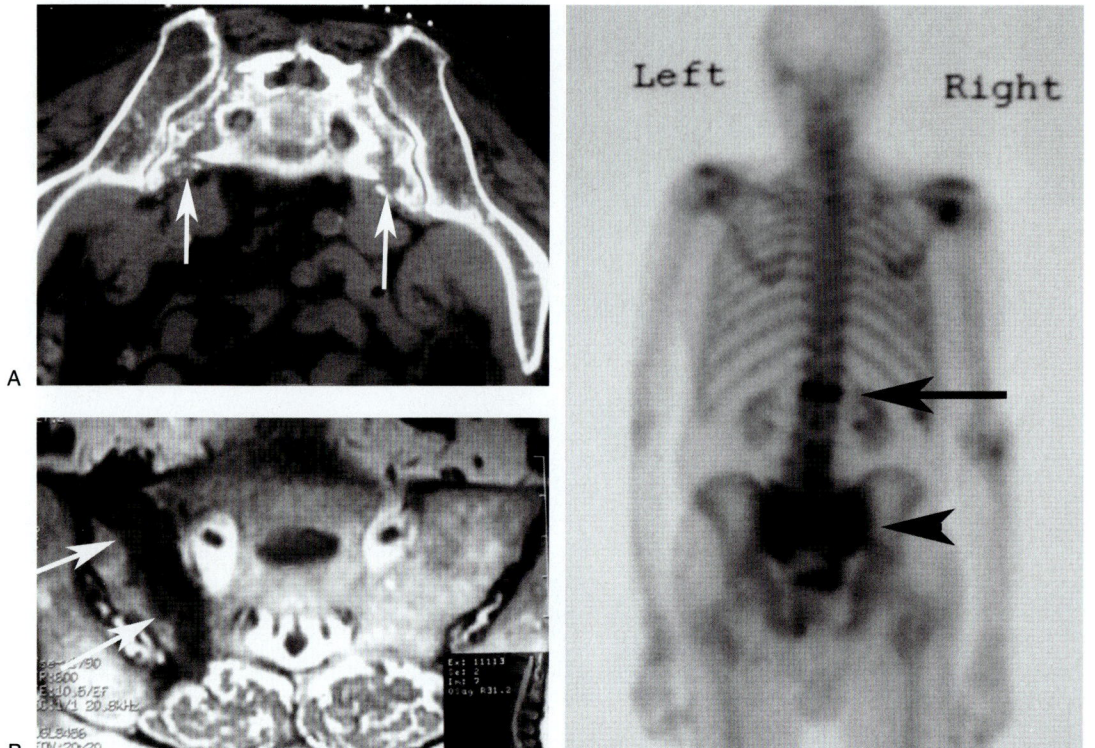

Figure 2.20. **(A)** Axial CT demonstrates bilateral sacral wing fractures (white arrows). **(B)** Coronal T1 MR image shows a unilateral sacral wing fracture (white arrows). The dark signal in the fracture is consistent with marrow edema. **(C)** A bone scan demonstrates a sacral insufficiency fracture (black arrowhead) associated with a vertebral compression fracture (black arrow).

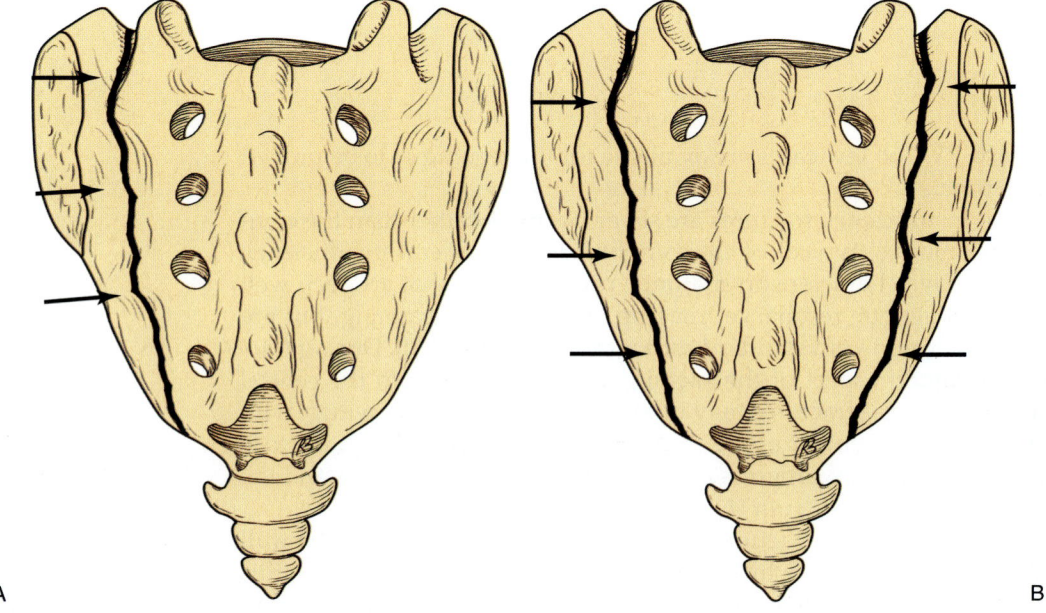

Figure 2.21. **(A)** Drawing of the sacrum demonstrates a unilateral sacral wing fracture (black arrows). **(B)** This drawing shows the bilateral sacral wing fracture (black arrows).

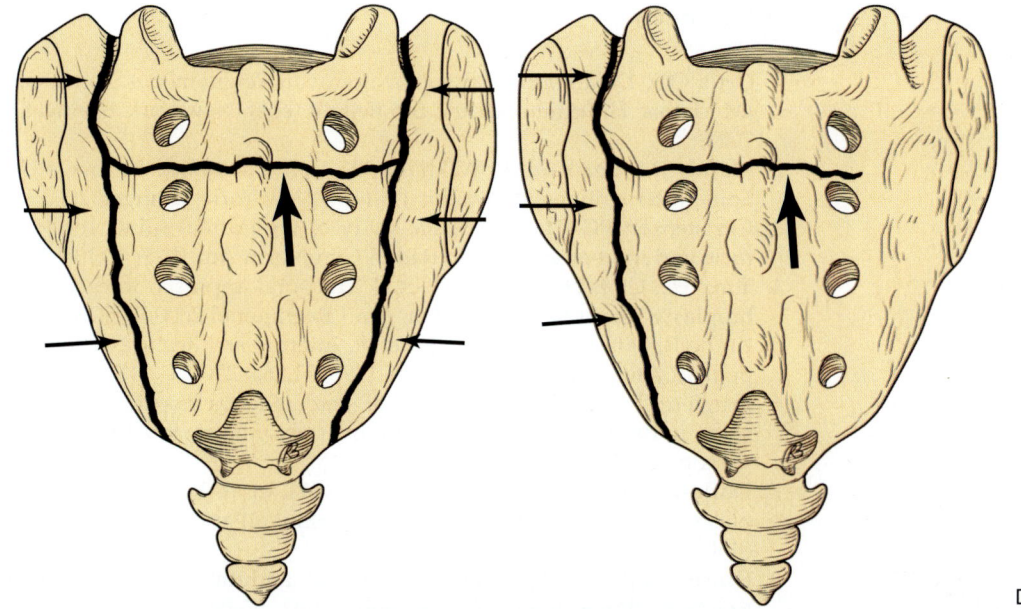

Figure 2.21. *Continued* **(C)** The fracture can extend through the central sacral region (large black arrow) connecting fractures through the lateral alar regions (smaller arrows). **(D)** This drawing shows a fracture limited to one sacral wing and extending into the central sacral body (black arrows). It spares the other sacral wing.

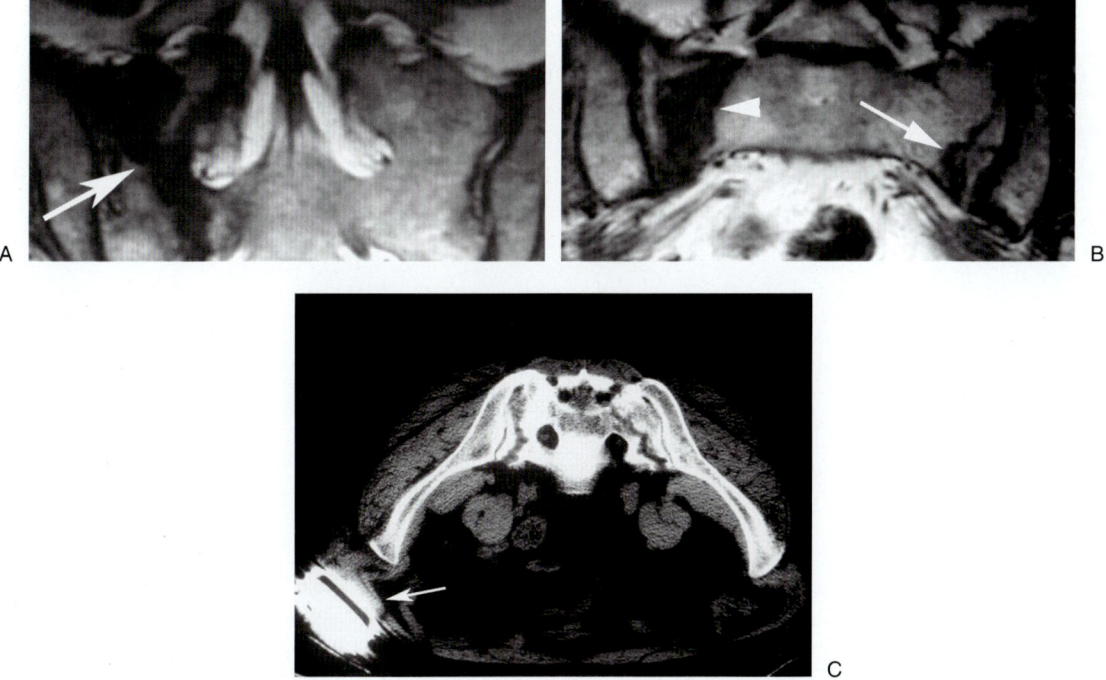

Figure 2.22. **(A)** Coronal T1 MR image shows the initial presenting sacral fracture that involves only one sacral wing (white arrow). **(B)** The same patient 2 months later has a repeat scan that now reveals another fracture extending into the opposite sacral wing (white arrow). The initial fracture (white arrowhead) is still seen. **(C)** A CT scan at the time of treatment with PS demonstrates the bilateral sacral wing fractures. Note that the patient has a pain pump (white arrow) in place and has had disabling pain throughout the course of this 6-month period.

References

1. Ortiz OO, Deramond H. Spine anatomy. In Percutaneous Vertebroplasty, JM Mathis, H Deramond, and SM Belkoff (eds). New York: Springer, 2001: 7–24.
2. Mathis JM, Shaibani A, Wakhloo AK. Spine anatomy. In Image-Guided Spine Interventions, JM Mathis JM (ed). New York: Springer, 2003:1–26.
3. Christenson PC. The radiologic study of the normal spine: cervical, thoracic and lumbar and sacral. Radiol Clin North Am 1977; 15:133–154.
4. Tong FC, Cloft HJ, Joseph GJ, et al. Transoral approach to cervical vertebroplasty for multiple myeloma. Am J Roentgenol 2000; 175:1322–1324.
5. Kothe R, O'Holleran JD, Liu W, et al. Internal architecture of the thoracic pedicle. An anatomic study. Spine 1996; 21:264–270.
6. Brugieres P, Gaston A, Heran F, et al. Percutaneous biopsies of the thoracic spine under CT guidance: transcostovertebral approach. J Comput Assist Tomogr 1990; 14:446–448.
7. Dufresne AC, Brunet E, Sola-Martinez MT, et al. Percutaneous vertebroplasty of the cervico-thoracic junction using an anterior route. J Neuroradiol 1998; 25:123–126.
8. Panjabi MM, Goel V, Oxland T, et al. Human lumbar vertebrae. Quantitative three-dimensional anatomy. Spine 1992; 17:299–306.
9. Lasjaunias P, Berenstein A. Surgical Neuroangiography. New York: Springer, 1990.
10. Nevitt MC, Ross PD, Palermo L, et al. Association of prevalent vertebral fractures, bone density, and alendronate treatment with incident vertebral fractures: effect of number and spinal location of fractures. Bone 1999; 25:613–619.
11. Cooper C, O'Neill T, Silman A. The epidemiology of vertebral fractures. Bone 1993; 14:S89–S97.
12. Eyheremendy EP, De Luca SE, Sanabria E. Percutaneous pediculoplasty in osteoporotic compression fractures. J Vasc Intervent Radiol 2004; 15: 869–874.

3

The Medical Management of Bone Health and Osteoporosis

Michele F. Bellantoni

Definition of Osteoporosis and Impact on Public Health

At the 2000 National Institutes of Health (NIH) Consensus Conference, osteoporosis was defined as a skeletal disorder characterized by compromised bone strength predisposing to an increased risk of fracture (1). As are many medical conditions associated with aging, osteoporosis is common, underrecognized as a public health concern, underdiagnosed, and inadequately treated by medical providers (2). The current estimates of 8 million osteoporotic women and 2.5 million osteoporotic men in the United States are expected to increase by about 40% by 2020, with estimated direct costs in 2002 dollars of $12.2 to $17.9 billion (3).

Yet recent clinical trials have shown that public health interventions and medical practices for the diagnosis, prevention, and treatment of osteoporosis are effective. The U.S. Surgeon General's Report of 2004 on Bone Health and Osteoporosis (4) was published in two forms: one for patient information and a separate guide for medical professionals, with the goal of addressing the lack of public awareness and neglect by medical providers that osteoporosis, or bone fragility with aging, is preventable and treatable, and not an inevitable consequence of aging.

Bone Metabolism Changes with Aging, Disease, and Environmental Influences

Throughout life, bone is a metabolically active body organ with a complex physiology that is a function of aging, gender, ethnicity, nutrition, physical activity, environmental exposures, and disease (Tables 3.1 and 3.2).

Physiology and Genetics

Men and women usually achieve peak bone mass by approximately age 30 years, but that peak bone mass can be influenced by genetic factors. Genetically based diseases can result in osteoporosis by young

Table 3.1. Determinants of Peak Bone Mass.

Parameter	Normal Peak Bone Mass	Low Peak Bone Mass
Genetics	Vitamin D and lipoprotein 5 receptors	Homocysteinuria
Metabolism	Normal gastrointestinal motility/absorption	Gastrointestinal malabsorption/celiac disease
	Euthyroid state	Hyperthyroid states/Graves' disease
		Sex hormone deficiency
		Amenorrhea
		Hypothalamic-pituitary disease
Body mass	Body mass Index >20 kg/m^2	Anorexia nervosa
Weight-bearing exercise	Physical activity 3 hours weekly	Trauma-induced immobility
Nutrition	Calcium intake, 1,000 mg daily	Inadequate calcium and vitamin D intake
	Vitamin D intake, 400 IU daily	Phosphate-containing sodas
Medications	Estrogen-containing oral contraceptives	Steroid medications
		Phenytoin
		Warfarin
Environmental exposures	Fluorinated drinking water	Tobacco use
		Excessive alcohol intake

Table 3.2. Determinants of Bone Loss with Aging.

Parameter	Positive Impact on Bone Health	Contributors to Bone Loss
Genetics	Vitamin D and lipoprotein 5 receptors	Excessive calcium excretion in urine
Metabolism	Estrogen synthesis in adipose tissue	Menopause
		Age-related testosterone deficiency in men
		Hyperparathyroidism
		Renal failure
Body mass index	>24 kg/m^2	<20 kg/m^2 (or cycled weight loss/gain)
Weight-bearing exercise	Walking 30 minutes daily Resistance training	Immobility secondary to hemiparesis from stroke or prolonged bed rest for medical illness
Medical conditions	None	Rheumatoid arthritis
Nutrition	Calcium intake, 1,200–1,500 mg daily	Inadequate calcium and vitamin D intake
	Vitamin D intake, 600–800 IU daily	Phosphate-containing sodas
Medications	Hormone replacement therapy	Steroid medications
	Antiresorptive agents	Phenytoin
	Thiazide diuretics	Gonadotropin antagonists
	Calcium carbonate antacids	Phosphate-binding antacids
Environmental exposures	Sunlight exposure	Tobacco use
		Excessive alcohol intake

adulthood (5). For example, homocysteinuria, a metabolic defect in cobalamin metabolism, produces impairments in cross-linking of collagen that result in fragile bone. Genetic variants in vitamin D receptors and lipoprotein receptor-related protein 5 and vitamin D are known to result in strong bone, whereas others result in fracture syndromes (6). Calcium excretion by the kidney is mediated genetically, and excess calcium loss in urine results in the formation of kidney stones and predisposes to demineralization of bone when dietary intake of calcium is insufficient to compensate for the urinary losses.

Environmental Factors

Environmental influences also are important to bone development. In children, low dietary calcium intake (7), vitamin D intake of less than 200 IU, consumption of carbonated beverages such as soda (8), and physical activity of less than 3 hours per week (9) all have been shown to contribute to low bone mass. Body weight is highly correlated with bone mass, and anorexia nervosa results in low peak bone mass (10). Skin is able to synthesize a precursor of vitamin D when exposed to ultraviolet light, but circulating vitamin D levels are known to decrease when sun exposure is limited, as during winter months, in northern climates, and in home-bound older adults who have limited dietary intake of dairy products fortified with vitamin D.

Aging

On average, men achieve greater bone size, although a quantitative computed tomography (CT) study has shown that women have greater trabecular bone mass by volume (11). After peak bone mass is achieved, little bone loss occurs in healthy adults until advanced age or, in women, menopause. With aging, the balance of bone formation to bone resorption is altered greatly by decreases in postpubertal circulating levels of sex hormones. Most common and most important is the universal menopause in women (12), but osteoporosis also results from androgen deprivation in men with aging.

Disease States

Disease states that alter gastrointestinal absorption of calcium and vitamin D (13); hepatic (14) and renal metabolism (15) of vitamin D; the endocrine systems of the hypothalamus and pituitary, thyroid, parathyroid (16), adrenal, and pancreatic glands; and the paracrine functions of the bone marrow all regulate bone formation and/or bone resorption and contribute to disease-related osteoporosis. A recently discovered hormone from fat cells, leptin, also has been shown to have effects on bone (17). Calcitriol, or 1,25-dihydroxyvitamin D_3, is the metabolically active hormone that increases intestinal absorption of calcium and phosphorus. Because dietary forms and skin-derived precursors of vitamin D are metabolized in the liver and kidney, severe impairments in renal function result in calcitriol deficiency, malabsorption of calcium through the gut, hypocalcemia, and ultimately a compensatory rise in parathyroid hormone and active bone resorption.

Celiac disease, one cause of gastrointestinal malabsorption, has a prevalence of 1 in 266 adults and may present solely as osteoporosis in approximately 15% of cases (13). Hyperthyroidism and hyperparathyroidism result in excessive bone resorption, and excess secretion of cortisol associated with clinical depression has been associated with osteopenia. Bacterial infections, such as periodontal disease and osteomyelitis, can produce localized bone loss. The alterations in molecular growth factors associated with rheumatoid arthritis and multiple myeloma are thought to result in osteopenia even without systemic glucocorticoid therapies. Repetitive weight loss is another risk for bone loss, although attention to nutrition and physical activity may limit this risk. Medical therapies of corticosteroids, anticoagulants that impair vitamin K metabolism (such as warfarin), and anticonvulsants that impair vitamin D metabolism (such as phenytoin, valproic acid, and carbamazepine) may impair bone formation, whereas antiestrogens used for breast cancer treatment in women and antiandrogens used for prostate cancer treatment in men result in excessive bone resorption.

Bone Strength and Fracture

Bone strength is achieved through a combination of three-dimensional architecture and the mineralization of the bone matrix proteins. Vitamin K is essential for the carboxylation of bone matrix proteins, whereas vitamin B complex mediates collagen cross-linking. The systemic hormones that regulate blood calcium levels, such as parathyroid hormone and calcitonin, do so, in part, through their mediation of bone mineralization. Calcium is an important mediator of cell communications in multiple body tissue, and, because bone serves as the reservoir of this mineral, limited dietary intake results in increased circulation of parathyroid hormone and bone demineralization (18).

The coupling of bone formation to bone resorption is controlled locally by signaling proteins under the control of the systemic hormones and growth factors (Figure 3.1). Macrophage colony-stimulating factor and receptor activator of nuclear factor kappa B ligand (RANKL) are osteoblastic-derived proteins that bind to receptors on the osteoclast precursors and stimulate bone resorption (19). In contrast, a third protein, osteoprotegerin, binds RANKL and prevents osteoclastic activity (20). The systemic hormones and local growth factors that stimulate bone resorption regulate the amounts of RANKL and osteoprotegerin. For example, estrogen deficiency results in an increase in RANKL. A second signaling pathway involves lipoprotein receptor-related protein 5 (21).

When bone resorption exceeds bone formation, bone fragility occurs, putting the skeletal system at risk for fracture, even when the injuring force is relatively minor, such as that from a fall (22). The risk of a fall increases with sensory deficits (such as inadequate vision and hearing), neurologic impairments (such as peripheral neuropathy, Parkinson's

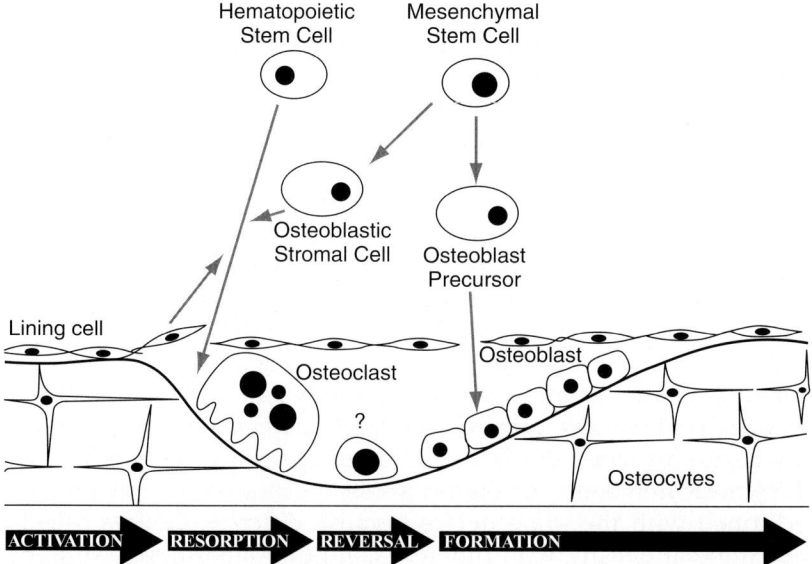

Figure 3.1. Systemic and local mediators of bone formation and bone resorption. (From Bone Health and Osteoporosis: A Report of the Surgeon General. Rockville, MD: U.S. Department of Health and Human Services, 2004.)

disease, and stroke), and loss of muscle strength from deconditioning (such as results from a bed-bound state, the most severe form of disuse, which results in rapid bone loss).

Assessing Bone Health and Osteoporosis Screening

The U.S. Preventive Task Force recommends assessment of bone mass/density for all women aged 65 years or older or those aged 60 years or older who have one or more osteoporosis risk factors (Table 3.1) (23). The National Osteoporosis Foundation guidelines recommend an initial assessment at age 70 years for men with no risk factors other than advanced age (24). All adults receiving systemic glucocorticoids and all young adults with sex hormone deficiency for whatever cause should be assessed, including women treated with antiestrogens and men treated with androgen deprivation. Bone fracture that occurs from a fall at standing height and age-related height loss of more than 1.5 inches suggest fragility fractures for which osteoporosis or other metabolic bone disorders may be an underlying cause.

Diagnostic Tools

Dual energy x-ray absorptiometry (DEXA) of the central skeleton is the most commonly used diagnostic procedure for assessing bone mineral density. The technology requires less than 30 minutes to measure multiple sites of spine, hip, and forearm; involves low-dose radiation comparable with background environmental exposures; and can be used to monitor osteoporosis treatments. The World Health Organization (25) has established definitions for normal, osteopenia, and osteoporosis based on standard deviations from peak bone health (Table 3.2). The International Society for Clinical Densitometry (26) has established standards that include assessment of at least three lumbar vertebral bodies, three hip sites (total hip, femoral neck, and trochanter), and the proximal third of the nondominant arm radius (27). This society also has established standards for DEXA diagnosis of osteoporotic versus normal in premenopausal women and men aged 50 years and older (Table 3.3). Pitfalls in DEXA technology include assessment of the spine in older adults who may have degenerative changes or dense vertebra from compression fractures and assessment in limited positioning of the hip due to arthritic conditions. Recently, some DEXA devices have been upgraded to assess vertebral deformity associated with vertebral compression fractures, termed an *instant vertebral assessment* (28), that may be useful when the DEXA spine image shows deformity. Serial DEXA measurements for monitoring osteoporosis treatments should be performed with the same device because different devices calculate bone mineral density with different computer algorithms. An appropriate interval for testing is every 2 years. Exceptions are made for individuals with high bone turnover (such as that related to untreated hyperparathyroidism, uncontrolled hyperthyroidism, and drugs that reduce sex hormone levels) or low bone formation (such as that related to systemic glucocorticoid use). For these high-risk groups, a yearly DEXA measurement is recommended.

Single x-ray absorptiometry devices and ultrasound devices are portable and often used to assess forearm and heel sites in community settings such as health fairs and nursing facilities (29). With aging, discordance of bone loss between the axial and appendicular skeleton is common, with vertebral bone loss occurring at more accelerated rates (11). Thus, limiting assessment to a forearm or heel scan may be insufficient for assessing bone health in an adult who is in the early stages of sex hormone deficiency or glucocorticoid use. At present, the heel ultrasound devices report a T-score that is not comparable to DEXA.

Table 3.3. International Society for Clinical Densitometry Criteria for Diagnosis by DEXA.

Status	Women		Men ≥50 Years Old (T-scores)*
	Premenopausal (Z-scores)	Postmenopausal (T-scores)	
Normal		−1.0 or above	−1.0 or above
Osteopenia		Between −1.0 and −2.5	
Osteoporosis	Low bone mineral density with secondary causes or risk factors	−2.5 or below	−2.5 or below[†]

* Diagnosis in men <50 years old should not be made on the basis of densitometric criteria alone.
† Plus clinical risk factors in men 50 to 64 years old.

For example, a T-score of −1.8 in heel ultrasound may predict a fracture risk equivalent to a DEXA T-score of −2.5 (30). However, ultrasound is useful in identifying older adults who may benefit from full DEXA assessment, especially those in a nursing home environment and those with a physical dependence that may limit full DEXA assessment.

Compared with DEXA, quantitative computerized tomography of the spine results in less artifact from spinal deformity but has higher levels of radiation and cost and, in general, has been used less widely in clinical practice. However, high-resolution computerized tomography is emerging as a novel technology for assessing the trabecular architecture of bone and has the potential for better prediction of bone strength and fracture risk than DEXA (31).

Medical Evaluation

Standard

The medical evaluation for the underlying cause of osteoporosis begins with a careful history of medical, family, medication, and social factors to assess risks for low peak bone mass, rapid adult bone loss, and medical diagnoses and treatments associated with osteoporosis. One study identified secondary causes of osteopenia in 51% of men and 41% of women studied (32). Tannenbaum et al. (32) found that, in women, the most common secondary causes were vitamin D deficiency (20%), hypercalciuria (10%), and gastrointestinal malabsorption (7%).

The medical history should elicit information about fractures (including peripheral sites of the forearm and ankle), disease states (such as rheumatoid arthritis, kidney stones, hyperthyroidism, gastrointestinal malabsorption, multiple myeloma, depression, and renal insufficiency), and surgical interventions (such as gastric stapling, partial gastrectomy, and small bowel resection) that may have resulted in impaired absorption of nutrients. A family history of fractures and disease states also should be obtained. Assessment of the patient's reproductive function should include the age of pubertal development, evaluation for prolonged amenorrhea after menarche in women, the age of cessation of menses in postmenopausal women, and evidence of sexual dysfunction in men.

The medication and nutritional history should determine exposure to medications that contain sex hormones, antiestrogens (such as aromatase inhibitors), medroxyprogesterone acetate (which can cause a hypoestrogen state in premenopausal women), systemic glucocorticoid, vitamin K–depleting anticoagulants (such as warfarin), antiseizure medications that impair vitamin D (such as phenytoin), and thyroxine supplements. The nutritional assessment should also determine routine dietary sources of calcium, vitamin D, vitamin B complex, and nutritional supplements.

Other information obtained should include a social history and systems review. The social history should include assessment of physical activity, history of smoking, and intake of alcohol, phosphate-containing beverages (such as sodas), and caffeine. The systems review should address sensory deficits and physical function (including a history of falls) and longitudinal changes in body weight. Bone pain is often caused by degenerative or inflammatory processes distinct from osteoporosis, although diffuse bone and muscle pain is associated with vitamin D deficiency.

The routine annual physical examination of all adults should include measurement of height, with loss of 1.5 or more inches prompting assessment for asymptomatic vertebral compression, and examination of the spine for kyphosis. Practical examinations that identify clinically significant kyphosis include assessment of whether the occiput can be positioned against the wall and whether the distance from the ribs to the pelvis is less than four finger breadths. Examinations to assess the risk of a fall include vision and hearing assessment, observation of gait, and neurologic assessment for balance, peripheral sensation, and muscle strength.

All patients about to undergo pharmacologic therapy for osteoporosis should receive basic laboratory screening for calcium, phosphorus, creatinine, alkaline phosphatase, albumin, and globulin and a complete blood count as a screen for multiple myeloma. A serum 25-hydroxyvitamin D level is recommended for older adults who limit sun exposure and dietary intake of vitamin D and for adults with conditions that predispose to gastrointestinal malabsorption. A 24-hour urine collection for calcium is recommended for patients with a history of kidney stones to assess for hypercalciuria. This evaluation can determine inadequate dietary intake of calcium when levels are low, but patient compliance is challenging.

Expanded Diagnostics

More extensive diagnostics are recommended when the degree of osteopenia as defined by the DEXA scan is greater than expected, when a fracture occurs without a substantial risk thereof based on history, or when serial DEXA scans show continued bone loss despite an adequate treatment plan. For men, measurement of the serum testosterone level is useful. For premenopausal women with menstrual irregularities, measurements of gonadotropin levels may uncover premature menopause. Measuring estrogen levels in postmenopausal women has no diagnostic utility. Elevations in serum intact molecule parathyroid hormone with normal serum 25-hydroxyvitamin D levels are diagnostic for asymptomatic primary hyperparathyroidism and may occur in the presence of normal serum calcium. Measurement of 1,25-dihydroxyvitamin D_3 levels is needed for patients with severe renal insufficiency. Urine and serum protein electrophoresis tests assess monoclonal gammopathy associated with multiple myeloma. The presence of serum antiglidian antibodies (such as endomysial antibody) suggests celiac disease, although small-bowel biopsy for villous atrophy is the gold standard for diagnosis. To assess adequately the hypothalamic–pituitary–adrenal regulation of cortisol, a 24-hour urine collection for cortisol or a dexamethasone suppression test is recommended. It is also recommended that the serum thyroid-stimulating hormone levels of patients receiving thyroxine supplements be maintained within normal range, as a suppressed level may cause bone resorption.

In addition, biochemical markers of bone turnover can be measured to assess a patient for a high bone-turnover state such as hyperparathyroidism, thyrotoxicosis, or sex-hormone-deficient states (33). In general, markers are not used to monitor treatments, except for individuals in high bone-turnover states.

Prevention and Treatment

Nutrition and Bone Health

The current U.S. recommended dietary allowances of daily elemental calcium are, for adults aged 19 to 50 years, 1,000 mg; and for adults more than 50 years old, 1,200 mg (34). The current recommended dietary allowance for vitamin D is 400 IU for adults aged 50 to 70 years and 600 IU for adults more than 70 years old, although the clinical guidelines followed in Canada include 800 IU for individuals more than 50 years old (35). A recent study has found that higher doses of vitamin D (such as 1,300 IU daily) may reverse bone pain and muscle weakness associated with aging (36).

The average American diet that excludes dairy products achieves only 300 mg of elemental calcium because little vitamin D is present naturally in other foods. With increased awareness of bone health, calcium and vitamin D fortification of fruit juices, breakfast cereals, skim milk puddings, and yogurts is increasing (Table 3.4). On average, 8 oz of calcium-fortified fruit juice contains 300 mg of elemental calcium, comparable with the level in milk.

There are multiple commercial formulations of calcium and vitamin D to supplement dietary sources. Although there are subtle differences in absorption, in general, all are clinically effective (37). Calcium

Table 3.4. Calcium-Enriched Foods.

Food	Serving Size (mg equivalent)	Calcium (mg)
Tofu	½ cup (400 mg)	434
Low-fat yogurt	8 oz (300–400 mg)	300
Fortified orange juice	1 cup (300–400 mg)	300
Fortified soy milk	1 cup (300–400 mg)	300
Skim, 1%, or 2% milk	1 cup (300–400 mg)	321
Fortified cereal	¾ cup (300–400 mg)	Varies by brand
Fortified oatmeal	1 packet (300–400 mg)	350
Cheddar, Monterey, or provolone cheese	1 oz (200–300 mg)	206
Spinach (cooked)	1 cup (200–300 mg)	237
Pizza	1 slice (100–200 mg)	100
Mustard greens (cooked)	1 cup (100–200 mg)	104
Cottage cheese	1 cup (100–200 mg)	138
Frozen yogurt or pudding	½ cup (100–200 mg)	152
American, feta, or mozzarella cheese	1 oz (100–200 mg)	174

Source: United States Department of Agriculture Nutrient Database for Standard Reference, http://www.nal.usda.gov/fnic/foodcomp.

carbonate tablets provide the greatest concentration of calcium per tablet (500 to 600 mg), although they are associated with more gas, bloating, and constipation than calcium citrate supplements (300 to 325 mg per tablet). Chewable tablets, powders that dissolve in beverages, calcium-enriched candies and chocolates, and liquid preparations offer a wide range of personal choice. Nutritional labels on commercial packages report the number of tablets per serving and the amount of elemental calcium. Many calcium supplements also contain 125 to 200 IU of vitamin D. Multiple vitamins marketed for older adults and women may also include 200 to 450 mg of elemental calcium per tablet. Gastrointestinal absorption of calcium is maximal at 600 mg, hence the need to ingest calcium-enriched dietary sources and supplements throughout the day.

Vitamin K, vitamin B complex with folate, and vitamin A also are essential for bone health. The daily U.S. recommended dietary allowances are vitamin K, 90 µg for women and 120 µg for men; vitamin B complex and folate, 400 IU; and vitamin A, 2,000 IU. Vitamin A in excess of 2,500 IU may increase risk of fracture. Older adults for whom warfarin has been prescribed should not take calcium or vitamin supplements that contain vitamin K.

Trace elements, such as magnesium, copper, zinc, and boron, play a role in bone metabolism, but there is inadequate evidence to support the routine use of dietary supplements to achieve intakes beyond those achieved through a well-balanced diet (38). Plants such as soy contain substances with estrogen-like activity. However, a recent randomized trial of a commercially prepared soy protein supplement showed that it did not prevent menopausal loss of bone density (39).

Although the effects of caffeine and alcohol on bone have not been well described, recommendations include limiting intake to two or less exposures of each of these substances daily. Carbonated beverages also should be limited to two or less daily, and they should not be ingested at the same time as calcium-enriched foods or supplements because they may impair calcium absorption (8).

Physical Activity

Exercise has been shown to increase bone mass and morphology during childhood bone development, prevent bone loss with aging, and reduce the risk of falls that result in fracture (40). In young adults, low-magnitude strains achieved through walking can maintain bone (40). Bed rest results in 1% loss of bone per week, which can be recovered at a rate of 1% per month when weight-bearing activity resumes (41), but building bone requires high-magnitude and novel, not customary, physical activity. Increases in the level or amount of such physical activity can raise issues of concern, including endurance loading and fatigue microdamage secondary to repetitive high-impact exercise (such as jogging), nerve entrapment syndromes of the spine and extremities secondary to poor body mechanics, and vertebral compression fractures secondary to flexion exercises of the spine in patients with severe osteopenia. Walking in appropriate footwear for

30 minutes daily is a safe and reasonable exercise prescription. Many community centers offer Tai Chi, of proven benefit for the prevention of falls. The management of newly diagnosed osteoporosis should include a physical therapy referral for instruction in proper technique for resistance exercise; for assessments of gait, balance, and leg-length discrepancies; for fitting of assistive devices to improve gait disorders; and for balance exercise to prevent falls.

Devices that convey vibrations to bone are under investigation and, if proved effective, potentially can be useful particularly for individuals with impaired mobility, such as stroke victims.

Prevention After Menopause and in High-Risk Conditions

Bone loss occurs in all women in the setting of estrogen deficiency. The lower the bone mass in a postmenopausal woman, the greater the risk of future fracture. Women begin menopause with different levels of bone mass, and women lose bone at different rates. The best predictor of early menopausal bone loss is low body weight. Thus, there will be differences among women in short- and long-term fracture risks (11).

A multidisciplinary approach to bone health after menopause is recommended, including advice about nutrition, physical activity, and healthy behaviors; medical assessment of osteoporosis risk by the primary medical provider; and appropriate referrals for DEXA before age 65 years for women with additional risk. The optimal daily calcium intake is 1,500 mg in combination with 400 to 600 IU of vitamin D. The diet should include more than five daily servings of fresh fruits and vegetables to achieve adequate vitamin B complex, folate, and vitamin K levels. Healthy behaviors include avoiding phosphate-containing beverages and limiting caffeine and alcohol use. Maintenance of a healthy body weight and of a body mass index of 24 to 25 kg/m^2 without cycled weight gain and loss is optimal. Walking 30 minutes daily in appropriate footwear and performing resistance exercises with a proper technique complete the behavioral approaches to optimal bone health.

Clinical trials of antiresorptive therapies of estrogens, selective estrogen receptor modulators (such as raloxifene) (42), and oral bisphosphonates (such as alendronate [43] and risedronate [44]) have shown prevention of menopausal bone loss and preservation of the microarchitecture of trabecular bone. The Women's Health Initiative Study, published in 2003, dramatically halted the routine medical practice of prescribing estrogens to postmenopausal woman for preventive health purposes (45). Although the Women's Health Initiative Study documented that conjugated estrogen reduced the rate of hip and symptomatic vertebral fractures by approximately one third, the adverse events of thromboembolic disorders, cardiovascular endpoints of myocardial infarction and stroke, and breast cancer outweighed the benefits to bone health (46). Raloxifene and alendronate therapies have been shown to result in statistically significant reductions in the incidence of vertebral fractures in postmenopausal women with normal or mild bone loss (42,43). However, the low incidence of bone fractures in healthy women under the age of 70 years may limit the clinical utility of these therapies for women with osteopenia and normal bone density.

Bisphosphonate therapies are used to prevent osteoporosis in high-risk patients, including hypogonadal men (47), adults treated with systemic glucocorticoids (48), and those with primary hyperparathyroidism (49). Because of the risk of falls, stroke patients should be considered for preventive therapies. Patients receiving systemic glucocorticoids and antiseizure medications that impair vitamin D metabolism should receive at least 1,000 IU of vitamin D daily.

For early postmenopausal women treated with estrogen or selective estrogen receptor modulators, the inhibition of bone loss erodes rapidly after discontinuation of drug therapy. Thus, maintenance may require long-term therapy. In contrast, bisphosphonates are deposited in bone and may have long-term effects after routine administration ceases (50). Clinical trials are underway to determine whether a drug holiday may be feasible after several years of oral bisphosphonate therapy.

Pharmacologic Therapies for the Treatment of Established Osteoporosis

Age-related fracture risk and bone mineral density should be considered before recommending pharmacologic intervention. A 50-year-old woman with bone mineral density within the World Health Organization's (51) definition of osteoporosis has a 2.5% risk of fracture within 5 years, whereas a 65-year-old woman with the same bone density has a 13% 5-year fracture risk (52). The number of osteoporotic women needed to be treated with pharmacologic therapy at age 50 to prevent one fracture is 100, but the number of older women is only 19 (52). Recently, the cost-effectiveness of alendronate therapy for osteopenic postmenopausal women with femoral neck T-scores better than −2.5 and no history of clinical fractures or other bone mineral density–independent risk factors for fracture has been questioned (53). It is expected that future recommendations for pharmacologic therapy will advocate intervention when the 5-year fracture rate is 10% at 1 year based on a combination of age, a few easily identified clinical risk factors, and bone mineral density (54).

Attention to adequate calcium and vitamin intake is needed to achieve normal bone architecture and strength in the setting of all pharmacotherapies. Indeed, one early study of fluoride had unfavorable results, likely secondary to inadequate mineralization of bone from excessive doses and vitamin D deficiency (55).

Until recently, the principal action of all drug therapies, including estrogens, selective estrogen receptor modulators, bisphosphonates, and calcitonin, was to decrease active bone resorption. Recently, synthetic derivatives of parathyroid hormone have offered an anabolic approach, although fracture data to date show no greater benefit, and long-term safety and efficacy data are lacking (56). Novel osteoporosis treatments under development are targeting the signaling pathways that couple bone resorption to bone formation and stimulate bone matrix protein synthesis.

Based on large clinical trials with fracture outcomes, the first-line treatment for established osteoporosis is oral bisphosphonates (44,46–48). Bisphosphonates, although limited in gastrointestinal absorption, are bone specific and have little systemic effects, hence their overall more desirable benefit-to-risk profile compared with estrogens and selective estrogen receptor modulators. The mechanism of action is impairment in cholesterol synthesis, although specific to osteoclasts secondary to the hydroxyapatite side chains. Current U.S. FDA-approved agents in this class include alendronate and risedronate in daily and once-weekly formulations and ibadronate in a once-monthly dose. Withdrawal of alendronate was shown to have no significant loss of bone density after 7 years (57). The most common adverse reactions are gastrointestinal and occur less frequently when dose intervals are less frequent than daily. Osteonecrosis with long-term oral bisphosphonates has been reported rarely (58). For patients who have had several years of oral bisphosphonate therapy and who have low biochemical markers of active bone resorption, clinicians are now considering at least a 1-year drug-free holiday with serial monitoring at 3, 6, and 12 months and resumption of bisphosphonate therapy when markers increase.

Treatment failure is difficult to assess because the pharmacologic intervention studies show that the various agents have a 30% to 60% efficacy in preventing fractures. Trials of oral bisphosphonate suggest that an adequate clinical response is achieved if serial bone density testing using the same DEXA device shows no loss of bone mineral density.

Intravenous administration of more potent bisphosphonates (such as zolendronic acid) may extend the dosing interval to once yearly and may offer therapy to those who do not tolerate oral therapy (59). The long-term benefits and risks of this approach are as yet unknown, and this intervention should be reserved for those who cannot tolerate standard oral therapies.

Selective estrogen receptor modulators, although effective antiresorptive agents, and estrogen are considered second-line therapies because of the systemic adverse effects that promote thrombosis. Of less concern with selective estrogen receptor modulators are the antiestrogen effects of hot flushes and vaginal atrophy. Long-term cardiovascular effects of raloxifene are currently under large-scale clinical investigation in a study analogous to the Women's Health Initiative Study of conjugated estrogen (45). Other trials are assessing the potential of raloxifene to prevent breast cancer in high-risk women (60). Newer compounds in this class are under development, with the goals of estrogenic effects on bone and the temperature-regulating center of the brain, antiestrogen effects on the breast and uterus, and no effect on the clotting cascades that result in thromboembolic events, myocardial infarction, and stroke. Testosterone replacement therapy for men 50 years of age or older is not recommended at present because of the potential adverse effects on the prostate gland, nor are there synthetic testosterone-like compounds analogous to selective estrogen receptor modulators.

Calcitonin, administered subcutaneously or intranasally, has weaker antiresorptive properties than the agents listed above, but without the systemic allergic reaction as an adverse effect. However, fracture data show that this compound offers no benefit in the prevention of hip fracture (61). With the increase in alternative therapies, calcitonin is used rarely in the clinical management of osteoporosis. Worldwide, strontium is available as an antiresorptive agent (62). It is too soon to determine how its risk-to-benefit profile compares with that of bisphosphonates. An in vitro study of statins, prescribed to impair hepatic metabolism of cholesterol, suggested that they may be effective antiresorptive agents with a mechanism of action similar to that of bisphosphonates (63). Cohort studies have shown fewer hip fractures with statin therapy, although these studies had no control for body weight, a strong predictor of bone mass (64,65). Clinical trials are needed to determine whether statins may be useful in the treatment of osteoporosis.

Anabolic agents that increase bone formation over resorption are in development. Parathyroid hormone derivatives synthesized by recombinant techniques are currently FDA approved or in clinical trials. Current data support their efficacy for the prevention of vertebral fractures (66), but no clinical trials have reported hip fracture endpoints. The bone mineral density increases are greater than those of bisphosphonates as a class, but the fracture data are insufficient for recommending parathyroid hormone derivatives over bisphosphonates as a first-line therapy. Safety, ease of administration, and cost of drugs are issues. At present there are insufficient data to support combination therapy with antiresorptive agents (67).

References

1. Kilbanski A, Adams-Campbell L, Bassford T, et al. Osteoporosis prevention, diagnosis, and therapy. JAMA 2001; 285(6):785–795.
2. Bellantoni M. Approach to the diagnosis and management of the elderly patient. In Kelley's Textbook of Internal Medicine. HD Humes (ed). Philadelphia: Lippincott Williams & Wilkins, 2000.
3. Tosteson ANA. Economic impact of fractures. In Osteoporosis in Men: The Effects of Gender on Skeletal Health. ES Orwell (ed). San Diego: Academic Press, 1999:15–27.
4. U.S. Department of Health and Human Services. Bone Health and Osteoporosis: A Report of the Surgeon General. Rockville, MD: U.S. Department of Health and Human Services, 2004.
5. Byers PH. Disorders of collagen biosynthesis and structure. In The Metabolic and Molecular Bases of Inherited Disease, 8th Ed. C Scriver, AL Beaudet, WA Sly, et al (eds). New York: McGraw-Hill, 2001:5241–5285.
6. Favus MJe. Primer on the Metabolic Bone Diseases and Disorders of Mineral Metabolism. Washington, DC: American Society for Bone and Mineral Research, 2003.
7. Welten DC, Kemper HCG, Post GB, et al. Relative validity of 16-year recall of calcium intake by a dairy questionnaire in young Dutch adults. J Nutr 1996; 126(11):2843–2850.

8. Wyshak G. Teenaged girls, carbonated beverage consumption, and bone fractures. Arch Pediatr Adolesc Med 2000; 154(6):610–613.
9. Specker B. Are activity and diet really important for children's bones? Nutr Today 2002; 37(2):44–49.
10. Zipfel S, Seibel MJ, Lowe B, et al. Osteoporosis in eating disorders: a follow-up study of patients with anorexia and bulimia nervosa. J Clin Endocrinol Metab 2001; 86(11):5227–5233.
11. Riggs BL, Khosla S, Melton LJ, III. Sex steroids and the construction and conservation of the adult skeleton. Endocr Rev 2002; 23(3):279–302.
12. Riggs BL, Khosla S, Melton LJ, III. A unitary model for involutional osteoporosis: estrogen deficiency causes both type I and type II osteoporosis in postmenopausal women and contributes to bone loss in aging men. J Bone Miner Res 1998; 13(5):763–773.
13. Stenson WF, Newberry R, Lorenz R, et al. Increased prevalence of celiac disease and need for routine screening among patients with osteoporosis. Arch Intern Med 2005; 165(4):393–399.
14. Crawford BAL, Kam C, Donaghy AJ, et al. The heterogeneity of bone disease in cirrhosis: a multivariate analysis. Osteoporos Int 2003; 14(12):987–994.
15. Cunningham J, Sprague SM, Cannata-Andia J, et al. Osteoporosis in chronic kidney disease. Am J Kidney Dis 2004; 43(3):566–571.
16. Bilezikian JP. Primary hyperparathyroidism. In Primer on the Metabolic Bone Diseases and Disorders of Mineral Metabolism. MJ Favus (ed). Washington, DC: American Society for Bone and Mineral Research, 2003.
17. Cock TA, Auwerx J. Leptin: cutting the fat off the bone. Lancet 2003; 362(9395):1572–1574.
18. Heaney RP. Constructive interactions among nutrients and bone-active pharmacologic agents with principal emphasis on calcium, phosphorus, vitamin D and protein. J Am Coll Nutr 2001; 20(5 Suppl):403S–409S.
19. Khosla S. Minireview: the OPG/RANKL/RANK system. Endocrinology 2001; 142(12):5050–5055.
20. Jorgensen HL, Kusk P, Madsen B, et al. Serum osteoprotegerin (OPG) and the A163G polymorphism in the OPG promoter region are related to peripheral measures of bone mass and fracture odds ratios. J Bone Miner Metab 2004; 22(2):132–138.
21. Boyden LM, Mao J, Belsky J, et al. High bone density due to a mutation in LDL-receptor–related protein 5. N Engl J Med 2002; 346(20):1513–1521.
22. Nevitt MC, Cummings SR, Hudes ES. Risk factors for injurious falls: a prospective study. J Gerontol 1991; 46(5):M164–M170.
23. Nelson HD, Helfand M, Woolf SH, et al. Screening for postmenopausal osteoporosis: a review of the evidence for the U.S. Preventive Services Task Force. Ann Intern Med 2002; 137(6):529–541; appendix E-541–E-543.
24. Binkley NC, Schmeer P, Wasnich RD, et al. What are the criteria by which a densitometric diagnosis of osteoporosis can be made in males and non-Caucasians? J Clin Densitom 2002; 5(Suppl):S19–S27.
25. Kanis JA, Melton LJ, III, Christiansen C, et al. The diagnosis of osteoporosis. J Bone Miner Res 1994; 9(8):1137–1141.
26. Leib ES, Lewiecki EM, Binkley N, et al. Official positions of the International Society for Clinical Densitometry. J Clin Densitom 2004; 7(1):1–6.
27. Hamdy RC, Petak SM, Lenchik L. Which central dual x-ray absorptiometry skeletal sites and regions of interest should be used to determine the diagnosis of osteoporosis? J Clin Densitom 2002; 5(Suppl):S11–S17.
28. Greenspan SL, von Stetten E, Emond SK, et al. Instant vertebral assessment: a noninvasive dual x-ray absorptiometry technique to avoid

misclassification and clinical mismanagement of osteoporosis. J Clin Densitom 2001; 4(4):373–380.
29. Grampp S, Genant HK, Mathur A, et al. Comparisons of noninvasive bone mineral measurements in assessing age-related loss, fracture discrimination, and diagnostic classification. J Bone Miner Res 1997; 12(5):697–711.
30. Frost ML, Blake GM, Fogelman I. Can the WHO criteria for diagnosing osteoporosis be applied to calcaneal quantitative ultrasound? Osteoporos Int 2000; 11(4):321–330.
31. Pistoia W, Van Rietbergen B, Lochmuller EM, et al. Image-based microfinite-element modeling for improved distal radius strength diagnosis: moving from "bench" to "bedside." J Clin Densitom 2004; 7(2):153–160.
32. Tannenbaum C, Clark J, Schwartzman K, et al. Yield of laboratory testing to identify secondary contributors to osteoporosis in otherwise healthy women. J Clin Endocrinol Metab 2002; 87(10):4431–4437.
33. Looker AC. The skeleton, race, and ethnicity [editorial]. J Clin Endocrinol Metab 2002; 87(7):3047–3050.
34. Standing Committee on the Scientific Evaluation of Dietary Reference Intakes FaNBIoM. Dietary Reference Intakes for Calcium, Phosphorous, Magnesium, Vitamin D, and Fluoride. Washington, DC: National Academies Press, 1997.
35. Brown JP, Josse RG, Scientific Advisory Council of the Osteoporosis Society of Canada. 2002 clinical practice guidelines for the diagnosis and management of osteoporosis in Canada. Can Med Assoc J 2002; 167(10 Suppl):S1–S34.
36. Heaney RP. Functional indices of vitamin D status and ramifications of vitamin D deficiency. Am J Clin Nutr 2004; 80(6 Suppl):1706S–1709S.
37. Heaney RP, Dowell MS, Bierman J, et al. Absorbability and cost effectiveness in calcium supplementation. J Am Coll Nutr 2001; 20(3):239–246.
38. U.S. Department of Agriculture, U.S. Department of Health and Human Services. Dietary Guidelines for Americans 2005. Washington, DC: U.S. Government Printing Office, 2005.
39. Kreijkamp-Kaspers S, Kok L, Grobbee DE, et al. Effect of soy protein containing isoflavones on cognitive function, bone mineral density, and plasma lipids in postmenopausal women: a randomized controlled trial. JAMA 2004; 292(1):65–74.
40. Beck BR, Snow CM. Bone health across the lifespan—exercising our options. Exerc Sport Sci Rev 2003; 31(3):117–122.
41. Leblanc AD, Schneider VS, Evans HJ, et al. Bone mineral loss and recovery after 17 weeks of bed rest. J Bone Miner Res 1990; 5(8):843–850.
42. Ettinger B, Black DM, Mitlak BH, et al. Reduction of vertebral fracture risk in postmenopausal women with osteoporosis treated with raloxifene: results from a 3-year randomized clinical trial. JAMA 1999; 282(7):637–645.
43. Black DM, Thompson DE, Bauer DC, et al. Fracture risk reduction with alendronate in women with osteoporosis: the Fracture Intervention Trial. J Clin Endocrinol Metab 2000; 85(11):4118–4124.
44. Harris ST, Watts NB, Genant HK, et al. Effects of risedronate treatment on vertebral and nonvertebral fractures in women with postmenopausal osteoporosis: a randomized controlled trial. Vertebral Efficacy with Risedronate Therapy (VERT) Study Group. JAMA 1999; 282(14):1344–1352.
45. Austin PC, Mamdani MM, Tu K, et al. Prescriptions for estrogen replacement therapy in Ontario before and after publication of the Women's Health Initiative Study. JAMA 2003; 289(24):3241–3242.
46. Rossouw JE, Anderson GL, Prentice RL, et al. Risks and benefits of estrogen plus progestin in healthy postmenopausal women: principal results

from the Women's Health Initiative randomized controlled trial. JAMA 2002; 288(3):321–333.
47. Orwoll E, Ettinger M, Weiss S, et al. Alendronate for the treatment of osteoporosis in men. N Engl J Med 2000; 343(9):604–610.
48. Reid DM, Hughes RA, Laan RFJM, et al. Efficacy and safety of daily risedronate in the treatment of corticosteroid-induced osteoporosis in men and women: a randomized trial. J Bone Miner Res 2000; 15(6):1006–1013.
49. Chow CC, Chan WB, Li JKY, et al. Oral alendronate increases bone mineral density in postmenopausal women with primary hyperparathyroidism. J Clin Endocrinol Metab 2003; 88(2):581–587.
50. Uusi-Rasi K, Sievanen H, Heinonen A, et al. Effect of discontinuation of alendronate treatment and exercise on bone mass and physical fitness: 15-month follow-up of a randomized, controlled trial. Bone 2004; 35(3):799–805.
51. WHO Study Group. Assessment of fracture risk and its application to screening for postmenopausal osteoporosis. Report of a WHO Study Group. WHO Tech Rep Ser 1994; 843:1–129.
52. Rosen CJ, Black DM, Greenspan SL. Vignettes in osteoporosis: a road map to successful therapeutics. J Bone Miner Res 2004; 19(1):3–10.
53. Schousboe JT, Nyman JA, Kane RL, et al. Cost-effectiveness of alendronate therapy for osteopenic postmenopausal women. Ann Intern Med 2005; 142(9):734–741; appendix W-157–W-163.
54. Kanis JA, Black D, Cooper C, et al. A new approach to the development of assessment guidelines for osteoporosis. Osteoporos Int 2002; 13(7):527–536.
55. Pak CYC, Zerwekh JE, Antich P. Anabolic effects of fluoride on bone. Trends Endocrinol Metab 1995; 6(7):229–234.
56. Reginster JY. Treatment of postmenopausal osteoporosis. BMJ 2005; 330(7496):859–860.
57. Bagger YZ, Tanko LB, Alexandersen P, et al. Alendronate has a residual effect on bone mass in postmenopausal Danish women up to 7 years after treatment withdrawal. Bone 2003; 33(3):301–307.
58. Odvina CV, Zerwekh JE, Rao DS, et al. Severely suppressed bone turnover: a potential complication of alendronate therapy. J Clin Endocrinol Metab 2005; 90(3):1294–1301.
59. Reid IR, Brown JP, Burckhardt P, et al. Intravenous zoledronic acid in post-menopausal women with low bone mineral density. N Engl J Med 2002; 346(9):653–661.
60. Fabian CJ, Kimler BF. Selective estrogen-receptor modulators for primary prevention of breast cancer. J Clin Oncol 2005; 23(8):1644–1655.
61. Chesnut CH, III, Silverman S, Andriano K, et al. A randomized trial of nasal spray salmon calcitonin in postmenopausal women with established osteoporosis: the Prevent Recurrence of Osteoporotic Fractures Study. Am J Med 2000; 109(4):267–276.
62. Meunier PJ, Roux C, Seeman E, et al. The effects of strontium ranelate on the risk of vertebral fracture in women with postmenopausal osteoporosis. N Engl J Med 2004; 350(5):459–468.
63. Sugiyama M, Kodama T, Konishi K, et al. Compactin and simvastatin, but not pravastatin, induce bone morphogenetic protein-2 in human osteosarcoma cells. Biochem Biophys Res Commun 2000; 271(3):688–692.
64. Bauer DC, Mundy GR, Jamal SA, et al. Use of statins and fracture: results of 4 prospective studies and cumulative meta-analysis of observational studies and controlled trials. Arch Intern Med 2004; 164(2):146–152.

65. Rejnmark L, Olsen ML, Johnsen SP, et al. Hip fracture risk in statin users—a population-based Danish case–control study. Osteoporos Int 2004; 15(6): 452–458.
66. Neer RM, Arnaud CD, Zanchetta JR, et al. Effect of parathyroid hormone (1-34) on fractures and bone mineral density in postmenopausal women with osteoporosis. N Engl J Med 2001; 344(19):1434–1441.
67. Black DM, Greenspan SL, Ensrud KE, et al. The effects of parathyroid hormone and alendronate alone or in combination in postmenopausal osteoporosis. N Engl J Med 2003; 349(13):1207–1215.

4

Surgical Options for Vertebral Compression Fractures

Aleksandar Curcin and Richard Henrys

Osteoporotic vertebral compression fractures (VCFs) rarely require surgical treatment. From the surgeon's perspective, a primary concern is confirming the absence of a neoplastic or infectious cause for the fracture. The decision to recommend surgical treatment depends on whether the spine is stable or unstable, and on the presence of a neurologic deficit. Stable VCFs usually are amenable to nonsurgical treatment. Unstable VCFs and/or VCFs resulting in neurologic deficit may require surgery.

Primary Considerations

Fracture Classification

There have been several classification systems devised to describe VCFs. In simplest terms, a VCF is a fracture in which the vertebral body partially collapses. A more concrete definition of a VCF has been suggested to include a 20% or 4-mm reduction of individual vertebral body height (1). Denis (2) has classified four types of VCFs based on morphology and stability (Figure 4.1). The most commonly encountered VCF is type B, which involves the superior endplate. Vertebral compression fractures typically present with involvement of the anterior vertebral cortex; however, VCFs may involve predominately the lateral cortex. The most important radiographic hallmark of these fractures is maintenance (no disruption) of the posterior vertebral cortex (the middle column).

Fracture Biomechanics

Vertebral compression fractures can be caused by several different force vectors (Figure 4.2). The intrinsic alignment of the spine (kyphosis or lordosis) also has a direct influence on what type of fracture will result from a given loading scenario. Axial loads on the spine typically result in burst-type fractures in the cervical and lumbar spine because those regions are normally in lordosis, whereas in the thoracic spine (which

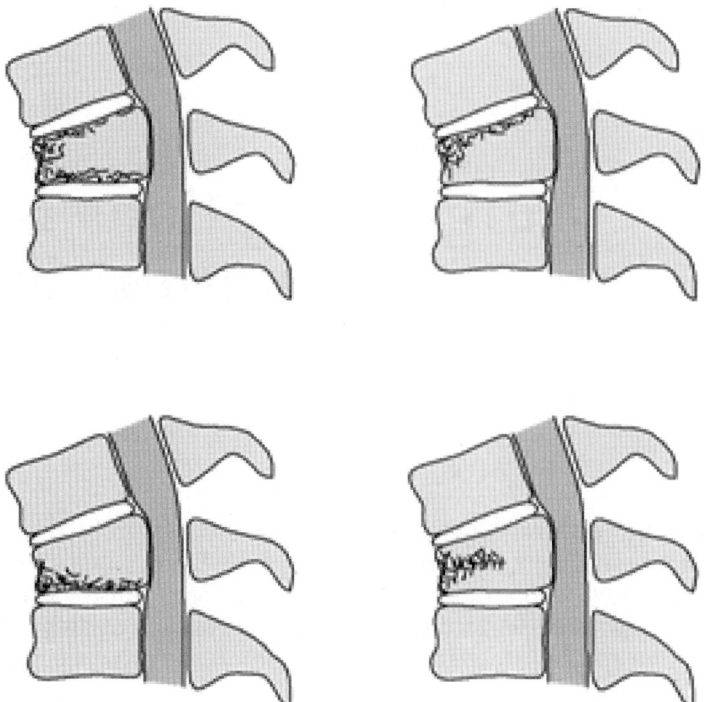

Figure 4.1. Four types of VCF as described by Denis. (From Denis [2], with permission.)

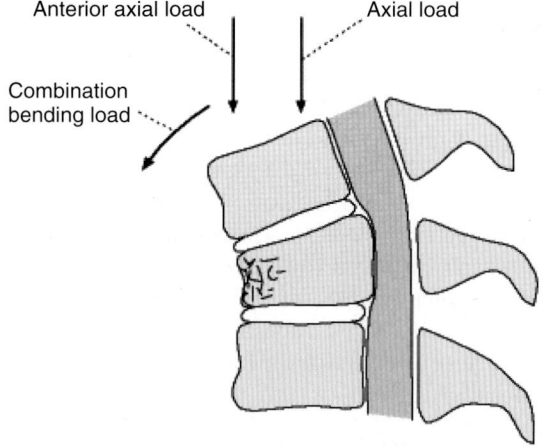

Figure 4.2. Force vectors contributing to VCF. (From J.M. Mathis, H. Deramond, and S.M. Belkoff [eds], Percutaneous Vertebroplasty. New York: Springer, 2002, with permission.)

has normal kyphosis), axial loads result in VCFs. Vertebral compression fractures in the lumbar and cervical regions typically are caused by a flexion mechanism.

Fractures in Weakened Bone

In patients with healthy bone stock, VCFs typically result from a substantial force that imparts considerable energy to the spine. These types of fractures are seen in falls from a moderate height, skiing accidents, or relatively minor vehicular trauma. With appropriate treatment, these fractures rarely collapse to a greater extent than that seen on immediate postinjury radiographs. In patients with compromised bone density (e.g., those with osteoporosis), minor trauma (e.g., sitting down hard on a chair) or even activities of daily living (e.g., bending over to make a bed) can result in a VCF. Radiographs of these fractures obtained in the immediate postinjury period may reveal a minor amount of collapse in the involved vertebra. However, these fractures often continue to collapse (3).

Spinal Instability

For any patient with a spinal injury, a critical question in evaluation and treatment is whether the spine is stable. Clinical instability of the spine has been defined by White and Panjabi (4) as "the loss of the ability of the spine, under physiologic loads, to maintain its pattern of displacement so that there is no initial or additional neurologic deficit, no major deformity, and no incapacitating pain." These authors have described detailed systems for assessing spinal stability. Although an extensive discussion of such an assessment is beyond the scope of this text, the reader is encouraged to consult this reference if caring for a patient for whom spinal instability becomes a concern.

Quick Assessment

Although precise definitions and criteria for spinal instability have been described, it is often helpful in daily clinical practice to be able to refer to quick "rules of thumb" in assessing a thoracic or thoracolumbar VCF for instability. The four essential parameters to consider are the amount of anterior collapse, the degree of segmental kyphosis, the presence of adjacent fractures, and the presence of weakened posterior restraints. Anterior collapse is assessed by using the uninjured vertebrae above and below the fracture as guidelines for normal height comparison. If a fractured vertebra has more than 50% loss of height or collapse of the anterior vertebral cortex, relative to the height of the adjacent vertebrae, it should be considered as potentially unstable (5). Segmental kyphosis should be measured to include the fractured segment. For example, the segmental kyphosis in an L1 superior endplate fracture would be measured from the superior endplate of T12 to the inferior endplate of L1. If segmental kyphosis measures more than 25°, the fracture should be considered potentially unstable. Multiple adjacent fractures may have a greater impact on spinal stability than would an isolated fracture. Multiple adjacent fractures, whether acute or a combination of acute and previous fractures, should be scrutinized carefully and considered as potentially unstable. If the clinician suspects that a fracture has weakened the posterior column restraints (e.g., has stretched the posterior ligaments or facet joints), it should be considered potentially unstable. The presence of more than two of these indicators of potential instability should serve as the impetus to apply more stringent criteria for instability, to follow the patient closely with serial examinations and radiographs, and to seek early surgical consultation.

Successive Fracture and Progressive Deformity

In the uninjured, stable spine, there is a balance of forces acting about the spinal column's axis of rotation. In Figure 4.3, the lever arm z (uninjured spine) is acted upon by the weight of the body and is counteracted by the posterior column restraints acting at the lever arm 3z. Note the relative increase in the anterior lever arm once a VCF develops. At this point, there is relatively less force counteracting the anterior collapse of the spinal column. In patients with osteoporotic bone, this situation is complicated by the fact that the fractured vertebral body continues to collapse, which increases the anterior lever arm even more. As a result of the increased anterior lever arm, less force is required to produce subsequent fractures and a progressive kyphotic deformity.

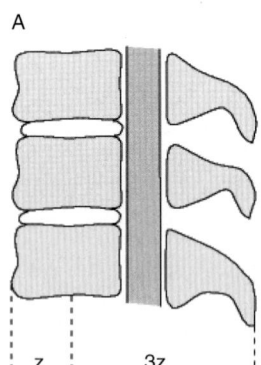
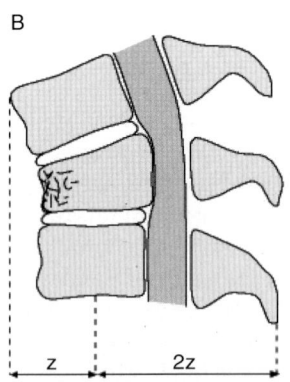
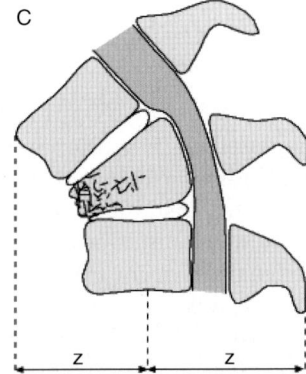

Figure 4.3. Biomechanical loading of the spine. **(A)** The lever arm z (uninjured spine) is acted on by the weight of the body and is counteracted by the posterior column restraints acting at a lever arm 3z. **(B)** Once a VCF has developed, there is a relative increase in the anterior lever arm, which results in relatively less force counteracting the anterior collapse of the spinal column. **(C)** In patients with osteoporotic bone, this situation is complicated by the fact that the fracture continues to collapse, which increases the anterior lever arm even more. As a result of the increased anterior lever arm, less force is required to produce subsequent fractures and a progressive kyphotic deformity. (From J.M. Mathis, H. Deramond, and S.M. Belkoff [eds], Percutaneous Vertebroplasty. New York: Springer, 2002, with permission.)

Surgical Treatment

Indications

For patients with osteoporotic VCFs, *absolute* indications for surgical treatment include spinal cord or cauda equina compression with neurologic deficit, progressive deformity (kyphosis or scoliosis) leading to pulmonary compromise, and progressive spinal deformity resulting in an imbalance of the trunk and torso. Patients with any one of these indications are counseled that surgical intervention is necessary to correct and reverse the damage caused by the fracture. *Relative* indications include intractable pain (including patients with persistent pain after percutaneous cement augmentation) and correction of spinal deformity for cosmesis. Patients falling into the "relative indications" category are advised that surgery may help alleviate their pain and correct an unsightly "hunchback" deformity. However, the risk:benefit ratio must be weighed carefully in these situations, and the patient's comorbid medical conditions are important factors in this decision process.

Options

For most patients with persistently painful VCFs, minimally invasive percutaneous vertebral augmentation with bone cement is an excellent treatment option. Many studies suggest that these techniques result in substantial pain relief for patients with painful osteoporotic and neoplastic VCFs (6–11). Percutaneous vertebral augmentation is discussed at length elsewhere in this text.

Open surgical treatment can be categorized as anterior approach, posterior approach, and combined anteroposterior approach procedures. Each of these approaches has its particular indications and challenges relative to the treatment of VCF.

Anterior Approach

An anterior approach to the spine is indicated for direct decompression of neural elements, anterior column structural reconstruction, and occasionally for osteotomy or anatomic release as correction for severe deformity. Vertebral compression fractures resulting in a neurologic deficit are generally uncommon; however, neurologic deficit can occur acutely or in an indolent fashion secondary to progressive collapse, deformity, instability, and stenosis. Patients presenting with neurologic deficit from fixed anterior impingement on the spinal cord or cauda equina most likely will require direct anterior decompression. Neural function recovery will be influenced by many factors, including how long the neural elements were compressed and which neural elements have been injured. Lee and Yip (12) retrospectively studied the results of 497 patients with osteoporotic VCFs. Ten patients suffered spinal cord compression and canal compromise resulting in neurologic deficit requiring surgery. These patients underwent anterior decompression via thoracotomy or retroperitoneal approach and reconstruction with iliac crest or fibular strut graft. All patients returned to independent ambulation with an assistive device, but none regained full lower extremity strength.

Anterior column structural reconstruction can be achieved by the use of autograft, allograft, metallic or synthetic vertebral body replacement, or polymethylmethacrylate cement. However, it often is difficult to maintain correction because of settling of the graft or implant into weakened osteoporotic bone. This phenomenon is complicated further by modulus mismatch between the local bone and the selected graft or implant. The goal is to provide the best modulus match of elasticity of bone while maintaining sufficient strength. The use of a substance with a higher modulus than that of osteoporotic bone likely will result in vertebral fractures adjacent to the construct, a phenomenon known as the *topping off/bottoming off syndrome*. Adding anterior instrumentation may improve results (13), but anterior screw fixation points in osteoporotic bone tend to be poor, and some anterior instrumentation can carry additional risks and complications.

Posterior Approach

A posterior approach to the spine is used in conjunction with pedicle screw instrumentation. In addition to providing spinal stabilization, the posterior approach occasionally can result in indirect neural decompression (Figure 4.4). In certain cases, the posterior approach may be combined with osteotomy for deformity correction. The strongest point of fixation for posterior instrumentation is the pedicle. However, in osteoporotic bone, pedicle screws are prone to pull-out because the mechanical strength of osteoporotic bone is substantially less than that of normal bone. Anterior cortical purchase of the vertebral bodies and

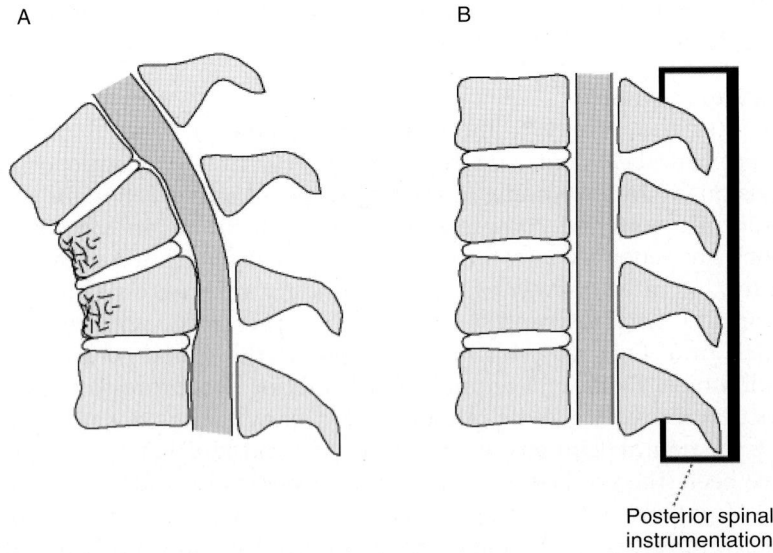

Figure 4.4. (A,B) Indirect decompression achieved as a result of restoring spinal alignment. (From J.M. Mathis, H. Deramond, and S.M. Belkoff [eds], Percutaneous Vertebroplasty. New York: Springer, 2002, with permission.)

anterior cortex fixation of the sacrum may increase pull-out strength. There are several biomechanical, cadaveric studies of screw designs that enhance pull-out strength, such as expandable and conical screws (14,15). Augmenting pedicle screws with polymethylmethacrylate (or calcium apatite cement) or coating them with hydroxyapatite also is shown to enhance pull-out strength (16–18). Cement augmentation of the most cephalad and caudal vertebral bodies included in the pedicle screw construct is probably the most common practice, even though to our knowledge there are no scientific studies to support this technique. The use of sublamina wires and lamina hooks to augment pedicle screw fixation has been shown to be comparable to cement augmentation (19). Using longer constructs with multiple sites of fixation and avoiding ending these constructs within kyphotic segments likely will decrease the number of failures seen in these osteoporotic patients (20). As with anterior procedures, modulus mismatch is also a concern and may result in topping/bottoming off syndrome. In an attempt to address this problem, some surgeons have advocated combining posterior instrumentation techniques with prophylactic vertebroplasty or kyphoplasty at the level adjacent to an instrumented construct. Sun and Liebschner (21) have demonstrated in a cadaveric model that vertebral bodies at risk for fracture required 20% fill of polymethylmethacrylate to enhance their strength and to lower fracture risk. To our knowledge, there have not been any short- or long-term studies evaluating outcomes of prophylactic cement augmentation.

Anterior correction of severe kyphosis from fractures that occur at the thoracolumbar junction would require taking down of the diaphragm, resulting in significant morbidity. However, in some of these cases a posterior approach in conjunction with pedicle subtraction *(eggshell)* osteotomy may achieve sufficient correction to avoid the extensive anterior surgery. In addition to correcting spinal alignment and balance, a pedicle subtraction osteotomy and instrumentation may result in indirect decompression of the neural elements (22).

Combined Approach
A combined anteroposterior approach is very effective in achieving complete neural decompression and restoring three-column integrity and stability. In addition, decreased hardware failure, increased fusion rates, and increased deformity correction may be achieved. Combined approaches, however, represent an extensive amount of surgery and resultant stress on multiple organ systems. This stress sometimes can be mitigated in part by staging the anterior and posterior portions of the surgery 1 week apart. Nevertheless, given the comorbidities in this patient population, combined approaches very rarely are indicated or applicable.

Summary and Conclusions

Patient morbidity and mortality are reduced when osteoporosis prevention regimens, including lifestyle modification and the use of pharmacologic agents, are implemented. All patients should be educated about their risk factors and options for reducing the risk of fracture. They should also be informed about the value of regular exercise and adequate calcium and vitamin D intake. Treatment decisions should be based on each individual patient's medical history and personal preferences. Patients with unstable spines should not be considered for treatment with PV, and a subspecialty consultation should be obtained. When surgery is indicated, the clinician must keep in mind the problems of instrumentation fixation in the osteoporotic spine.

References

1. Black DM, Palermo L, Nevitt MC, et al. Defining incident vertebral deformity: a prospective comparison of several approaches. The Study of Osteoporotic Fractures Research Group. J Bone Miner Res 1999; 14(1): 90–101.
2. Denis F. The three column spine and its significance in the classification of acute thoracolumbar spinal injuries. Spine 1983; 8:817–831.
3. Lyritis GP, Mayasis B, Tsakalakos N, et al. The natural history of the osteoporotic vertebral fracture. Clin Rheumatol 1989; 8(Suppl 2):66–69.
4. White AAI, Panjabi MM. Clinical Biomechanics of the Spine, 8th Ed. Philadelphia: Lippincott Williams & Wilkins, 1990.
5. Garfin SR, Blair B, Eismont FJ, et al. Thoracic and upper lumbar spine injuries. In Skeletal Trauma: Fractures, Dislocations, Ligamentous Injuries, 2nd Ed. BD Browner, JB Jupiter, AM Levine, et al (eds). Philadelphia: WB Saunders Co, 1998:947–1034.
6. Cortet B, Cotten A, Boutry N, et al. Percutaneous vertebroplasty in the treatment of osteoporotic vertebral compression fractures: an open prospective study. J Rheumatol 1999; 26(10):2222–2228.
7. Garfin SR, Yuan HA, Reiley MA. New technologies in spine: kyphoplasty and vertebroplasty for the treatment of painful osteoporotic compression fractures. Spine 2001; 26(14):1511–1515.
8. Heini PF, Walchli B, Berlemann U. Percutaneous transpedicular vertebroplasty with PMMA: operative technique and early results. A prospective study for the treatment of osteoporotic compression fractures. Eur Spine J 2000; 9(5):445–450.
9. Jensen ME, Evans AJ, Mathis JM, et al. Percutaneous polymethylmethacrylate vertebroplasty in the treatment of osteoporotic vertebral body compression fractures: technical aspects. Am J Neuroradiol 1997; 18(10): 1897–1904.
10. Martin JB, Jean B, Sugiu K, et al. Vertebroplasty: clinical experience and follow-up results. Bone 1999; 25(Suppl 2):11S–15S.
11. Spivak JM, Johnson MG. Percutaneous treatment of vertebral body pathology. J Am Acad Orthop Surg 2005; 13(1):6–17.
12. Lee YL, Yip KM. The osteoporotic spine. Clin Orthop 1996; 323:91–97.
13. Kaneda K, Asano S, Hashimoto T, et al. The treatment of osteoporotic-posttraumatic vertebral collapse using the Kaneda device and a bioactive ceramic vertebral prosthesis. Spine 1992; 17(Suppl 8):S295–S303.
14. Kwok AWL, Finkelstein JA, Woodside T, et al. Insertional torque and pull-out strengths of conical and cylindrical pedicle screws in cadaveric bone. Spine 1996; 21(21):2429–2434.
15. Cook SD, Salkeld SL, Stanley T, et al. Biomechanical study of pedicle screw fixation in severely osteoporotic bone. Spine J 2004; 4(4):402–408.

16. Sanden B, Olerud C, Larsson S. Hydroxyapatite coating enhances fixation of loaded pedicle screws: a mechanical in vivo study in sheep. Eur Spine J 2001; 10(4):334–339.
17. Sarzier JS, Evans AJ, Cahill DW. Increased pedicle screw pullout strength with vertebroplasty augmentation in osteoporotic spines. J Neurosurg Spine 2002; 96(3):309–312.
18. Wuisman PI, Van Dijk M, Staal H, et al. Augmentation of (pedicle) screws with calcium apatite cement in patients with severe progressive osteoporotic spinal deformities: an innovative technique. Eur Spine J 2000; 9(6):528–533.
19. Tan JS, Kwon BK, Dvorak MF, et al. Pedicle screw motion in the osteoporotic spine after augmentation with laminar hooks, sublaminar wires, or calcium phosphate cement: a comparative analysis. Spine 2004; 29(16): 1723–1730.
20. Hu SS. Internal fixation in the osteoporotic spine. Spine 1997; 22(Suppl 24):43S–48S.
21. Sun K, Liebschner MA. Biomechanics of prophylactic vertebral reinforcement. Spine 2004; 29(13):1428–1435.
22. Saita K, Hoshino Y, Kikkawa I, et al. Posterior spinal shortening for paraplegia after vertebral collapse caused by osteoporosis. Spine 2000; 25(21): 2832–2835.

5
Patient Evaluation and Selection

M.J.B. Stallmeyer and Gregg H. Zoarski

Vertebral compression fractures (VCFs) can occur as a result of osteoporosis, malignant primary bone tumors, osteolytic metastases, and some benign bone tumors such as vertebral hemangiomas. Percutaneous vertebroplasty (PV) has emerged as an effective technique for treatment of painful VCFs. At present, the safety and effectiveness of PV in treating asymptomatic but abnormal vertebral bodies remains unproven and controversial (1). When considering whether a patient is an appropriate candidate for PV, it is important to distinguish the pain caused by VCFs from numerous other causes of back pain. Careful adherence to clinical and imaging selection criteria is crucial to procedural success; when patients are properly selected, PV may provide substantial pain relief and/or improved mobility in 75% to 92.4% of patients with osteoporotic fractures (1–9) and in 50% to 86% of patients with pathologic VCFs secondary to neoplasm (1,3,5,10–15).

Disease Processes Causing Vertebral Compression Fractures

Osteoporosis

The most common cause of VCF is osteoporosis, which may be related to aging (primary osteoporosis) or result from chronic steroid use or androgen deprivation therapy (secondary osteoporosis). It is estimated that 10 million Americans over age 50 years have osteoporosis, with another 34 million at risk on the basis of low bone mass (16). Direct care costs for osteoporotic fractures range from $12.2 to $17.9 billion each year (17). More than 700,000 symptomatic VCFs come to medical attention in the United States each year. These result in 150,000 hospital admissions and 161,000 physician office visits (18). More than 4% of patients with osteoporotic spine fractures due to minimal trauma become functionally dependent, and 1.9% require nursing home placement (19,20). With aging of the population, the burden of osteoporosis on the health care system is expected to increase substantially.

Primary osteoporosis is characterized by diminished bone mass involving both cortical and trabecular bone, with increased susceptibility to microfracture and thus gross insufficiency fracture. The axial skeleton, femoral neck, and wrist are most commonly affected. The majority of VCFs due to primary osteoporosis occur in postmenopausal women (21,22). The radiographic prevalence of thoracic or lumbar vertebral compression deformity has been reported to be as high as 26% in women over age 50 years when defined as a loss of more than 15% of vertebral body height (22). The frequency of vertebral compression deformity, which may or may not be symptomatic, increases with age in postmenopausal women, from 500 per 100,000 person-years in women 50–54 years of age to 2,960 per 100,000 person-years in women older than 85 (22). The age-adjusted prevalence of osteoporosis in Hispanic and Asian women is similar to that found in Caucasian women, while that of African-American women is lower (23); nevertheless, the rate of bone loss in all ethnic groups increases with age. The incidence of primary osteoporosis in elderly men is also significant: Cooper et al. (24) found an age-adjusted incidence of VCFs in men of 81 per 100,000 person-years, slightly more than half that of women (153 per 100,000) in the same study population.

About 20% of women and more than 50% of men with osteoporosis have a secondary cause of bone loss (25–27). One of the most frequent causes is long-term corticosteroid use, which decreases bone formation and accelerates bone resorption by osteoclasts (28). Patient populations at risk for steroid-induced insufficiency fracture include patients with asthma or chronic obstructive pulmonary disease (COPD), rheumatoid arthritis, malignancies such as lymphoma and multiple myeloma, transplant patients (26), and patients with inflammatory bowel disease (29,30). Osteoporosis is also an important side effect of androgen deprivation therapy for prostate cancer (31).

Vertebral compression fractures, which are the most frequently occurring type of osteoporosis-related fracture, are associated with significant morbidity and mortality. They have been associated with difficulty in performing activities of daily living and impaired psychosocial performance; patients may curtail their activity level due to fear of additional fractures and become unable to care for themselves (20,32–38). Furthermore, there is increased mortality in patients who have had osteoporotic VCFs compared with age-matched controls, with mortality increasing with both the number of fractures (39) and the duration of follow-up (40). The kyphotic deformities caused by VCFs are associated with pulmonary dysfunction, including significantly decreased vital capacity and forced expiratory volume (32), constipation, and alterations in balance.

Although osteoporosis is a systemic disease, most osteoporotic VCFs are located at or near the thoracolumbar junction (Figure 5.1). Most occur "spontaneously" (46%) or after only minimal trauma (36%).

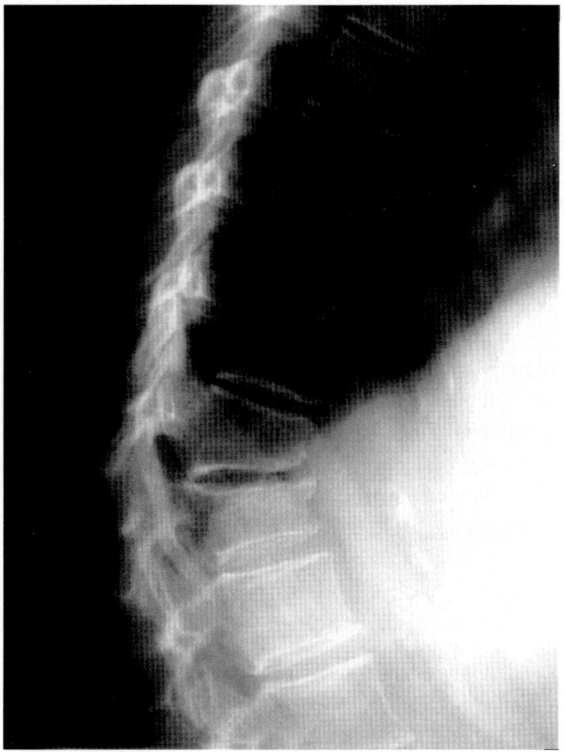

Figure 5.1. Lateral radiograph of the lumbar spine showing adjacent osteoporotic thoracolumbar VCFs that occurred when this patient lifted a bag of groceries. (From J.M. Mathis, H. Deramond, and S.M. Belkoff [eds], Percutaneous Vertebroplasty. New York: Springer, 2002, with permission.)

Because a history of clear antecedent trauma is often lacking, a correct diagnosis is made in only 43% of first visits to a health care provider (41). Patients typically present with acute pain and tenderness over the spine at or near the level of radiographic compression deformity. Radiculopathy is rare but has been reported (42); severe neurologic deficit or spinal cord compression is even more unusual but does occur (43).

Magnetic resonance imaging (MRI) is extremely useful in the evaluation of osteoporotic VCFs, especially when fractures of different ages are present. Magnetic resonance imaging demonstrates characteristic changes in marrow signal that vary with the age of the fracture (44–46). Acute and subacute fractures less than 30 days old typically demonstrate signal changes consistent with bone marrow edema: the marrow is hypointense in signal on T1-weighted images and hyperintense on T2-weighted and short tau inversion recovery (STIR) sequences (Figure 5.2). About 1 month following fracture, the majority of osteoporotic VCFs become isointense to normal bone marrow on T1- and T2-

weighted sequences (Figure 5.2). Fully healed compression fractures may demonstrate a return of normal marrow signal (Figure 5.3) or may appear hypointense on both T1- and T2-weighted sequences when there is significant sclerosis. Cuenod et al. (47) described a band of T2-hyperintense signal subjacent to the fractured endplate in 48% of acute osteoporotic VCFs (Figure 5.3). Additionally, subacute blood products may be found beneath the endplates of the affected vertebra. Acute and subacute fractures may become isointense to normal vertebrae following administration of gadolinium contrast.

The finding of bone marrow edema on MRI is extremely helpful in predicting which patients are most likely to respond favorably to treatment. In a retrospective review of a large series of patients treated with PV for osteoporotic VCFs, Alvarez et al. (9) demonstrated marked to complete pain relief in 68.4% and moderate pain relief in 27.6% of patients demonstrating typical T1-hypointense, T2-hyperintense changes on MRI. They found no significant pain relief in 78.6% of patients in whom these findings were absent. When MRI signal changes suggestive of healing with sclerosis are seen, a confirmatory computed tomography (CT) scan should be obtained; in such cases needle placement and injection of polymethylmethacrylate (PMMA) cement may be impossible or may yield suboptimal clinical and radiographic results (Figure 5.4).

In some cases of benign osteoporotic VCF there may be retropulsion of bone into the spinal canal; this usually occurs at the level of the superior endplate but may also occur along the inferior endplate (47) (Figures 5.2 and 5.3). In Kummell's disease, thought to be a result of avascular necrosis, a fluid collection forms along the superior endplate following osteoporotic VCF (48–50) (Figure 5.5). Magnetic resonance imaging of patients with Kummell's disease demonstrates a fluid collection that borders the superior endplate and that is hypointense on T1-weighted images and markedly hyperintense on T2-weighted sequences. Adjacent inflammatory changes in the vertebral body that would be expected in osteomyelitis are absent (44).

Plain radiographs, often the first study obtained when an osteoporotic VCF is suspected, will demonstrate diffuse osteopenia and may reveal more than one vertebral compression deformity. This makes exact localization of symptomatic levels by plain films alone unreliable, except perhaps when sequential films have been obtained (Figure 5.2). Thin-section (3 mm or less) CT with sagittal reconstructions is the best modality for determining whether a fracture line extends through the endplates or posterior wall of the vertebral body (Figure 5.2). These are important findings when PV is considered, as it may increase the risk of cement extrusion into the disc or spinal canal.

Bone scintigraphy may also aid in differentiating acute from chronic fractures and should be considered for patients unable to undergo MRI. A study by Maynard et al. (51) suggested that increased tracer uptake at the level of a vertebral compression fracture is highly predictive of a positive clinical response following PV; these authors achieved subjective pain relief in 26 out of 28 (93%) patients in their series. Of 44 patients with positive bone scan findings in the series of Alvarez et al.

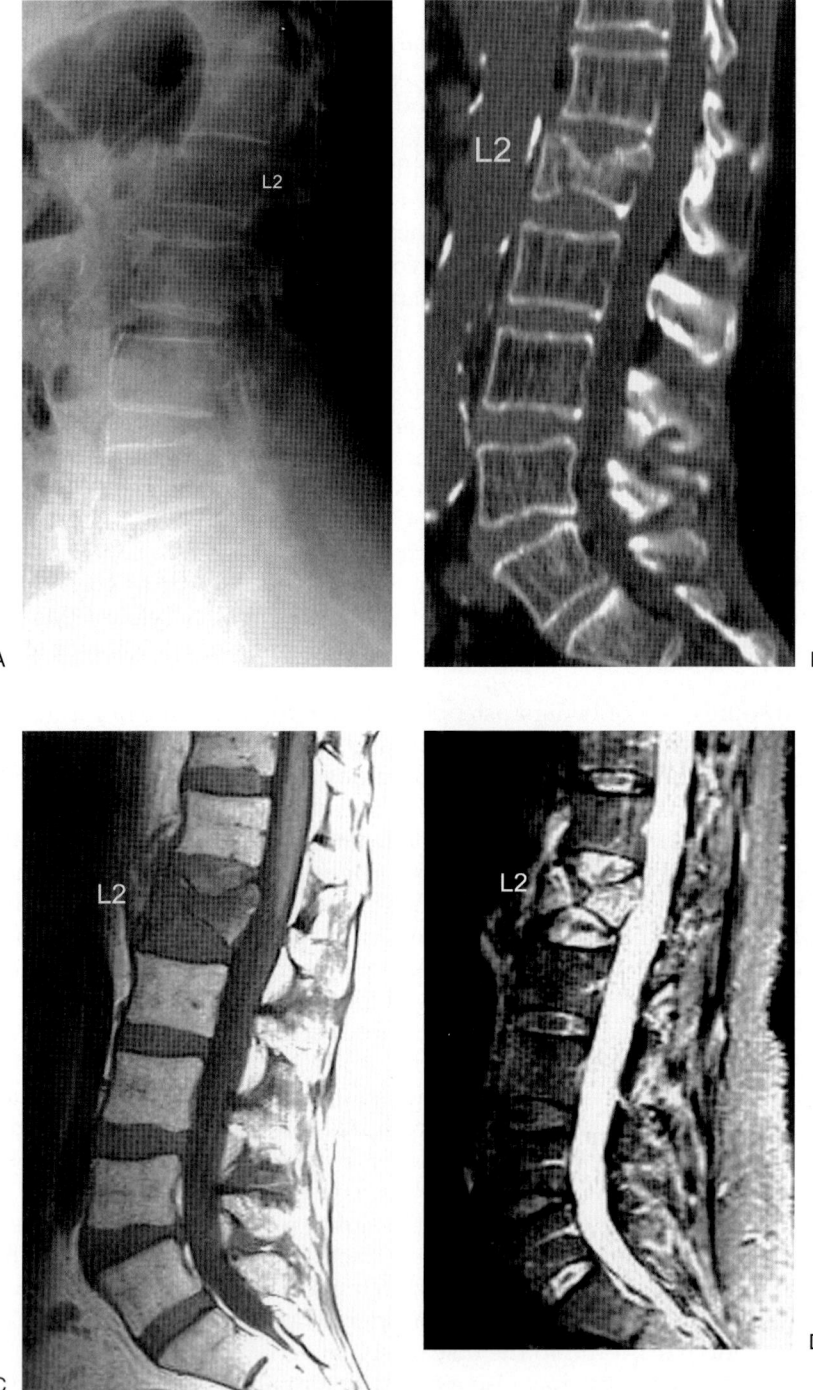

Figure 5.2. This 70-year-old woman with primary osteoporosis presented with severe focal back pain and urinary retention. **(A)** Lateral spine radiograph demonstrates a mild compression deformity at L2. **(B)** CT sagittal reconstruction shows a compression fracture at L2 with fracture lines extending through the posterior wall and inferior endplate. **(C)** Sagittal T1-weighted and **(D)** STIR MR images show edema signal in the L2 vertebral body, consistent with acute fracture. Note retropulsion of the superior endplate of L2. Remaining vertebral bodies show normal signal on MRI.

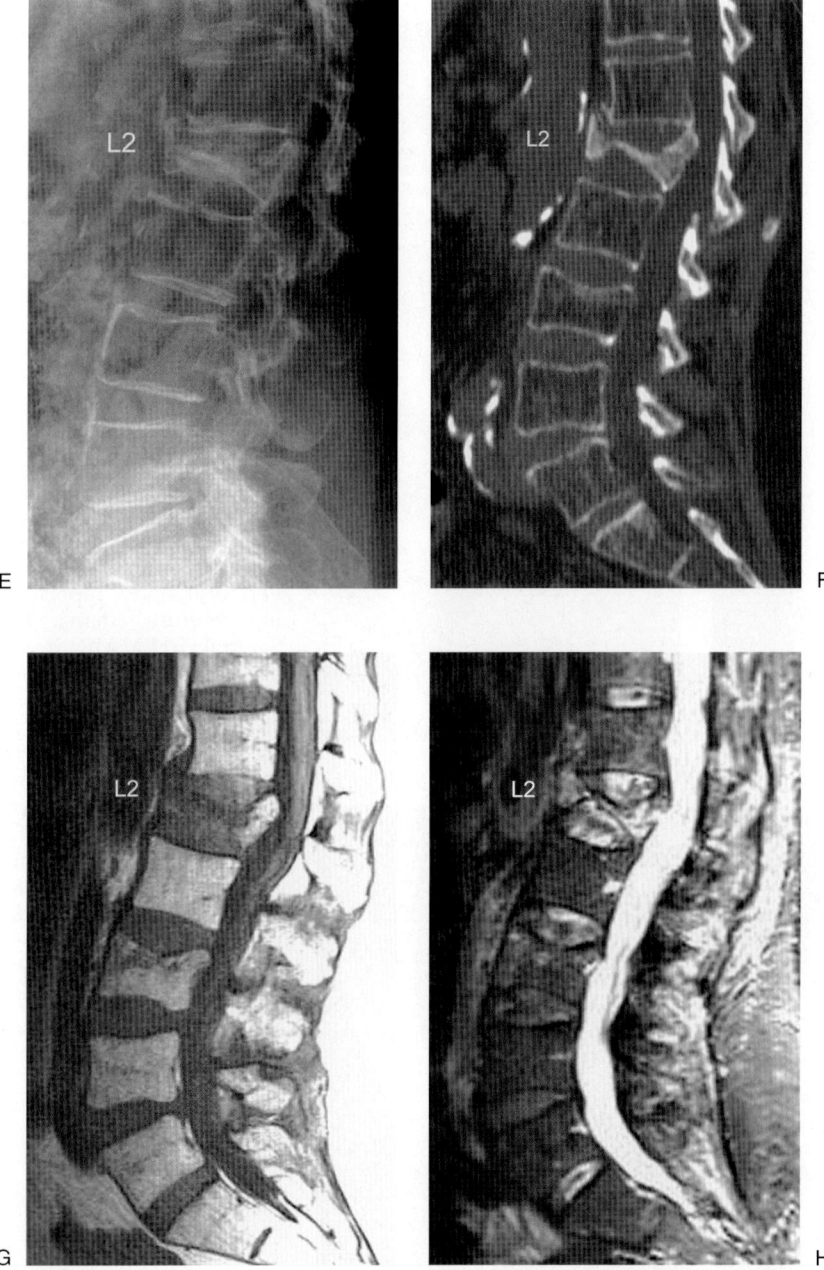

Figure 5.2. *Continued* Three months later, **(E)** lateral spine radiograph, **(F)** CT sagittal reconstruction, **(G)** sagittal T1-weighted MR image, and **(H)** STIR sagittal image show progression of the L1 vertebral body fracture to vertebra plana. Note persistent edema signal in L1 and worsening local kyphotic deformity. T1-weighted and STIR sagittal MR images demonstrate new edema signal and within L3, representing a new compression fracture.

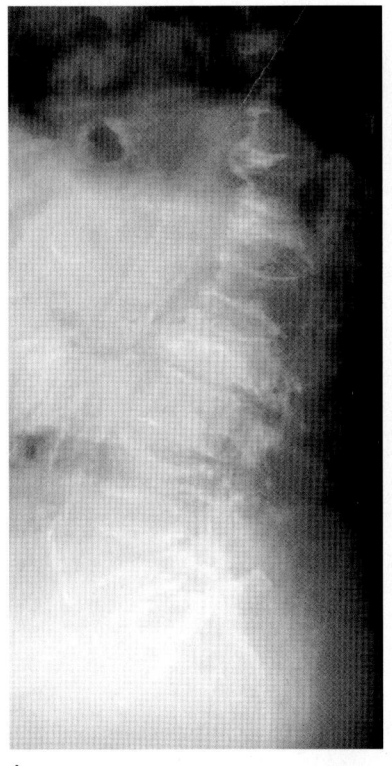
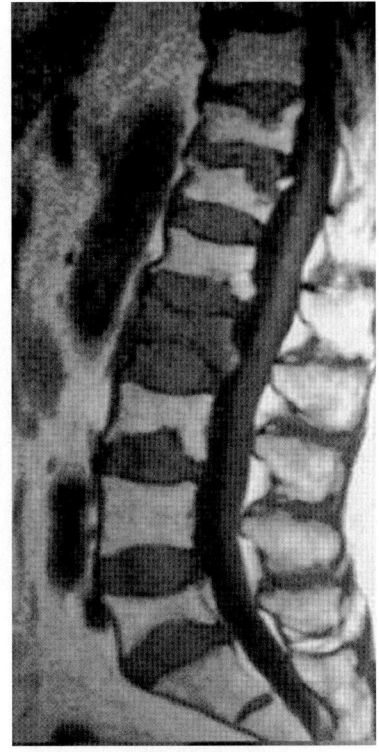
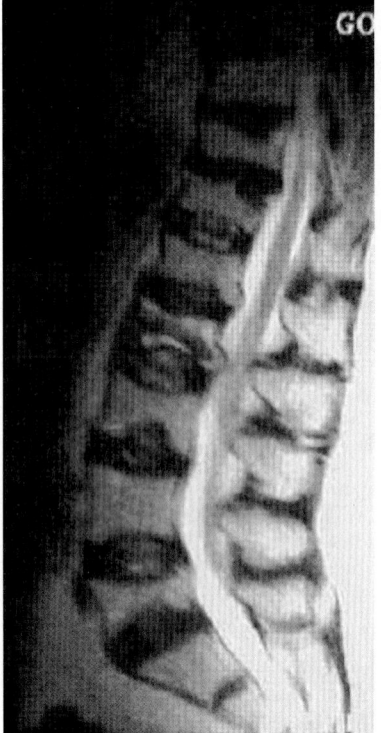

Figure 5.3. This patient with osteoporosis and multiple lower thoracic and lumbar vertebral compression deformities complained of focal pain and tenderness. **(A)** Lateral spine radiograph. **(B)** Sagittal T1-weighted MR image showing acute and chronic osteoporotic compression fractures. The acutely compressed L2 vertebra showed hypointense marrow signal. Other compressed vertebrae showed normal marrow signal, indicating old, healed fractures. **(C)** T2-weighted MR image showing heterogeneously increased signal in the L2 vertebral body, representing fracture edema. **(D)** Sagittal STIR MR image showing prominent hyperintense signal in L2 with characteristic location to the upper portion of the vertebral body. On examination under fluoroscopy, L2 was the most painful level. (From J.M. Mathis, H. Deramond, and S.M. Belkoff [eds], Percutaneous Vertebroplasty. New York: Springer, 2002, with permission.)

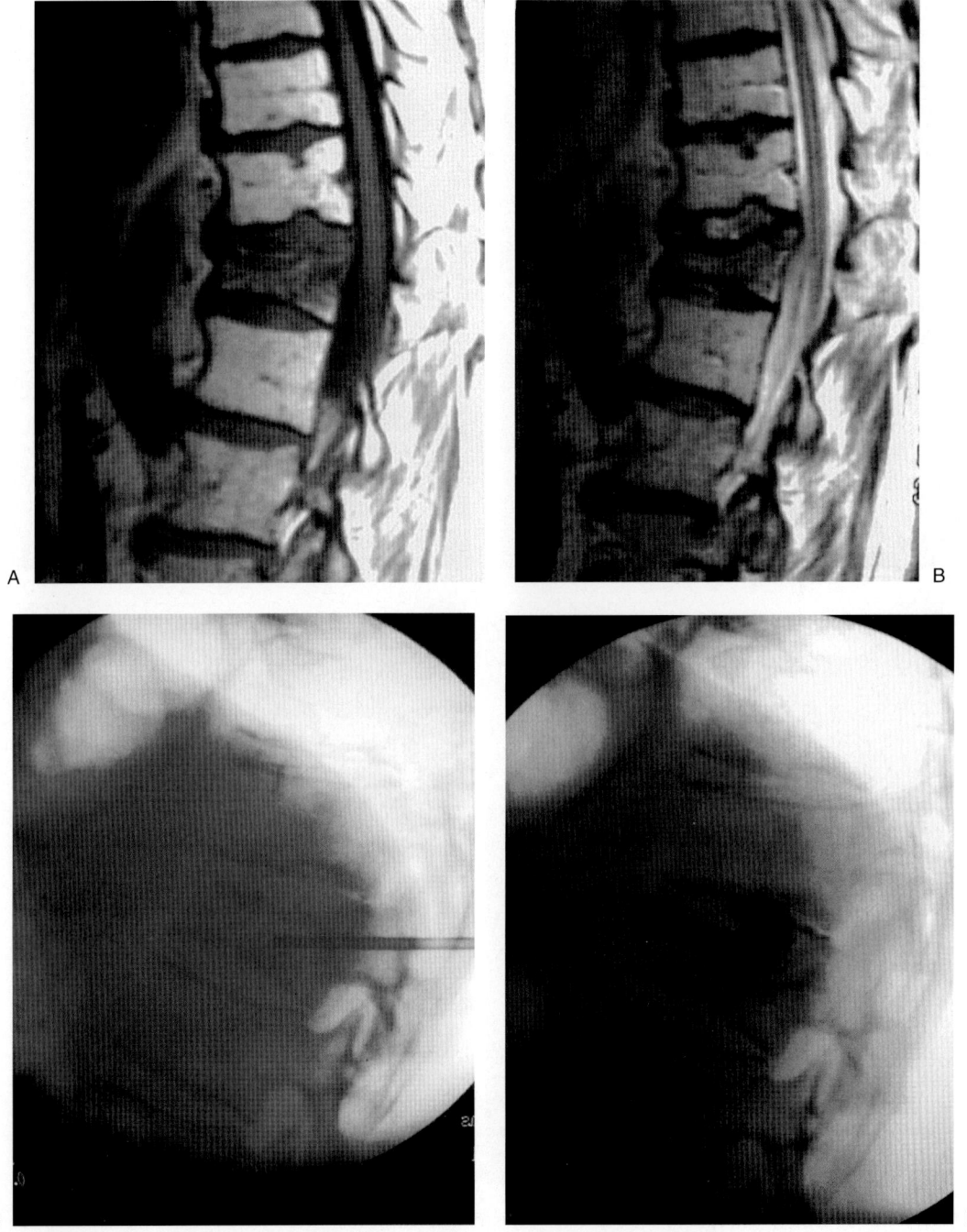

Figure 5.4. This 68-year-old man had long-standing thoracolumbar compression fracture and back pain. Sagittal T1-weighted **(A)** and T2-weighted **(B)** images show hypointense signal in the fractured T12 vertebral body, indicating sclerosis rather than edema. **(C)** Lateral radiograph shows increased density of T12 compared with neighboring vertebral bodies. Placement of needles for cement injection was very difficult because of increased bone density. **(D)** Lateral view after PV shows relatively little intraosseous deposition of cement and minor extrusion into the disc space. (From J.M. Mathis, H. Deramond, and S.M. Belkoff [eds], Percutaneous Vertebroplasty. New York: Springer, 2002, with permission.)

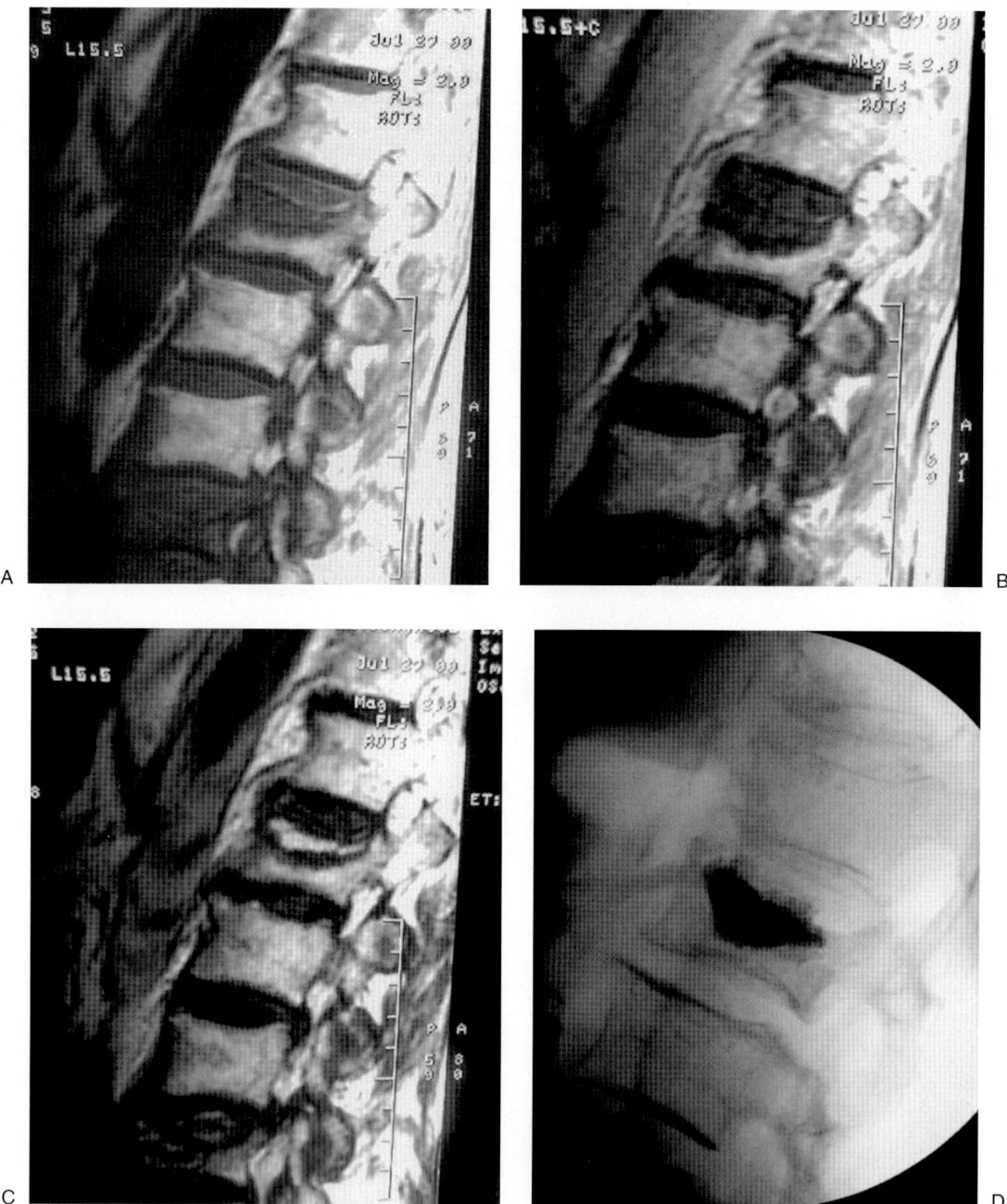

Figure 5.5. Kummell's disease (avascular necrosis of the superior endplate). This 95-year-old woman had a painful L1 compression fracture. **(A)** T1-weighted MR image showing markedly diminished signal along upper vertebral endplate. **(B)** Postcontrast T1-weighted MR image showing no enhancement within the abnormal region of the vertebra. **(C)** T2-weighted MR image showing compression fracture of L1 with fluid along the superior endplate and subjacent sclerotic bone. **(D)** Lateral image after PV showing deposition of cement in the region of avascular necrosis and fluid accumulation. The patient reported substantial pain relief. (From J.M. Mathis, H. Deramond, and S.M. Belkoff [eds], Percutaneous Vertebroplasty. New York: Springer, 2002, with permission.)

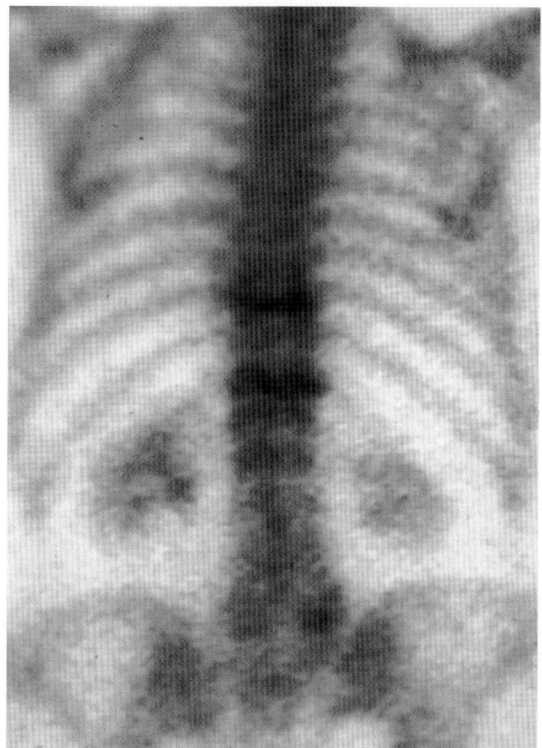

Figure 5.6. Tc-99m–labeled MDP radionuclide bone scan image, posterior view, showing increased uptake at the levels of acute T10 and T12 osteoporotic VCFs. (From J.M. Mathis, H. Deramond, and S.M. Belkoff [eds], Percutaneous Vertebroplasty. New York: Springer, 2002, with permission.)

(9), 28 described marked to complete pain relief, while 16 reported partial pain relief. Of note, the majority of patients in this series also had abnormal findings on MRI. Although this study did not explicitly compare the predictive value of MRI and scintigraphy, of the four patients with increased uptake on bone scan but normal bone marrow signal on MRI, only one patient was considered a treatment success. This is consistent with the finding that a bone scan may show elevated tracer uptake for up to 12 months following fracture; bone scintigraphy should be interpreted with this fact in mind (Figure 5.6).

Malignant Compression Fractures

Common causes of malignant VCFs include osteolytic metastases and multiple myeloma. As with osteoporotic compression fractures, patients usually present with acute pain and tenderness over the spine at or very near the level of radiographic deformity. An antecedent history of malignancy is often known at the time of presentation, and these lesions tend to have certain imaging features that distinguish them from benign VCFs.

Plain film and CT imaging of malignant bone lesions often reveals focal lytic lesions within the affected vertebral body, with destruction or focal rarefaction of bony trabeculae. Expansion of the contours of the bone and the presence of additional lesions at other levels favor a malignant etiology. If a potentially malignant lesion is located in the posterior aspect of the vertebral body, thin-section (1-mm) CT images are usually helpful in evaluating the integrity of the posterior wall of the vertebral body and pedicles prior to performing vertebroplasty (Figure 5.7). Posterior wall involvement or pedicle destruction is not an absolute contraindication to PV; in one early series by Deramond et al. (5), partial or complete destruction of the posterior vertebral body wall was present in over 50% of patients with malignant lesions treated with PV, and successful treatment of lytic lesions involving the pedicles has been reported (52,53). Where tumor mass has destroyed the usual bony landmarks of the posterior vertebral body wall or pedicles, intrathecal injection of myelographic contrast prior to performing vertebroplasty may help in visualizing any tumor displacement into the spinal canal as cement is injected (54).

Bone scintigraphy may demonstrate increased uptake, but may be normal or equivocal, particularly in multiple myeloma. Foci of increased uptake within the spine on F-18 fluorodeoxyglucose (FDG) positron emission tomography (PET) is highly suggestive of spinal metastatic disease, even when lesions are single (55).

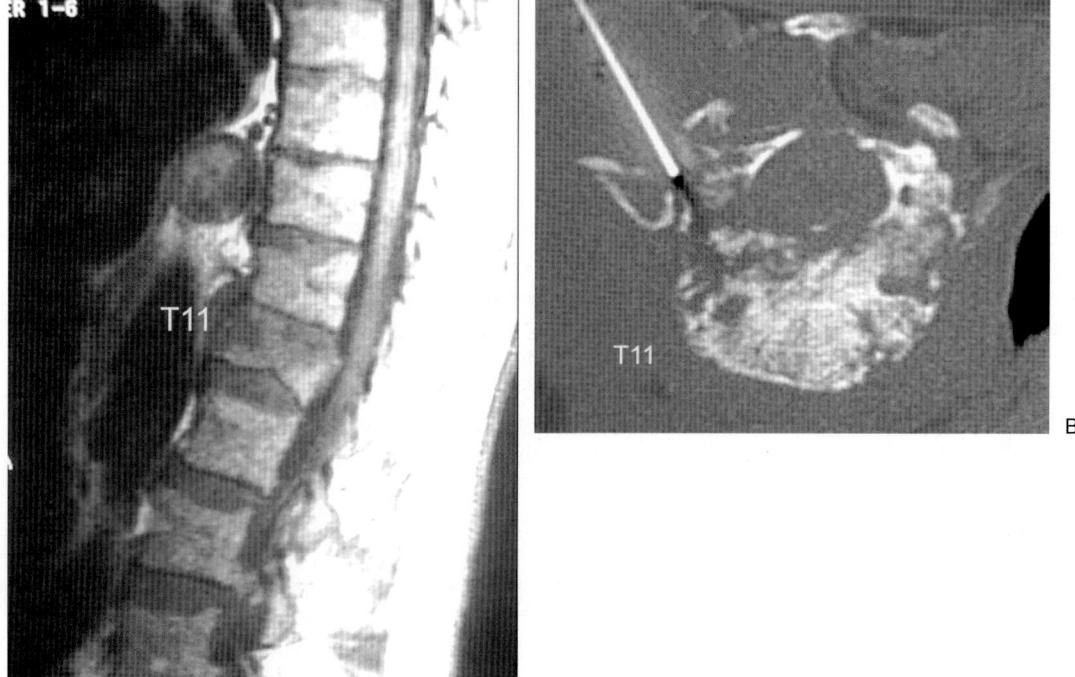

Figure 5.7. Malignant compression fracture. **(A)** Sagittal T1-weighted image and **(B)** thin-section axial CT image demonstrate diffuse tumor infiltration of T11 with destruction of the posterior wall of the vertebral body.

Magnetic resonance imaging findings suggestive of malignant compression fracture include heterogeneous marrow signal or bright enhancement (Figure 5.8). Short tau inversion recovery sequences with fat suppression are particularly helpful in identifying edema within malignant VCFs; heterogeneous or diffuse vertebral hyperintensity on STIR and T2-weighted sequences is typical of malignant disease (46). While some authors have reported that malignant compression fractures demonstrate hypointense or isointense signal compared with adjacent vertebrae on diffusion-weighted MR sequences (56–58), other authors have disputed this finding (59). Other findings that favor the diagnosis of malignant VCF include abnormal signal in the posterior elements, expansion of the contour of the vertebral body or posterior elements, and an associated epidural or extravertebral soft tissue mass (46,47). In some patients, however, imaging findings remain equivocal, particularly in patients with hematopoietic malignancies, who often demonstrate a diffuse pattern of bone marrow infiltration (60). In patients with multiple myeloma, distinguishing VCFs due to tumor infiltration versus those caused by steroid treatment (secondary osteoporosis) can be difficult. While the distribution of lesions in myeloma is often similar to that seen in benign osteoporotic fracture, upper thoracic involvement has been suggested to favor the diagnosis of myeloma (61). In cases where the etiology of a compression fracture is in question, biopsy can easily be performed coaxially through the vertebroplasty needle prior to injection of cement.

Symptomatic spinal cord compression at the level of a VCF is a clear contraindication to PV; even a small amount of cement extravasation or displacement of tumor into the spinal canal as cement is injected could worsen symptoms or could make decompressive surgery technically more difficult. Percutaneous vertebroplasty may be considered after the stenotic canal has been decompressed. Radiculopathy without cord compression is not a contraindication to PV; in these patients, however, tumor infiltration of the pedicle may make needle placement more difficult or could increase the risk of cement extravasation as the needle is withdrawn.

Vertebral Hemangiomas

Vertebral hemangiomas (VHs) are common benign vascular lesions of the spine found in 5%–11% of patients at autopsy. Approximately two-thirds are solitary and about one-third are multiple (62); the majority (about 60%) are found in the thoracic region (63,64). Most VHs are asymptomatic and only come to attention when discovered incidentally during a radiologic examination. Rarely, VHs become painful either with or without an associated compression fracture. Some exhibit aggressive characteristics such as expansion of the contours of the vertebral body and extension of tumor outside the vertebrae and into the epidural space. Either of these features may produce nerve root impingement or spinal cord compression (64–66). Cement injection in these cases may be performed for pain relief, strengthening of the bone, and devascularization of the hemangioma (67–69).

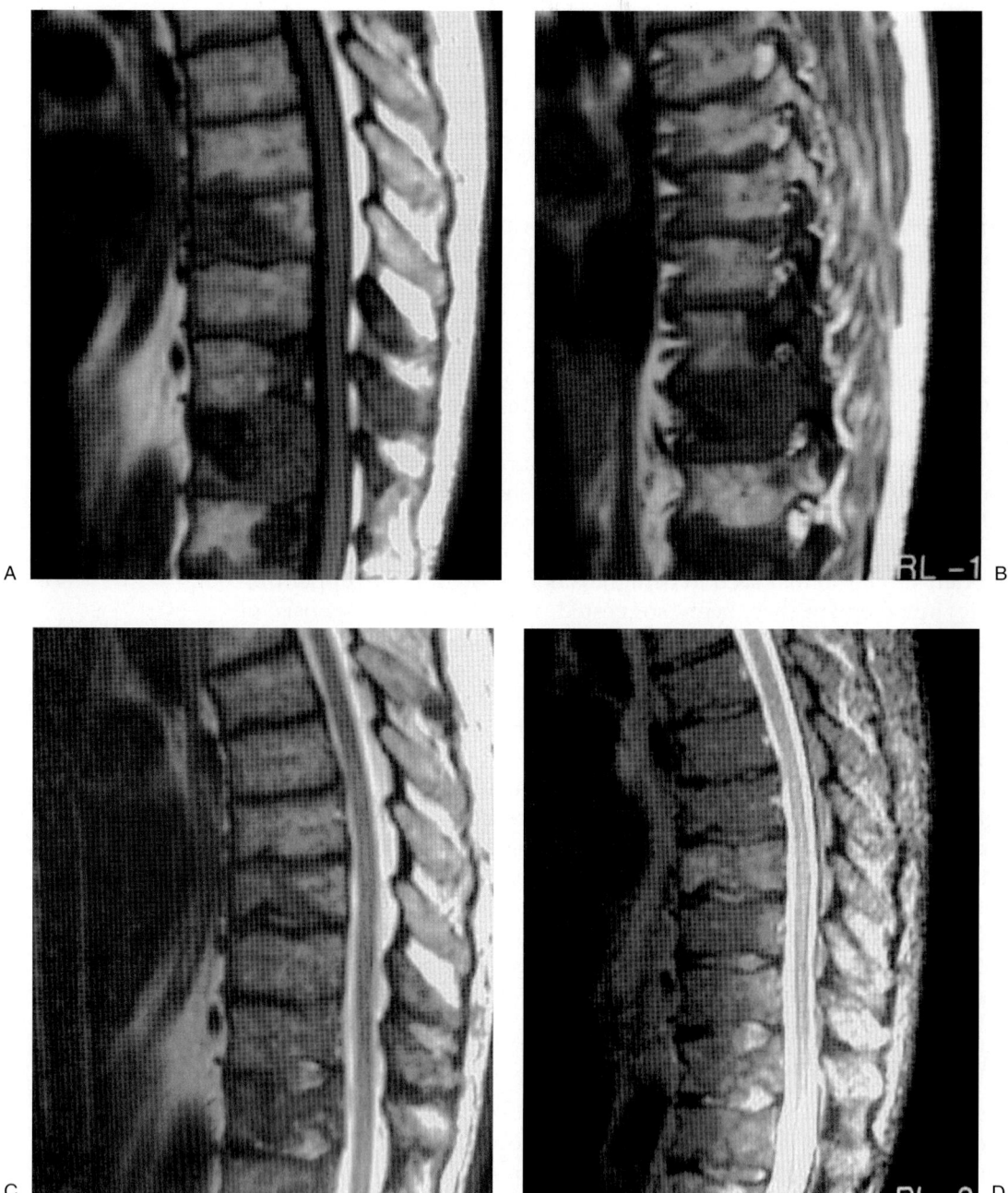

Figure 5.8. This 51-year-old man had metastatic adenocarcinoma. **(A)** Sagittal T1-weighted MR image showing multiple hypointense foci of marrow replacement within lower thoracic vertebrae. **(B)** T1-weighted MR image showing foci of marrow replacement within multiple pedicles. **(C)** T2-weighted MR image showing intermediate but heterogeneous signal throughout the vertebral bodies. **(D)** Sagittal STIR MR image showing increased signal intensity within metastatic foci. The more homogeneous high signal represented edema from a partial pathologic compression fracture of a midthoracic vertebra. (From J.M. Mathis, H. Deramond, and S.M. Belkoff [eds], Percutaneous Vertebroplasty. New York: Springer, 2002, with permission.)

Plain films of VHs reveal a coarse, thickened, vertically striated trabecular pattern within the vertebral body, sometimes with bulging of the posterior cortical margin. Extension of tumor into the pedicles may occur. Thin-section (1-mm) CT imaging is useful in evaluating for involvement of the pedicles (which may modify needle trajectory), in determining the integrity of the posterior wall of the vertebral body, and in identifying encroachment upon the spinal canal (70,71) (Figure 5.9).

Magnetic resonance imaging of VHs typically demonstrates a circumscribed, mottled lesion that is predominantly hyperintense to normal bone marrow on both T1- and T2-weighted sequences (72,73). Histologically, hyperintense signal within the lesion corresponds to fat tissue and not to a hemorrhagic component, while more hypointense striations correspond to thickened bony trabeculae. Aggressive hemangiomas, however, may appear hypointense on T1- and T2-weighted MR sequences when vascular channels predominate (74); these will also tend to enhance more densely than normal bone marrow (Figure 5.9).

Injection of PMMA cement or the acrylic cement n-butyl cyanoacrylate into VHs has been performed for analgesia and reduction of intraoperative blood loss (75–77). In particular, preoperative injection of PMMA into VHs has been found to reduce the risk of massive hemorrhage associated with decompressive laminectomy and resection of VHs bulging into the epidural space (75–77). Percutaneous vertebroplasty can be performed safely in this setting (77), as long as frank spinal cord compression is not present.

Patient Selection

Appropriate patient selection is essential to achieving clinical success with PV. Because more than 80% of the population will suffer from back pain at some point in life (78–80), practitioners of PV commonly receive inquiries regarding patients with other etiologies of back pain such as degenerative disc disease, spinal stenosis, facet arthropathy, and sacroiliac joint dysfunction. Physicians practicing PV need an efficient screening mechanism to avoid being overwhelmed by requests to see patients for whom treatment is not indicated.

Indications

The primary indication for PV is alleviation of pain associated with VCFs caused by osteoporosis, hemangioma, or tumor invasion. Best clinical success is generally achieved in patients with pain and tenderness on palpation that is localized to the level of radiographic compression deformity or vertebral marrow infiltration.

The timing of treatment has liberalized as clinical experience with PV has broadened. In early published and unpublished treatment series, most patients had been allowed to fail conventional medical therapy (analgesics, bracing, and bed rest) for at least several months

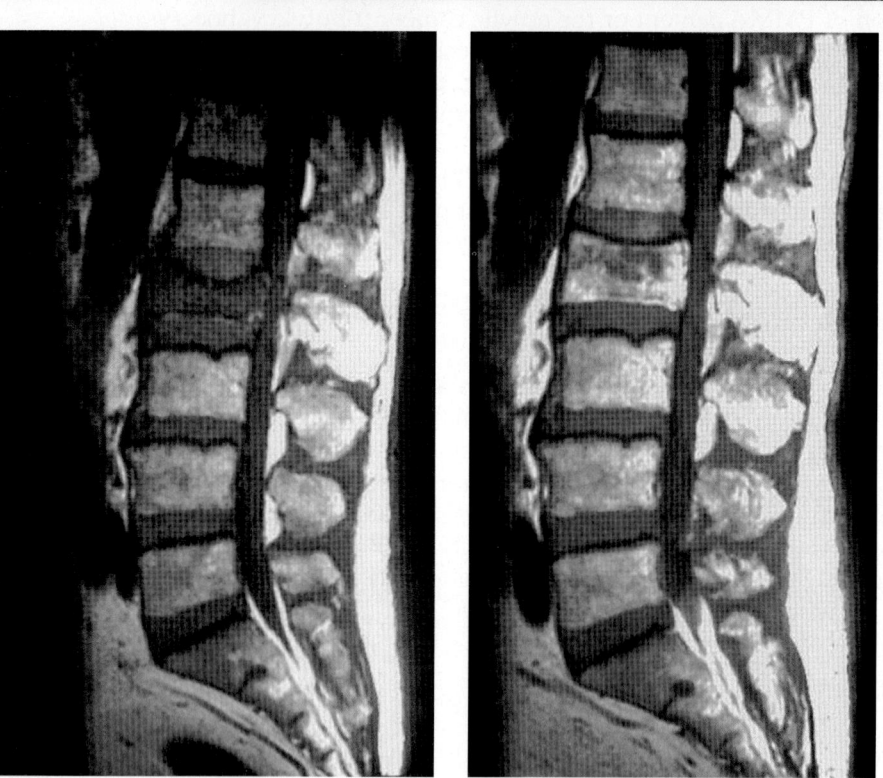

Figure 5.9. Vertebral hemangioma. This patient had focal back pain and tenderness. **(A)** Lateral radiograph showing coarse vertical trabecular striations characteristic of VH. **(B)** Axial CT through L2 confirmed trabecular thickening typical of VH. Expansion of posterior cortex resulted in narrowing of the spinal canal. **(C)** Sagittal T1-weighted MR image showing deformity and hypointense signal within L2. **(D)** Postcontrast T1-weighted image showing enhancement of L2 VH. Again, note expansion of posterior cortical margin. (From J.M. Mathis, H. Deramond, and S.M. Belkoff [eds], Percutaneous Vertebroplasty. New York: Springer, 2002, with permission.)

prior to vertebroplasty (4,8). More recent series have advocated treatment as early as a few weeks (2) or even within days of the occurrence of a painful VCF if pain is so severe as to require parenteral narcotics and hospitalization. Late treatment (after 6 months) is less likely to be successful in completely relieving pain; however, investigators have reported symptomatic improvement with PV performed even years after the initial injury (9,81).

At present, there is no definable role for prophylactic treatment of osteoporotic vertebrae thought to be at high risk for collapse (1). Current data suggest that even patients with severe kyphosis and pulmonary compromise due to prior osteoporotic compression fractures are unlikely to benefit significantly from the procedure in the absence of local pain and tenderness. Although some have advocated a role for prophylactic PV in patients with sentinel pain or signal changes on MRI suggestive of microfracture, these indications are neither widely accepted nor approved as an indication, and no studies have been undertaken to substantiate the utility of performing vertebroplasty for prophylaxis. This indication may change in the future as additional research is performed.

Treatment of painful tumor infiltration without fracture seems more reasonable; however, the increased risk of cement leakage, particularly where cortical breakthrough of tumor is present, should be considered. At this time, there is likely insufficient data to evaluate the efficacy of vertebroplasty for this particular indication. For patients with malignant infiltration, it is not clear whether PV should be performed prior to radiation therapy or reserved for patients who have already received maximal doses of therapeutic radiation. In our experience, vertebroplasty does not adversely impact upon the effects of radiation given subsequent to PMMA injection, and irradiation has not been shown to alter the integrity of cured PMMA (82). Percutaneous vertebroplasty likely dislodges some marrow elements into the bloodstream as PMMA is injected (83). This has raised a concern that PV may promote the dissemination of metastases. While only theoretical, these concerns suggest that vertebroplasty should probably be performed after rather than before an effective dose of radiation therapy.

Younger patients with normal bone mineral density and traumatic VCFs are generally not considered candidates for PV, as it is expected they will heal well without intervention. However, PV has been performed successfully in some patients with burst fracture and disabling back pain refractory to bracing and analgesics; for these patients, successful pain relief was obtained by injection of cement into the clefts of the burst fracture (84). Percutaneous vertebroplasty should certainly be considered for young patients with irreversible underlying metabolic abnormality, such as those with secondary osteoporosis receiving steroid treatment for inflammatory bowel disease, asthma, or COPD and those who have received a transplant. Multiple vertebral fractures have been successfully and appropriately treated in a 36-year-old woman with systemic lupus erythematosus, eliminating debilitating pain and the need for narcotic analgesics (85). Percutaneous vertebroplasty also resulted in rapid relief of pain for a 25-year-old man with collapse of L2 due to previously radiated Langerhans cell histiocytosis (86).

Kyphoplasty, a modification of the standard vertebroplasty procedure, utilizes a balloon bone tamp to attempt to elevate the fractured endplates and restore vertebral body height, thus reducing kyphotic deformity. Height restoration has been demonstrated ex vivo (87), but was often incomplete under conditions simulating physiologic axial loads (88). Recent reports (88–91) describe success in partially restoring vertebral body height in clinical use in both benign and malignant compression fractures. Average height restoration with kyphoplasty has been reported as approximately 3 mm, with a trend (at least anecdotally) toward better height restoration in patients with more recent fractures (90,92). At least 8 mm of residual vertebral height is required for introduction of the required cannulas, which may limit treatment of vertebra plana and other severe compression fractures by this technique. Remarkable height restoration, up to 106% of expected normal vertebral height, has also been observed in many patients undergoing PV alone for dynamically mobile fractures (93,94).

Contraindications

The role of this PV in stabilizing VCFs in the absence of local pain and tenderness, that is, asymptomatic VCFs, and in prophylactic treatment of patients with osteoporotic vertebrae thought to be at high risk for collapse remains unproven.

Active infection is a contraindication to PV; osteomyelitis, discitis, and epidural abscess are absolute contraindications. Emergent performance of PV is rarely, if ever, required, and treatment of patients with fever or sepsis should be postponed until they are afebrile and leukocytosis has resolved. It is also necessary to correct any significant coagulopathy prior to placement of a large-bore bone needle in the vicinity of the spinal canal.

Fractures with greater than 70% loss of vertebral height are technically difficult to treat: the operator may find it challenging or impossible to achieve a satisfactory needle placement within the remaining vertebral body. However, even in severe collapse, vertebral body height is typically better preserved along the lateral aspects of the vertebral body than centrally. Preprocedure evaluation with CT scanning including sagittal and coronal reconstructions may help in selecting a region of the vertebra with adequate residual height to permit treatment by PV. Successful treatment of a small series of patients with greater than 65% to 70% loss of vertebral body height in low thoracic or lumbar vertebrae has been reported (95); the operators used a bilateral transpedicular approach and positioned bone needles in the lateral aspects of the vertebral bodies. Another report described successful PV in a series of 37 patients with 48 severe osteoporotic compression fractures, also with less than one-third of original vertebral body height remaining (96). Complete pain relief was obtained in 47% of patients, while partial pain relief was obtained in 50%. In these series there was a significant incidence of cement leakage into the adjacent disc (35%) or paravertebral soft tissues (8%), but these were asymptomatic. Despite these encouraging results, treating a true vertebra plana may be technically impossible.

Percutaneous vertebroplasty above the level of T5 or T6 is technically difficult: pedicles are typically small, and the orientation of the pedicles may be unfavorable for transpedicular needle placement. Vertebral access can often be obtained using smaller needles (typically 13 gauge or 16 gauge) or a parapedicular trajectory. Computed tomography, or combined fluoroscopic and CT guidance, may be used to plan a reasonably safe approach to these lesions. If appropriate precautions are taken, the risk of complications such as pedicle fracture, cement extravasation, or pneumothorax can be minimized (97).

Cervical vertebral lesions such as hemangiomas (98,99) and metastases may be treated by using smaller needles and a lateral or an anterolateral approach. An anterior trans-oral approach under general anesthesia with biplane fluoroscopic guidance was recently reported in the treatment of upper cervical pain due to myelomatous infiltration of the C2 vertebra; the patient was discharged pain free at 24 hours after the procedure and continued to be pain free at 6 month follow up (100).

At the present time, PV of traumatic compression fractures in young, otherwise healthy patients is not recommended, as the long term effects of vertebral PMMA injection are unknown. The majority of these patients have normal capability to heal the fracture within 4 to 6 weeks; in the interim, symptomatic relief can be obtained with oral analgesics, bed rest, and bracing.

Radiculopathy is not a contraindication to PV; however, the procedure may not improve these symptoms and may in some cases worsen them (101). As previously noted, significant spinal canal stenosis at the level of the compression fracture is at least a relative contraindication to PV. In such cases, preprocedure CT scan supplemented by sagittal and coronal reformatted images can aid in determining whether treatment is possible or advisable. In the case of osteoporotic VCFs, CT will usually reveal that the posterior vertebral body wall is intact. In some cases, however, a fracture line may extend into the posterior vertebral body wall (see Figure 5.2); this likely increases the risk for symptomatic extravasation; however, this has never been studied in a formal fashion. If the degree of retropulsion is so severe as to cause myelopathy, vertebroplasty should not be performed without prior surgical decompression (1).

In malignant compression fractures, the posterior wall of the vertebral body may be destroyed by tumor; it is generally accepted by most practitioners of vertebroplasty that this finding increases the risk of extravasation of cement or tumor displacement into the ventral epidural space and neural foramina (4,5,102–104). However, as long as tumor protrusion into the epidural space is not so severe as to produce cord compression or myelopathy, and appropriate needle placement can be obtained, PV can be performed safely in such patients (103).

In treatment of osteoporotic compression fractures, the risk of complication requiring surgical intervention ranges from 0% to 3% (2–5). Of patients treated with PV for neoplasm (e.g., lytic metastases), multiple myeloma, or lymphoma, surgical intervention for complications such as cord compression or unrelenting radiculopathy has been required in 2.7% to 5.4% (11). Less significant complications that do not require surgery have been reported in up to 10% of patients treated for malignant etiologies (5). In one large series of 258 patients with various etiologies of VCF (113 tumors, 78 hemangiomas, 67 osteoporotic collapse), there was only a single case of spinal cord compression requiring surgery (0.38%), and this occurred in a patient with tumor. Radicular pain occurred in 13 patients (5%), but only 3 required surgery (104). These results are encouraging and suggest the value of operator experience.

Screening of the Physician-Referred Patient

An appropriate clinical history, physical examination, and relevant imaging studies should be obtained as the first step in evaluation of the vertebroplasty candidate. This information is sought in order to differentiate the pain of compression fracture from other etiologies such as disc herniation, spinal cord or nerve root compression, discogenic back pain, facet arthropathy, or spinal stenosis. In our practice, all patients who have no contraindication are studied with MRI obtained just prior to treatment with PV.

Clinical history should include a discussion of the precipitating event leading to compression fracture. Commonly, the patient will report acute onset of pain following minimal trauma. Pain generally worsens with weight bearing and is often at least partially relieved by recumbency. Physical examination should demonstrate pain and tenderness corresponding closely to the level of radiographic fracture deformity. If multiple levels of VCF are present, successful identification of the target level(s) can often only be accomplished after thoughtful analysis of physical examination combined with MRI.

It is important to determine whether the etiology of a VCF might be due to underlying malignancy. Referring physicians' office notes aid considerably in deciding in advance whether a biopsy should be performed prior to cement injection.

Screening of the Self-Referred Patient

Initial evaluation of the self-referred patient is often more difficult, as this population tends to include not only patients for whom PV may be indicated, but also patients with other causes of subacute and chronic back pain. It is important to stress that disease processes such as disc herniation, spinal stenosis, or facet and sacroiliac joint arthropathy will not be helped by PV.

Preprocedure Consultation

Once imaging and clinical findings have been reviewed, and it has been determined that the patient may be an appropriate candidate for PV, a preprocedure consultation with the patient and interested family members may be arranged. Meeting with the family members involved in the patient's care is particularly important for elderly or debilitated patients. Alternatively, and especially in cases where patients must travel a long distance for treatment, telephone consultation with the patient and family prior to the day of the procedure is suggested to screen for allergies, anticoagulant medications, sleep apnea, or medical problems (e.g., COPD, congestive heart failure) that could lead to procedural difficulties. An MRI is performed prior to consultation, but on the same day. Often, PV is performed on the same day when appropriate.

It is helpful to begin by reviewing the history and clinical findings with the patient. Important points to discuss include the time of onset of symptoms, precipitating factors such as trauma, the premorbid status of the patient, impact on activities of daily living, and analgesic use. It is also helpful to know whether prior similar episodes of pain have occurred and, if so, how they resolved. A brief clinical examination can help identify the approximate location of pain and tenderness for correlation with imaging findings. This examination will also serve as an opportunity to evaluate the patient's overall condition and readiness to undergo PV, identify potential difficulties in prone positioning and unique sedation requirements, and allow discovery of contraindicated medications such as coumadin.

Most patients and families will be somewhat familiar with PV through the popular press or Internet searches. The consultation should nevertheless include a brief discussion of how the procedure is performed at your institution, as well as specific instructions about whether current medications should be taken on the day of the procedure, diet instructions, what to expect during the procedure, and information on postprocedure care, transport back to home or to a health care facility, and the expected course of recovery.

The preprocedure consultation is also a time to discuss potential treatment complications. If the procedure is performed by a trained operator with adequate fluoroscopic imaging and appropriate opacification of cement, serious clinical complications should be extremely rare. The most commonly encountered complication is localized pain and tenderness at the needle sites in the first 72 hours following the procedure, usually due to local bruising or hematoma. Minor bruising will resolve with only mild analgesics such as ibuprofen or acetaminophen, and bruising can be minimized with 5 minutes of manual compression over the dermatotomy incision following trocar removal. Dermatomal pain can sometimes occur, more commonly when PV is being performed for treatment of a malignant lesion, but will also often resolve without specific treatment. Patients with significant postoperative radicular pain may require a brief course of nonsteroidal anti-inflammatory drugs, oral steroids, or local steroid injections at the affected area (2,13). Serious potential complications include significant cement extravasation into epidural veins or into the spinal canal, with subsequent spinal cord or nerve root compression, and possible radiculopathy or paraplegia. Excessive cement extrusion into paravertebral veins may cause symptomatic pulmonary embolism (105,106), and a single case of paradoxical cerebral arterial embolism has been reported (107). Puncture of the lung with resultant pneumothorax may occur during inaccurate needle placement for an intended thoracic vertebroplasty. Infection complicating PV is rare, but has been reported (104).

Adequate visualization of cement during injection is a crucial factor for safe performance of PV. Several newer methacrylate preparations are packaged with premeasured amounts of radio-opacifying agents such as barium, tungsten, or tantalum to provide adequate visibility. Some operators, however, may still prefer to add radio-opacifying agents to one of the commercially available bone cements. With their addition, however, the cement injected is no longer the same medical device approved by the Food and Drug Administration. The operator should address this fact with the patient at the time of consultation.

Patient and Family Expectations

It is important to consider patient and family expectations during the consultation. If the patient is a good candidate for PV and the fracture is subacute, a good response can be expected; 80% to 90% of patients typically report significant pain relief. If, however, the fracture has been present for many months or years, the likelihood of substantial pain relief will be diminished (9,44). If a patient has multiple symptomatic VCFs, staging options should focus on treating the most painful compression fractures first. A thorough discussion of staging strategy may also prevent disappointment should the patient's pain not be significantly alleviated during the first treatment session.

No more than two, or perhaps three, levels should be treated at a single session in order to minimize the incidence of symptomatic complications related to venous extravasation of cement (105,106) or fat (83). Fat embolization, in particular, has been implicated as a cause of fatal pulmonary embolization in patients undergoing cemented hip arthroplasty (108); it should be noted, however, that much larger volumes of cement are utilized in hip arthroplasty than in PV.

Another concern in treating multiple levels in a single session is the potential cardiotoxic effect of free methylmethacrylate monomer. Injection of free monomer in concentrations similar to those for surgical patients undergoing cemented hip arthroplasty has been shown to produce hypotension, bradycardia, and depression of myocardial function in isolated perfused rabbit hearts (109) and in anesthetized dogs (110). A few cases of transient arterial hypotension have been reported in patients undergoing PV (111,112). A recent study of the cardiac effects of cement injection, however, found no significant association between PMMA injection during PV and systemic cardiovascular instability (113).

Patient Instructions

For vertebroplasty procedures performed during the morning, the patient should have had nothing by mouth (NPO) after midnight except for medications. If the procedure is scheduled for the afternoon, the patient should be NPO for a sufficient time (at least 4 hours in most institutions) to permit safe administration of medication for conscious sedation.

In general, patients are advised to take their usual medications with sips of water on the day of the procedure. Diabetics who will be NPO after midnight should be instructed to adjust their insulin dosage appropriately. Patients taking anticoagulants should discontinue their use at an appropriate interval before the procedure, but only following consultation with the primary care or prescribing physician.

Preprocedure Laboratory Studies

Routine examinations that should be performed before percutaneous vertebroplasty include a complete blood count, prothrombin time/partial thromboplastin time/International Normalized Ratio or activated clotting time, and platelet count. If intraosseous venography is contemplated, laboratory evaluation of blood urea nitrogen and creatinine levels may also be ordered.

Examination Under Fluoroscopy

Although in many cases it is possible to make a reasonable correlation between the general area of pain described by the patient and the level of VCF on imaging studies, it is always a good idea to localize painful vertebrae by examining the patient under fluoroscopy immediately prior to performing PV. This is especially true for patients with multilevel disease, who often have difficulty precisely localizing discomfort, and for patients reporting diffuse pain and tenderness.

Careful palpation over the posterior elements is performed to identify the most painful vertebral levels. Thumb pressure over each spinous process, or side-to-side movement of a spinous process, will often elicit tenderness in the setting of an acute VCF. Pressure and palpation over paravertebral muscles (i.e., parasagittal palpation) may also help to identify whether or not muscle spasm constitutes an additional component of the patient's pain.

Conclusions

Numerous studies have documented the safety and efficacy of PV. Technical skill alone will not guarantee consistently good outcomes; adherence to rigid patient selection criteria suggested by previous publications will help to ensure clinical success.

References

1. McGraw JK, Cardella J, Barr JD, Mathis JM, Sanchez O, Schwartzberg MS, Swan TL, Sacks MD, for the Society of Interventional Radiology Standards of Practice Committee. Society of Interventional Radiology quality improvement guidelines for percutaneous vertebroplasty. J Vasc Intervent Radiol 2003; 14(9):S311–S315.
2. Cyteval C, Sarrabere MP, Roux JO, Thomas E, Jorgensen C, Blotman F, Sany J, Taourel P. Acute osteoporotic vertebral collapse: open study on percutaneous injection of acrylic surgical cement in 20 patients. Am J Roentgenol 1999; 173(6):1685–1690.
3. Gangi A, Dietemann JL, Mortazavi R, Pfleger D, Kauff C, Roy C. CT-guided interventional procedures for pain management in the lumbosacral spine. RadioGraphics 1998; 18(3):621–633.
4. Jensen ME, Evans AJ, Mathis JM, Kallmes DF, Cloft HJ, Dion JE. Percutaneous polymethylmethacrylate vertebroplasty in the treatment of osteoporotic vertebral body compression fractures: technical aspects. Am J Neuroradiol 1997; 18(10):1897–1904.
5. Deramond H, Depriester C, Galibert P, Le Gars D. Percutaneous vertebroplasty with polymethylmethacrylate. Technique, indications, and results. Radiol Clin North Am 1998; 36(3):533–546.
6. McGraw JK, Lippert JA, Minkus KD, Rami PM, Davis TM, Budzik RF. Prospective evaluation of pain relief in 100 patients undergoing percutaneous vertebroplasty: results and follow-up. J Vasc Intervent Radiol 2002; 13(9 Pt 1):883–886.
7. Zoarski GH, Snow P, Olan WJ, Stallmeyer MJ, Dick BW, Hebel JR, De Deyne M. Percutaneous vertebroplasty for osteoporotic compression fractures: quantitative prospective evaluation of long-term outcomes. J Vasc Intervent Radiol 2002; 13(2 Pt 1):139–148.
8. Cortet B, Cotten A, Boutry N, Flipo RM, Duquesnoy B, Chastanet P, Delcambre B. Percutaneous vertebroplasty in the treatment of osteoporotic vertebral compression fractures: an open prospective study. J Rheumatol 1999; 26(10):2222–2228.
9. Alvarez L, Perez-Higueras A, Granizo JJ, deMiguel I, Quinones D, Rossi RE. Predictors of outcomes of percutaneous vertebroplasty for osteoporotic vertebral fractures. Spine 2004; 30(1):87–92.
10. Jensen ME, Kallmes DE. Percutaneous vertebroplasty in the treatment of malignant spine disease. Cancer J 2002; 8(2):194–206.
11. Cortet B, Cotten A, Boutry N, Dewatre F, Flipo RM, Duquesnoy B, Chastanet P, Delcambre B. Percutaneous vertebroplasty in patients with osteolytic metastases or multiple myeloma. Rev Rhum Engl Ed 1997; 64(3):177–183.
12. Cotten A, Dewatre F, Cortet B, Assaker R, Leblond D, Duquesnoy B, Chastanet P, Clarisse J. Percutaneous vertebroplasty for osteolytic metastases and myeloma: effects of the percentage of lesion filling and the leakage of methyl methacrylate at clinical follow-up. Radiology 1996; 200(2):525–530.
13. Weill A, Chiras J, Simon JM, Rose M, Sola-Martinez T, Enkaoua E. Spinal metastases: indications for and results of percutaneous injection of acrylic surgical cement. Radiology 1996; 199(1):241–247.
14. Kaemmerlen P, Thiesse P, Bouvard H, Biron P, Mornex F, Jonas P. [Percutaneous vertebroplasty in the treatment of metastases. Technic and results.] J Radiol 1989; 70(10):557–562.

15. Kaemmerlen P, Thiesse P, Jonas P, Bascoulergue Y, Lapras C, Duquesnel J. Percutaneous injection of orthopedic cement in metastatic vertebral lesions [letter]. N Engl J Med 1989; 321(2):121.
16. National Osteoporosis Foundation. America's Bone Health: The State of Osteoporosis and Low Bone Mass in Our Nation. Washington, DC: National Osteoporosis Foundation, 2002.
17. Tosteson AN, Hammond CS. Quality of life assessment in osteoporosis: health status and preference based measures. Pharmacoeconomics 2002; 20(5):289–303.
18. Riggs BL, Melton LJ 3rd.The worldwide problem of osteoporosis: insights afforded by epidemiology. Bone 1995; 17(Suppl 5):505S–511S.
19. U.S. Dept. of Health and Human Services, Public Heath Service, Office of the Surgeon General. Report of the Surgeon General's Workshop on Osteoporosis and Bone Health, December 12–13, 2002. Washington, DC: U.S. Department of Health and Human Services, 2002.
20. Greendale GA, Barrett-Connor E, Ingles S, Haile R. Late physical and functional effects of osteoporotic fracture in women: the Rancho Bernardo study. J Am Geriatr Soc 1995; 43(9):955–961.
21. Melton LJ 3rd. How many women have osteoporosis now? J Bone Miner Res 1995; 10(2):175–177.
22. Melton LJ 3rd, Kan SH, Frye MA, Wahner HW, O'Fallon WM, Riggs BL. Epidemiology of vertebral fractures in women. Am J Epidemiol 1989; 129(5):1000–1011.
23. U.S. Dept. of Health and Human Services, Public Heath Service, Office of the Surgeon General. Bone Health and Osteoporosis: A Report of the Surgeon General: Executive Summary. Washington, DC: U.S. Department of Health and Human Services, 2004.
24. Cooper C, Atkinson EJ, O'Fallon WM, Melton LJ 3rd. Incidence of clinically diagnosed vertebral fractures: a population-based study in Rochester, Minnesota, 1985–1989. J Bone Miner Res 1992; 7(2):221–227.
25. Fitzpatrick LA. Secondary causes of osteoporosis. Mayo Clin Proc 2002; 77(5):453–468.
26. Nolla JM, Gomez-Vaquero C, Romera M, Roig-Vilaseca D, Rozadilla A, Mateo L, Fiter J, Juanola X, Rodriguez-Moreno J, Valverde J, Roig-Escofet D. Osteoporotic vertebral fracture in clinical practice. 669 Patients diagnosed over a 10 year period. J Rheumatol 2001; 28(10):2289–2293.
27. Stein E, Shane E. Secondary osteoporosis. Endocrinol Metab Clin North Am 2003; 32(1):115–134.
28. Rehman Q, Lane NE. Effect of glucocorticoids on bone density. Med Pediatr Oncol 2003; 41(3):212–216.
29. Schulte CM. Review article: bone disease in inflammatory bowel disease. Aliment Pharmacol Ther 2004 (Suppl 20); 4:43–49.
30. Reinshagen M, von Tirpitz C. Osteoporosis and other extraintestinal symptoms and complications of inflammatory bowel diseases. Dig Dis 2003; 21(2):138–145.
31. Ross RW, Small EJ. Osteoporosis in men treated with androgen deprivation therapy for prostate cancer. J Urol 2002; 167(5):1952–1956.
32. Schlaich C, Minne HW, Bruckner T, Wagner G, Gebest HJ, Grunze M, Ziegler R, Leidig-Bruckner G. Reduced pulmonary function in patients with spinal osteoporotic fractures. Osteoporos Int 1998; 8(3):261–267.
33. Gold DT, Shipp KM, Lyles KW. Managing patients with complications of osteoporosis. Endocrinol Metab Clin North Am 1998; 27(2):485–496.
34. Leidig-Bruckner G, Minne HW, Schlaich C, Wagner G, Scheidt-Nave C, Bruckner T, Gebest HJ, Ziegler R. Clinical grading of spinal osteoporosis:

quality of life components and spinal deformity in women with chronic low back pain and women with vertebral osteoporosis. J Bone Miner Res 1997; 12(4):663–675.
35. Lyles KW, Gold DT, Shipp KM, Pieper CF, Martinez S, Mulhausen PL. Association of osteoporotic vertebral compression fractures with impaired functional status. Am J Med 1993; 94(6):595–601.
36. Huang C, Ross PD, Wasnich RD. Vertebral fracture and other predictors of physical impairment and health care utilization. Arch Intern Med 1996; 156(21):2469–2475
37. Nevitt MC, Ettinger B, Black DM, Stone K, Jamal SA, Ensrud K, Segal M, Genant HK, Cummings SR. The association of radiographically detected vertebral fractures with back pain and function: a prospective study. Ann Intern Med 1998; 128(10):793–800.
38. Lindsay R, Silverman SL, Cooper C, Hanley DA, Barton I, Broy SB, Licata A, Benhamou L, Geusens P, Flowers K, Stracke H, Seeman E. Risk of new vertebral fracture in the year following a fracture. JAMA 2001; 285(3):320–323.
39. Kado DM, Browner WS, Palermo L, Nevitt MC, Genant HK, Cummings SR. Vertebral fractures and mortality in older women: a prospective study. Study of Osteoporotic Fractures Research Group. Arch Intern Med 1999; 159(11):1215–1220.
40. Cooper C, Atkinson EJ, Jacobsen SJ, O'Fallon WM, Melton LJ 3rd. Population-based study of survival after osteoporotic fractures. Am J Epidemiol 1993; 137(9):1001–1005.
41. Patel U, Skingle S, Campbell GA, Crisp AJ, Boyle IT. Clinical profile of acute vertebral compression fractures in osteoporosis. Br J Rheumatol 1991; 30(6):418–421.
42. Heggeness MH. Spine fracture with neurological deficit in osteoporosis. Osteoporos Int 1993; 3(4):215–221.
43. Salomon C, Chopin D, Benoist M. Spinal cord compression: an exceptional complication of spinal osteoporosis. Spine 1988; 13(2):222–224.
44. Do HM. Magnetic resonance imaging in the evaluation of patients for percutaneous vertebroplasty. Top Magn Reson Imaging 2000; 11(4):235–244.
45. Yamato M, Nishimura G, Kuramochi E, Saiki N, Fujioka M. MR appearance at different ages of osteoporotic compression fractures of the vertebrae. Radiat Med 1998; 16(5):329–334.
46. Baker LL, Goodman SB, Perkash I, Lane B, Enzmann DR. Benign versus pathologic compression fractures of vertebral bodies: assessment with conventional spin-echo, chemical-shift, and STIR MR imaging. Radiology 1990; 174(2):495–502.
47. Cuenod CA, Laredo JD, Chevret S, Hamze B, Naouri JF, Chapaux X, Bondeville JM, Tubiana JM. Acute vertebral collapse due to osteoporosis or malignancy: appearance on unenhanced and gadolinium-enhanced MR images. Radiology 1996; 199(2):541–549.
48. Kummell H. Ueber traumatische ezkrankungen der wirbelsault. Dtsch Med Wochenschr 1895; 21:180–181.
49. Brower AC, Downey EF Jr. Kummell disease: report of a case with serial radiographs. Radiology 1981; 141(2):363–364.
50. Dupuy DE, Palmer WE, Rosenthal DI. Vertebral fluid collection associated with vertebral collapse. Am J Roentgenol 1996; 167(6):1535–1538.
51. Maynard AS, Jensen ME, Schweickert PA, Marx WF, Short JG, Kallmes DF. Value of bone scan imaging in predicting pain relief from percuta-

neous vertebroplasty in osteoporotic vertebral fractures. Am J Neuroradiol 2000; 21(10):1807–1812.
52. Gailloud P, Beauchamp NJ, Martin JB, Murphy KJ. Percutaneous pediculoplasty: polymethylmethacrylate injection into lytic vertebral pedicle lesions. J Vasc Intervent Radiol 2002; 13(5):517–521.
53. Martin JB, Wetzel SG, Seium Y, Dietrich PY, Somon T, Gailloud P, Payer M, Kelekis A, Ruefenacht DA. Percutaneous vertebroplasty in metastatic disease: transpedicular access and treatment of lysed pedicles—initial experience. Radiology. 2003; 229(2):593–597.
54. Sarzier JS, Evans AJ. Intrathecal injection of contrast medium to prevent polymethylmethacrylate leakage during percutaneous vertebroplasty. Am J Neuroradiol 2003; 24(5):1001–1002.
55. Bohdiewicz PJ, Wong CY, Kondas D, Gaskill M, Dworkin HJ. High predictive value of F-18 FDG PET patterns of the spine for metastases or benign lesions with good agreement between readers. Clin Nucl Med 2003; 28(12):966–970.
56. Chan JH, Peh WC, Tsui EY, Chau LF, Cheung KK, Chan KB, Yuen MK, Wong ET, Wong KP. Acute vertebral body compression fractures: discrimination between benign and malignant causes using apparent diffusion coefficients. Br J Radiol 2002; 75(891):207–214.
57. Baur A, Stabler A, Bruning R, Bartl R, Krodel A, Reiser M, Deimling M. Diffusion-weighted MR imaging of bone marrow: differentiation of benign versus pathologic compression fractures. Radiology 1998; 207(2):349–356.
58. Park SW, Lee JH, Ehara S, Park YB, Sung SO, Choi JA, Joo YE. Single shot fast spin echo diffusion-weighted MR imaging of the spine; is it useful in differentiating malignant metastatic tumor infiltration from benign fracture edema? Clin Imaging 2004; 28(2):102–108.
59. Castillo M, Arbelaez A, Smith JK, Fisher LL. Diffusion-weighted MR imaging offers no advantage over routine noncontrast MR imaging in the detection of vertebral metastases. Am J Neuroradiol 2000; 21(5):948–953.
60. Kim HJ, Ryu KN, Choi WS, Choi BK, Choi JM, Yoon Y. Spinal involvement of hematopoietic malignancies and metastasis: differentiation using MR imaging. Clin Imaging 1999; 23(2):125–133.
61. Lecouvet FE, Vande Berg BC, Maldague BE, Michaux L, Laterre E, Michaux JL, Ferrant A, Malghem J. Vertebral compression fractures in multiple myeloma. Part I. Distribution and appearance at MR imaging. Radiology 1997; 204(1):195–199.
62. Schmorl G, Junghanns H. The Human Spine in Health and Disease, 2nd Ed. New York: Grune and Stratton, 1971:325.
63. Laredo JD, Reizine D, Bard M, Merland JJ. Vertebral hemangiomas: radiographic evaluation. Radiology 1986; 161(1):183–189.
64. Krueger EG, Sobel GL, Weinstein C. Vertebral hemangioma with compression of the spinal cord. J Neurosurg 1961; 18:331–338.
65. McAllister VL, Kendall BE, Bull JW. Symptomatic vertebral haemangiomas. Brain 1975; 98(1):71–80.
66. Ghormley RK, Adson AW. Hemangioma of the vertebrae. J Bone Joint Surg 1941; 23:887–895.
67. Galibert P, Deramond H, Rosat P, LeGars D. Note preliminaire sur le traitement des angiomes vertebraux par vertebroplastie acrylique percutanee. [Preliminary note on the treatment of vertebral angioma by percutaneous acrylic vertebroplasty.] Neurochirurgie (France) 1987; 33(2):166–168.
68. Galibert P, Deramond H. La vertebroplastie percutanee comme traitement des angiomes vertebraux et des affections dolorigenes et fragilisantes du

rachis. [Percutaneous acrylic vertebroplasty as a treatment of vertebral angioma as well as painful and debilitating diseases.] Chirurgie 1990; 116(3):326–334; discussion, 335.
69. Deramond H. Darrasson R, Galibert P. Percutaneous vertebroplasty with acrylic cement in the treatment of aggressive spinal angiomas. Rachis 1989; 1:143–153.
70. Schnyder P, Fankhauser H, Mansouri B. Computed tomography in spinal hemangioma with cord compression. Report of two cases. Skel Radiol 1986; 15(5):372–375.
71. Yu R, Brunner DR, Rao KC. Role of computed tomography in symptomatic vertebral hemangiomas. J Comput Tomogr 1984; 8(4):311–315.
72. Friedman DP. Symptomatic vertebral hemangiomas: MR findings. Am J Roentgenol 1996; 167(2):359–364.
73. Ross JS, Masaryk TJ, Modic MT, Carter JR, Mapstone T, Dengel FH. Vertebral hemangiomas: MR imaging. Radiology 1987; 165(1):165–169.
74. Laredo JD, Assouline E, Gelbert F, Wybier M, Merland JJ, Tubiana JM. Vertebral hemangiomas: fat content as a sign of aggressiveness. Radiology 1990; 177(2):467–472.
75. Ng VW, Clifton A, Moore AJ. Preoperative endovascular embolisation of a vertebral haemangioma. J Bone Joint Surg Br 1997; 79(5):808–811.
76. Ide C, Gangi A, Rimmelin A, Beaujeux R, Maitrot D, Buchheit F, Sellal F, Dietemann JL. Vertebral haemangiomas with spinal cord compression: the place of preoperative percutaneous vertebroplasty with methyl methacrylate. Neuroradiology 1996; 38(6):585–589.
77. Cotten A, Deramond H, Cortet B, Lejeune JP, Leclerc X, Chastanet P, Clarisse J. Preoperative percutaneous injection of methyl methacrylate and N-butyl cyanoacrylate in vertebral hemangiomas. Am J Neuroradiol 1996; 17(1):137–142.
78. Lee P, Helewa A, Goldsmith CH, Smythe HA, Stitt LW. Low back pain: prevalence and risk factors in an industrial setting. J Rheumatol 2001; 28(2):346–351.
79. Wells N. Studies of Current Health Problems: Back Pain. London: Office of Health Economics, 1985:4–25.
80. Roland MO, Morrell DC, Morris RW. Can general practitioners predict the outcome of episodes of back pain? BMJ (Clin Res Ed) 1983; 286(6364):523–525.
81. Kaufmann TJ, Jensen ME, Schweickert PA, Marx WF, Kallmes DF. Age of fracture and clinical outcomes of percutaneous vertebroplasty. Am J Neuroradiol 2001; 22(10):1860–1863.
82. Murray JA, Bruels MC, Lindberg RD. Irradiation of polymethylmethacrylate: in vitro gamma radiation effect. J Bone Joint Surg Am 1974; 56(2):311–312.
83. Aebli N, Krebs J, Davis G, Walton M, Williams MJ, Theis JC. Fat embolism and acute hypotension during vertebroplasty: an experimental study in sheep. Spine 2002; 27(5):460–466.
84. Chen JF, Lee ST. Percutaneous vertebroplasty for treatment of thoracolumbar spine bursting fracture. Surg Neurol 2004; 62(6):494–500.
85. Mathis JM, Petri M, Naff N. Percutaneous vertebroplasty treatment of steroid-induced osteoporotic compression fractures. Arthritis Rheum 1998; 41(1):171–175.
86. Cardon T, Hachulla E, Flipo RM, Chastanet P, Rose C, Deprez X, Duquesnoy B, Delcambre B, Devulder B. Percutaneous vertebroplasty with acrylic cement in the treatment of a Langerhans cell vertebral histiocytosis. Clin Rheumatol 1994; 13(3):518–521.

87. Belkoff SM, Mathis JM, Fenton DC, Scribner RM, Reiley ME, Talmadge K. An ex vivo biomechanical evaluation of an inflatable bone tamp used in the treatment of compression fracture. Spine 2001; 26(2):151–156.
88. Belkoff SM, Jasper LE, Stevens SS. An ex vivo evaluation of an inflatable bone tamp used to reduce fractures within vertebral bodies under load. Spine 2002; 27(15):1640–1643.
89. Dudeney S, Lieberman IH, Reinhardt MK, Hussein M. Kyphoplasty in the treatment of osteolytic vertebral compression fractures as a result of multiple myeloma. J Clin Oncol 2002; 20(9):2382–2387.
90. Lieberman IH, Dudeney S, Reinhardt MK, Bell G. Initial outcome and efficacy of "kyphoplasty" in the treatment of painful osteoporotic vertebral compression fractures. Spine 2001; 26(14):1631–1638.
91. Theodorou DJ, Theodorou SJ, Duncan TD, Garfin SR, Wong WH. Percutaneous balloon kyphoplasty for the correction of spinal deformity in painful vertebral body compression fractures. Clin Imaging 2002; 26(1): 1–5.
92. Garfin SR, Yuan HA, Reiley MA. New technologies in spine: kyphoplasty and vertebroplasty for the treatment of painful osteoporotic compression fractures. Spine 2001; 26(14):1511–1515.
93. Hiwatashi A, Moritani T, Numaguchi Y, Westesson PL. Increase in vertebral body height after vertebroplasty. Am J Neuroradiol 2003; 24(2): 185–189.
94. McKiernan F, Jensen R, Faciszewski T. The dynamic mobility of vertebral compression fractures. J Bone Miner Res 2003; 18(1):24–29.
95. O'Brien JP, Sims JT, Evans AJ. Vertebroplasty in patients with severe vertebral compression fractures: a technical report. Am J Neuroradiol 2000; 21(8):1555–1558.
96. Peh WC, Gilula LA, Peck DD. Percutaneous vertebroplasty for severe osteoporotic vertebral body compression fractures. Radiology 2002; 223(1):121–126.
97. Kallmes DF, Schweickert PA, Marx WF, Jensen ME. Vertebroplasty in the mid- and upper thoracic spine. Am J Neuroradiol 2002; 23(7):1117–1120.
98. Feydy A, Cognard C, Miaux Y, Sola Martinez MT, Weill A, Rose M, Chiras J. Acrylic vertebroplasty in symptomatic cervical vertebral haemangiomas: report of 2 cases. Neuroradiology 1996; 38(4):389–391.
99. Dousset V, Mousselard H, de Monck d'User L, Bouvet R, Bernard P, Vital JM, Senegas J, Caille JM. Asymptomatic cervical haemangioma treated by percutaneous vertebroplasty. Neuroradiology 1996; 38(4):392–394.
100. Tong FC, Cloft HJ, Joseph GJ, Rodts GR, Dion JE. Transoral approach to cervical vertebroplasty for multiple myeloma. Am J Roentgenol 2000; 175(5):1322–1324.
101. Ratliff J, Nguyen T, Heiss J. Root and spinal cord compression from methylmethacrylate vertebroplasty. Spine 2001; 26(13):E300–E302.
102. Cotten A, Boutry N, Cortet B, Assaker R, Demondion X, Leblond D, Chastanet P, Duquesnoy B, Deramond H. Percutaneous vertebroplasty: state of the art. RadioGraphics 1998; 18(2):311–320; discussion, 320–323.
103. Shimony JS, Gilula LA, Zeller AJ, Brown DB. Percutaneous vertebroplasty for malignant compression fractures with epidural involvement. Radiology 2004; 232(3):846–853. Epub 2004 Jul 23.
104. Chiras J, Deramond H. Complications des vertebroplasties. In Echecs et Complications de la Chirurgie du Rachis: Chirurgie de Reprise. G Saillant, C Laville (eds). Paris, France: Sauramps Medical, 1995:149–153.

105. Jang JS, Lee SH, Jung SK. Pulmonary embolism of polymethylmethacrylate after percutaneous vertebroplasty: a report of three cases. Spine 2002; 27(19):E416–E418.
106. Padovani B, Kasriel O, Brunner P, Peretti-Viton P. Pulmonary embolism caused by acrylic cement: a rare complication of percutaneous vertebroplasty. Am J Neuroradiol 1999; 20(3):375–357.
107. Scroop R, Eskridge J, Britz GW. Paradoxical cerebral arterial embolization of cement during intraoperative vertebroplasty: case report. Am J Neuroradiol 2002; 23(5):868–870.
108. Parvizi, J. Holiday AD, Ereth MH, Lewallen DG. The Frank Stinchfield Award. Sudden death during primary hip arthroplasty. Clin Orthop 1999; 369:39–48.
109. Wong KC, Martin WE, Kennedy WF, Akamatsu TJ, Convery RF, Shaw CL. Cardiovascular effects of total hip placement in man. With observations on the effects of methylmethacrylate on the isolated rabbit heart. Clin Pharmacol Ther 1977; 21(6):709–714.
110. Wade Waters IW, Baran KP, Schlosser MJ, Mack JE, Davis WM. Acute cardiovascular effects of methyl methacrylate monomer: characterization and modification by cholinergic blockade, adrenergic stimulation and calcium chloride infusion. Gen Pharmacol 1992; 23(3):497–502.
111. Marx WF, Schweikert P, Jensen ME, Kallmes DF. Short Term Clinical Complication Rate of Percutaneous Vertebroplasty for Osteoporotic Compression Fractures: Analysis of 462 Treated Levels. Proceedings of the 40th Annual Meeting of the American Society of Neuroradiology, May 13–17, 2002, Vancouver, BC, Presentation 85, p 76.
112. Vasconcelos C, Gailloud P, Martin JB, Murphy KJ. Transient arterial hypotension induced by polymethylmethacrylate injection during percutaneous vertebroplasty. J Vasc Intervent Radiol 2001; 12(8):1001–1002.
113. Kaufmann TJ, Jensen ME, Ford G, Gill LL, Marx WF, Kallmes DF. Cardiovascular effects of polymethylmethacrylate use in percutaneous vertebroplasty. Am J Neuroradiol 2002; 23(4):601–604.

6
Biomechanical Considerations

Stephen M. Belkoff

Percutaneous vertebroplasty (PV) has enjoyed rapid acceptance as a procedure with which to stabilize vertebral compression fractures (VCFs) and to prevent fractures in vertebral bodies weakened by osteolytic tumors. The procedure is being performed with increasing frequency, and scientific investigations into basic questions regarding the clinical efficacy and technical aspects of the procedure are becoming more common. This chapter reviews the current body of knowledge regarding PV fundamental research and attempts to place into clinical perspective the results from that research.

Mechanism of Pain Relief

The augmentation and stabilization of vertebrae using acrylic cement as an open procedure (vertebroplasty) has been practiced for many years (1–10). However, the percutaneous introduction of cement into a vertebra was first reported in 1987 (11). The procedure consisted of injecting polymethylmethacrylate (PMMA) cement through a large-bore needle into a painful vertebral hemangioma that had aggressively consumed a C2 vertebra. The vertebral hemangioma was injected primarily to prevent subsequent collapse of the involved vertebra, but the procedure also reportedly resulted in marked pain relief (11). The procedure was quickly adapted to stabilize osteoporotic VCFs (12). Since the introduction of PV, retrospective and prospective studies have reported pain relief in approximately 90% of patients treated for osteoporotic VCFs (13–19) and in approximately 70% of patients treated for various tumors (20–23). Although the exact mechanism of pain relief is unknown and may differ in patients with osteoporotic VCFs and those with tumors, possible mechanisms include thermal, chemical, and mechanical factors (24,25). Histologic studies of retrieved specimens report a zone of necrosis around the cement. This zone has been attributed to thermal damage, cytotoxicity from the methylmethacrylate (MMA) monomer, and ischemia (26,27). Because the specimens describe a single point in time, one can only speculate as to the cause of the necrosis. Retrieved specimens from animal models did not indicate necrosis around the cement (28).

Thermal

It has been hypothesized that the heat of polymerization causes thermal necrosis of neural tissue and is therefore the mechanism responsible for pain relief (24). When PMMA polymerizes, heat is generated in the exothermic polymerization reaction (29). Concern about potential thermal tissue injury caused by the heat of polymerization has been the topic of orthopaedic investigations, with particular reference to arthroplasty (29–32). Thermal injury illustrates an Arrhenius relationship in which temperature magnitude and exposure time are both critical factors. Thermal necrosis of osteoblasts occurs when temperatures are higher than 50°C for more than 1 minute (33,34), but apoptosis occurs when osteoblasts are exposed to lower temperatures for longer periods of time (35). Some investigators have measured temperatures as high as 122°C during polymerization (36), but the volumes of cement required to generate such temperatures are substantially greater than those typically used in PV (35). Neural tissue may be more sensitive than osteoblasts to temperature (37).

A previous ex vivo study suggests that temperature is not a mechanism of pain relief (38). In that study, thermocouples were placed at three locations inside vertebral bodies (Figure 6.1) to assess the risk of thermal injury to interosseous nerves, periosteal nerves, and the spinal cord. The vertebral bodies received concurrent bipedicular injections totaling 10 mL of PMMA cement. Although temperatures exceeded 50°C for more than 1 minute at the anterior cortex and in the center of the vertebral body, the authors concluded that temperature was an

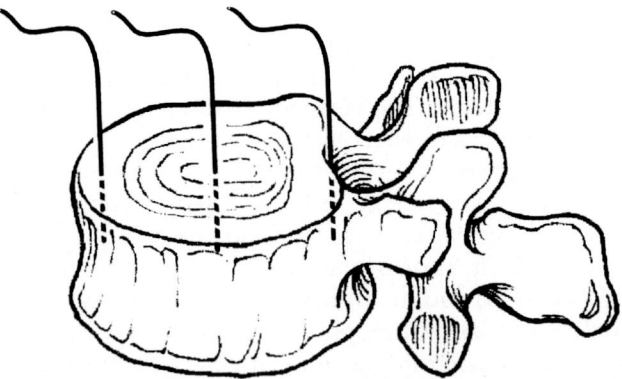

Figure 6.1. Schematic of a vertebral body instrumented with thermocouples to measure temperature elevation caused by polymerizing PMMA cement. Thermocouples were placed at the anterior cortex, at the centrum, and under the venus plexus of the spinal canal. (From J.M. Mathis, H. Deramond, and S.M. Belkoff [eds], Percutaneous Vertebroplasty. New York: Springer, 2002, with permission.)

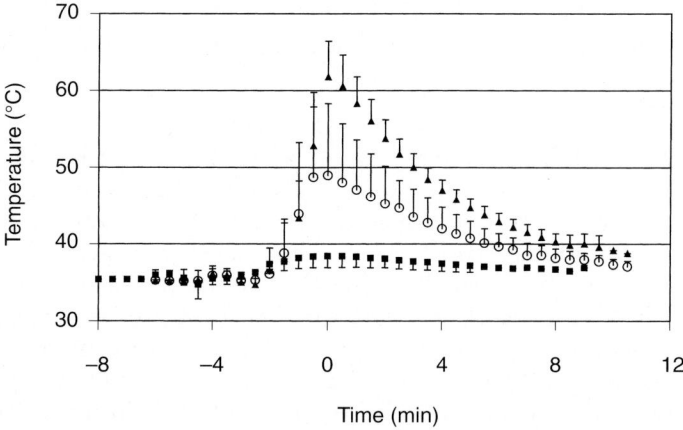

Figure 6.2. Typical temperature-versus-time response of a vertebral body injected with 10 mL of PMMA cement. Temperatures of 50°C for more than 1 minute cause necrosis of osteoblasts. (From J.M. Mathis, H. Deramond, and S.M. Belkoff [eds], Percutaneous Vertebroplasty. New York: Springer, 2002, with permission.)

unlikely mechanism of pain relief. The study was recently reconducted (39). To reflect the smaller volumes being injected in contemporary practice of PV, a 6-mL cement volume group was added to the previous study protocol (Figure 6.2). Another important change in the experimental design was that the cannulae were removed during cement polymerization to prevent inadvertent heat transfer through the cannulae into the bath. Even with smaller volumes injected (i.e., 6 mL), peak temperatures were higher and dwell times above 50°C were longer than those previously measured. For some specimens, peak temperatures were in excess of 110°C. Although the potential for thermal injury cannot be ruled out, the role of temperature remains unresolved. The ex vivo model did not account for active heat transfer secondary to blood profusion, which would be expected to remove much of the heat in vivo. In another study, temperatures measured in an in vivo goat model were below those needed to cause thermal injury (40). The low temperatures may be explained by the effect of blood profusion, but they also may be a consequence of the small volume of cement injected relative to that used in humans. The average volume of cement injected into the goat spines was 0.8 mL, an order of magnitude lower than the volume injected in the human cadaver studies. It is doubtful that the thermal energy and resulting temperature elevations can be scaled linearly based on the size of the vertebral bodies from the respective species. Until temperatures are measured in vivo in human patients, the risk of thermal injury during vertebroplasty will remain undetermined.

Temperature may, however, play a role in slowing tumor growth (31). A recent study indicated that apoptosis likely occurs in osteoblasts exposed to 48°C for 10 minutes or more (35). If similar results are found for tumor cells, apoptosis and diminished tumor cell proliferation may result from exposure to polymerizing PMMA.

Chemical

Methylmethacrylate monomer is cytotoxic (41), but it is unknown if concentrations present in vivo immediately after PV are sufficiently high to be neurotoxic and therefore a mechanism of pain relief (24). In vitro concentrations exceeding 10 mg/mL have been shown to be toxic to leukocytes and endothelial cells (41), yet there are no reports that suggest in vivo concentrations reach such magnitudes. During knee arthroplasty, blood serum levels immediately after cementation and tourniquet release have been measured as high as 120 µg/mL, but such levels typically are much lower (<2 µg/mL) and drop precipitously minutes after cementation (42). During total hip replacement, blood serum concentrations between 0.02 and 59 µg/mL have been measured (43). The volumes of cement used for hip and knee arthroplasty are two to three times larger than those typically used with PV, and the monomer concentrations measured for those procedures are 10 to 100 times less than MMA concentrations reported to be cytotoxic to tissue cultures (41). Even though the cement used with PV typically is prepared with a greater monomer-to-polymer ratio than that of cement used for arthroplasty, it seems unlikely that MMA toxicity is responsible for pain relief experienced with PV.

Cytotoxicity also has been implicated in the antitumoral effect noted clinically (44). However, a recent cell culture study (45) suggested that MMA monomer is cytotoxic to breast cancer cells in concentrations similar to those for leukocytes and endothelial cells (41). Thus, it also seems unlikely that MMA monomer leachate from cement injected during PV has an antitumoral role. Nevertheless, until intravertebral MMA concentrations are measured in vivo, the hypothetical cytotoxic effect of MMA monomer will remain in question.

Mechanical

Mechanical stabilization of the affected vertebral body appears to be the most likely mechanism of pain relief. As with fixation of fractures in other parts of the human skeleton, internal fixation (in the current case, by PV) likely stabilizes the fracture and prevents micromotion at the fracture site, thereby limiting painful nerve stimulation (46,47). In tumors, the pain relief mechanism may be more complex. If the vertebral body contains regions of instability resulting from osteolytic activity by the tumor, PV may prevent micromotion and subsequent pain. If the cement injected during PV has some antitumoral effect (44), then the pain associated with rapid tumor growth may be diminished. The antitumoral effect may be thermal or chemical, as mentioned above, but it also may result from ischemia caused by the mechanical displacement of tumor tissue by the cement and resulting hydrostatic pressure. Thus, injecting PMMA cement into tumors of the spine may have the triumvirate effect of vertebral body stabilization, pain relief, and tumor growth impediment.

Biomechanical Stabilization

Basic Biomechanics

The spine serves to transmit loads from the upper body through the pelvis into the lower extremities. The spine is conceptually divided into three columns: anterior, medial, and posterior. The medial and anterior columns serve to resist axial compressive loads (48) that increase in magnitude from the cervical region to the lumbar region. Because the center of gravity of the human body is located anterior to the spinal column, it creates a combined load resulting in axial compression and an anterior bending moment. For the spine to remain erect, tensile forces along the posterior column (i.e., paraspinous muscles and ligaments) need to act about the medial column, which serves as a fulcrum, while the anterior column acts to resist compression (Figure 6.3). During anterior flexion (e.g., bending over to tie a pair of shoes), the body's center of gravity moves anteriorly, increasing the bending moment on the spine and the compressive stresses on the anterior column. Bending over to pick up a load not only moves the center of

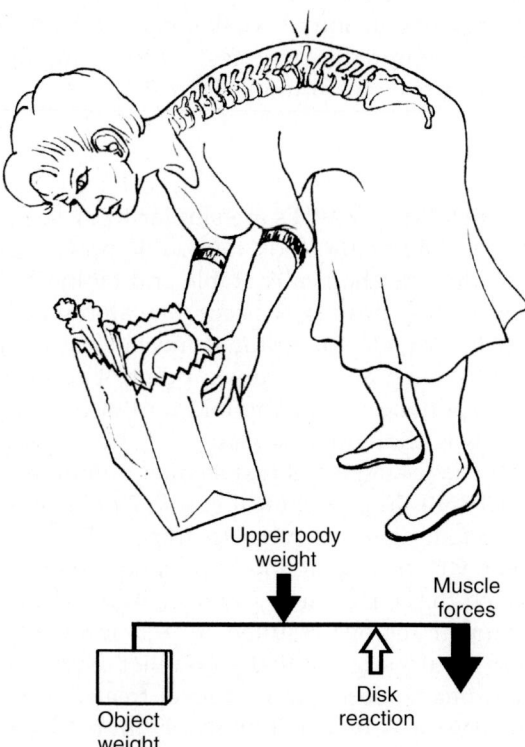

Figure 6.3. The body's center of gravity is anterior to the spine, creating an anterior bending moment and axial compression on the spine. Anterior flexion increases the anterior bending moment, thereby increasing the stresses on the spine and placing the spine at risk for fracture. (From J.M. Mathis, H. Deramond, and S.M. Belkoff [eds], Percutaneous Vertebroplasty. New York: Springer, 2002, with permission.)

gravity anteriorly, but it also increases the magnitude of the anteriorly located load, which, when combined with the increased moment arm, dramatically increases the compressive stresses on the anterior column. It is this excessive compressive stress that results in VCFs. By definition, VCFs exhibit disruption of the anterior column (48).

Compressive strength of vertebra is roughly related to the square of the vertebral bone mineral density (BMD) (49). When a patient's BMD is 2 standard deviations below the average for the sex-, height-, weight-, and race-matched young population, the patient is considered to be osteopenic. When BMD drops below 2.5 standard deviations, the patient is considered osteoporotic (50). In patients with osteoporosis, vertebral BMD might be half of what it was in their youth, which means the vertebral compressive strength may be as low as a one fourth of what it was in their previous young healthy condition.

Although many VCFs go undiagnosed (51,52), 700,000 VCFs are reported each year in the United States (53), 300,000 to 400,000 of which result in hospital admissions. Vertebral compression fractures that are diagnosed may be immediately radiographically apparent or may present with pain but little or no radiographically discernible deformity (54). The former fracture type is typically associated with an acute onset of pain during lifting, raising a window, and so forth, whereas the latter type suggests an initial weakening (perhaps as a result of microfractures) that reportedly progresses into radiographically diagnosable wedge fractures 6 to 16 weeks later (54).

Volume Fill

The goals of stabilization for VCFs are similar to those of stabilization for fractures in other sites in the body, namely, to prevent painful micromotion and provide a mechanically stable and biologically conducive environment for fracture healing to occur. The amount of strength and stability needed to provide the optimal mechanical environment for VCF healing is unknown and remains a point of controversy (55,56). Early in the PV experience, complete injection of the anterior column of the vertebrae was thought necessary (57), but recent clinical and experimental data have suggested that smaller volumes of cement may be sufficient (18,19,58). In one clinical study, 29 patients treated with PV received injected volumes ranging from 2.2 to 11.0 mL (mean, 7.1 mL) of cement; 90% of the patients experienced pain relief (13). Barr et al. (59) indicated that injection of 2 to 3 mL into the thoracic and 3 to 5 mL into the lumbar regions resulted in 97% moderate to complete pain relief. These results suggest that pain relief may be achieved with smaller volumes, but no correlation of level treated, volume injected, and clinical outcome was reported explicitly. In osteolytic metastases and myeloma, there is reportedly no correlation between the percentage of lesion filled and pain relief (60). A similar lack of relationship between cement dose and pain relief was suggested for osteoporotic compression fractures (61). A recent ex vivo study attempted to determine the relationship between cement volume injected and subsequent mechanical stabilization and found that only 2 mL of PMMA was needed to restore strength in osteoporotic vertebral bodies (Figure 6.4), but that larger volumes (4 to 8 mL) were needed to restore stiffness (62). Because the correlation between volume of cement injected and restoration of mechanical properties was very weak, another study was undertaken to correlate the cement volume as a percentage of vertebral body volume with the restoration of mechanical properties (58). In this manner, the geometry of the vertebral body was removed from the analysis. Although the resulting correlation was similarly weak, it suggested that an injection of cement on the order of 30% of the vertebral body volume restored stiffness. A computational model of vertebroplasty reported that only 14% volume fill was needed to restore stiffness (63). Considering the variation in the experimental data, the experimental results and computational results are not necessarily inconsistent. Mechanical property restoration is a function of the volume of cement injected, the density of the host bone, and, to a lesser extent, the location of the cement.

Postvertebroplasty stiffness is the mechanical parameter likely to be linked most closely with pain relief (62). Restoring initial strength might be expected to prevent refracture of the treated vertebra, whereas restoring initial vertebral body stiffness likely prevents micromotion and the pain associated with it. However, fully restoring prefracture stiffness to vertebral bodies may not be necessary or even desirable. As with other fractures, providing some mechanical stability, even less than that of the prefracture state, may be sufficient to allow healing (64). If the repair is too stiff, stress shielding may occur and impede fracture healing. If the repair is not stiff enough, excessive motion at the fracture site may occur, resulting in nonunion. Furthermore, the remaining cancellous bone in the vertebral body is still osteoporotic and at risk of fracture. Thus, it is not surprising that there are some reports of refracture around the cement injected during a previous vertebroplasty (55,65). Some clinicians might be inclined to fill the vertebral body maximally in hopes of preventing secondary fractures, but this increases the risk of extravasation and subsequent pulmonary complications and theoretically may prevent the endplates from deflecting, thereby increasing disc pressure and placing adjacent levels at increased risk of fracture (66). However, disc pressure measurements ex vivo do not support this hypothesis (67).

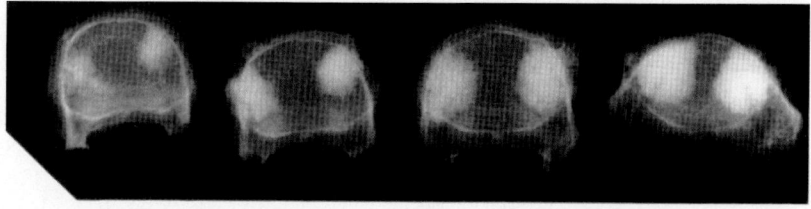

Figure 6.4. Radiograph of typical cement (Simplex P) distribution when 2, 4, 6, or 8 mL is injected into lumbar vertebrae. (From J.M. Mathis, H. Deramond, and S.M. Belkoff [eds], Percutaneous Vertebroplasty. New York: Springer, 2002, with permission.)

The volume and material properties of cement needed to achieve sufficient stabilization for healing and to prevent pain are yet unknown and can be determined definitively only by a prospective, controlled, randomized clinical study. Some of the conflicting opinions regarding the appropriate volume of cement needed for injection stem from the different goals of the procedure. Providing fracture stabilization to prevent pain and allow fracture healing may require a different cement volume than that needed to prevent fracture through prophylactic augmentation.

Unipedicular Injection

In another ex vivo study, Tohmeh et al. (47) found that vertebral body strength may be restored via a unipedicular injection of 6 mL of cement without risk of vertebral body collapse on the uninjected side (Figure 6.5). Both injection protocols in that study (6 mL unipedicular, 10 mL bipedicular) resulted in increased strength and restored stiffness to fractured vertebral bodies. These results (47), considered in conjunction with those of the previously mentioned volume-fill study (62), suggest that the injection of the appropriate cement volume is more important than the manner in which it is injected. The findings also were supported by a subsequent study in which injected volumes more closely reflect those in the contemporary practice of vertebroplasty. Despite results from a computational model to the contrary (63,68), a unipedicular injection of an appropriate volume of cement may allow adequate stabilization with the added benefit of reduced procedure time and risk associated with bilateral cannula placement. A similar ex

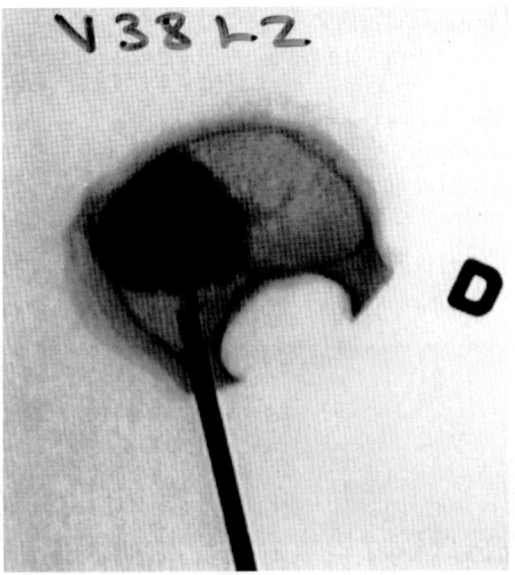

Figure 6.5. Typical distribution of cement after unipedicular injection of 6 mL of PMMA cement. (From J.M. Mathis, H. Deramond, and S.M. Belkoff [eds], Percutaneous Vertebroplasty. New York: Springer, 2002, with permission.)

vivo study (69) compared the compressive strength of vertebral bodies augmented prophylactically by a single posterolateral injection to those left unaugmented. Those investigators found that augmentation, even by modest (4.3 ± 1.6 mL) volumes of cement, increased vertebral body strength. Preliminary clinical outcome data on a limited number of patients in which the unipedicular procedure has been performed (59) support the ex vivo findings (47). However, it is unknown if unipedicular injections of volumes used in those ex vivo studies (47,54) would result in adequate mechanical stabilization clinically.

Kyphosis Reduction

Restoration of height lost as a result of VCF and correction of the resulting kyphosis have the potential benefit of reducing postfracture sequelae such as loss of appetite, reduced pulmonary capacity, and diminished quality of life (70–74). Vertebral body height measured ex vivo suggests that minimal height (i.e., 1 to 2 mm) is restored after PV (75–77). To increase height restoration, a new device, the inflatable bone tamp, has been developed (75,78). The procedure used to place and inflate the bone tamp has been termed *kyphoplasty* (see Chapter 8 for a detailed description). Ex vivo tests indicate that the tamp treatment restores significantly more height than does standard PV treatment and achieves restoration of mechanical properties similar to that of PV (75,78). A recent report (79) suggests that similar height restoration may be achieved clinically, whether performing kyphoplasty (80) or not. The controversy over height restoration is presented in the chapter on kyphoplasty (see Chapter 8).

Injection Pressure

Another controversy regarding vertebroplasty concerns the pressure needed to deliver the cement into the vertebral body. Some investigators (81) report that creating a void allows cement to be injected under lower pressure than would be the case if cement were injected directly into the vertebral body. If a lower pressure were required to deliver the cement, the argument goes, then a more viscous cement could be used. Cement with greater viscosity is less likely to extravasate and result in clinical complications (82). Concern over injection pressure really stems from the tactile feedback clinicians receive during injection. Approximately 95% of the pressure required for cement injection is to overcome the friction in the cannula. This pressure can be substantial, especially when injecting cements that are or have become viscous (83). Only approximately 5% of the injection pressure is a function of the infiltration parameters of the vertebral body (82). The required pressure at the tip of the cannula is only that needed to displace the marrow, fat, and blood products in the vertebral body. A bench study reported that rapid injections of cement were required to produce a measurable increase in intravertebral body pressure (83). In that study, the cement was injected at a rate well in excess of what would be deemed clinically safe. Even then, the measured pressure was only 6 to 10 mm Hg above ambient pressure, but the pressure in the syringe exceeded 18,000 mm Hg.

Altered Kinematics/Adjacent Fractures

There is much concern about the potential increased risk of fractures occurring in the levels adjacent to vertebral bodies that have been treated with vertebroplasty. Retrospective clinical studies report conflicting results (84,85). Taking into consideration that risk of a subsequent vertebral body fracture increases 12.6 times after the initial fracture and that compression fractures are most prevalent in the thoracolumbar junction (86), it is difficult to differentiate which fractures would have occurred had vertebroplasty not been performed. None of the current clinical studies has sufficient power to make such a differentiation.

From a mechanical perspective, it is theoretically unlikely that stress concentration would occur at a level adjacent to one that had received vertebroplasty. Vertebroplasty typically restores or nearly restores the native strength and stiffness of the vertebral body. Thus, by definition, no stress concentration results. Even if large volumes of cement were injected, thus increasing the strength and stiffness of the vertebral body, most spinal motion occurs at the level of the disc. Unless the mechanics of the disc are altered (i.e., damaged, filled with cement) or the demands for motion increased (compensation for fused levels), no alteration in normal spine kinematics would be expected. Adjacent fractures occur most often when several levels are fused. In this instance, the normal kinematics of the spine is altered. In the normal spine, motion occurs in the flexible disc. After fusion, the levels adjacent to the fused levels are required to compensate for the lost motion. The resultant excessive motion places increased stress on those levels and puts them at risk for fracture. Interestingly, vertebroplasty is one of the procedures used in orthopaedic surgery to reduce the risk of fracture in the adjacent level. Should cement leak into the disc, however, the adjacent level is at increased risk of fracture (87).

A recent biomechanical study investigated the effect of vertebroplasty and kyphoplasty on adjacent disc pressures (67). Although disc pressure was reduced dramatically when an adjacent level was fractured, once the level was treated with either kyphoplasty or vertebroplasty, disc pressure increased, but not back to the prefracture normal level. These findings support the conclusion that vertebroplasty and kyphoplasty do not increase the risk of adjacent fractures, a finding that is in opposition to computational models (66). An ex vivo study of two-level functional spine units (FSUs) reported the augmented FSU was 19% weaker than the unaugmented FSU, although the difference was not significant (88). The investigators suggested that vertebroplasty may place adjacent levels at risk of fracture (88). It should be noted that that study may have introduced some experimental bias by always augmenting the caudal level of the FSU. The authors also injected a high volume (8.8 mL, on average) of cement relative to common vertebroplasty practice. Despite the attempts to identify biomechanically the risks of adjacent fractures, the true risk may be identified only through a carefully controlled, prospective, randomized clinical study.

Materials and Tests

Cement Alterations

Since the publication of the first edition (89), several cements have received approval by the Federal Drug Administration (FDA) in the United States and by the Conformitè Europèene in Europe. Before this approval was given, many clinicians prepared their own mixtures of cement by altering the composition of PMMA cements that typically were approved for arthroplasty. Common alterations included (1) increasing the monomer-to-polymer ratio to increase working time and decrease viscosity (13,57,90), (2) adding radio-opacifiers to increase cement visualization under fluoroscopy (13,57,90), and (3) adding antibiotics (13). Altering an FDA-approved product is not considered off-label use; it creates a new device that needs to be FDA approved.

Monomer-to-Polymer Ratio
Increasing the monomer-to-polymer ratio decreases the compressive material properties of the cement (Figure 6.6) (91–93). Because cements altered for use with PV typically have monomer-to-polymer ratios of about 0.72 mL/g (compared with the manufacturer-recommended ratio of 0.5 mL/g), there likely is an increased amount of unreacted monomer available to enter the circulatory system (91–93). Even so, actual blood serum concentration during PV may be lower than that measured during total hip arthrodesis because the quantity of cement injected (<10 mL) is much smaller than that for hip arthrodesis (>40 mL) (41,42,94).

Radio-Opacification
Altering the concentration of radio-opacifiers significantly alters the material properties of the cement, as does the combined alteration of

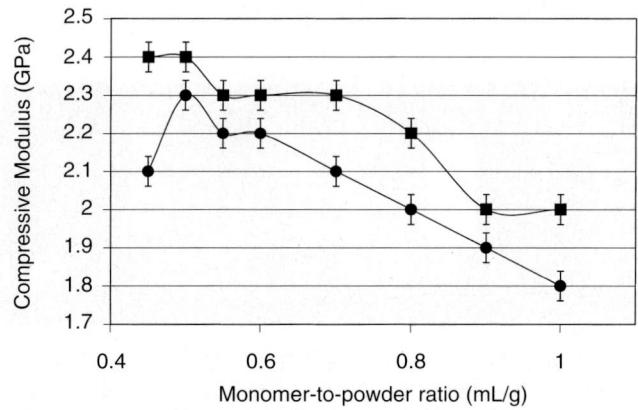

Figure 6.6. Cement compressive modulus as a function of the monomer-to-powder ratio for Simplex P. (From J.M. Mathis, H. Deramond, and S.M. Belkoff [eds], Percutaneous Vertebroplasty. New York: Springer, 2002, with permission.)

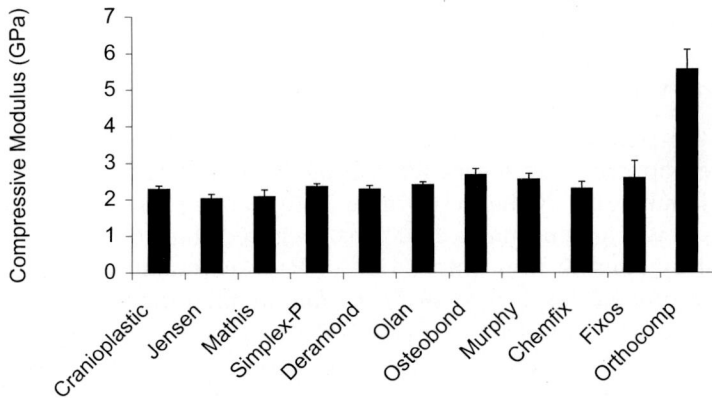

Figure 6.7. Relative compressive strengths for various cement recipes used in PV. (From J.M. Mathis, H. Deramond, and S.M. Belkoff [eds], Percutaneous Vertebroplasty. New York: Springer, 2002, with permission.)

monomer-to-polymer ratio and opacification (95). Although these modifications are statistically significant, they are of dubious clinical importance. In a recent study of tested cement recipes, the cement composition (Figure 6.7) that exhibited the minimum relative material properties (95) was the composition that has been used clinically during the past decade in the United States (13), but there have been no reports of complications associated with mechanical failure of that cement composition. Complications that have been reported are predominantly cement extravasation or the consequences of extravasation (13,96–98). The prevention of extravasation by means of adequate opacification and careful fluoroscopic visualization during cement injection is essential for the safe practice of PV (Figure 6.8). Thus, selecting a cement that can be injected easily and has proper opacification takes precedence over a cement that is unmodified and retains its original material properties.

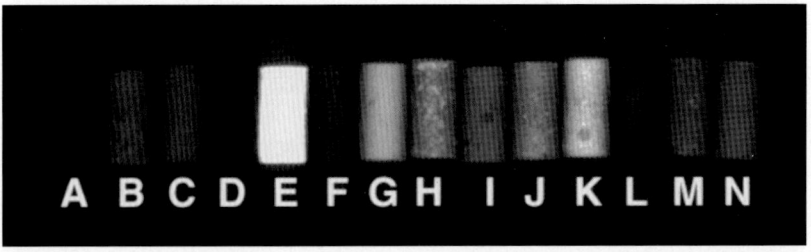

Figure 6.8. Radiopacities of various mixtures of cement: A, Simplex P; B, Simplex P with 20% by weight $BaSO_4$; C, Mathis recipe; D, Cranioplastic with 10 percent by weight $BaSO_4$; E, Fixos; F, Chemfix3; G, Orthocomp; H, Murphy recipe; I, Olan recipe; J, Simplex P with 30% by weight $BaSO_4$; K, Deramond recipe; L, Cranioplastic with 20% $BaSO_4$; M, Jensen recipe; N, Cranioplastic with 30% by weight $BaSO_4$ (see Jasper et al. [92] for composition details). (From J.M. Mathis, H. Deramond, and S.M. Belkoff [eds], Percutaneous Vertebroplasty. New York: Springer, 2002, with permission.)

Antibiotics

The efficacy of adding antibiotics to cement to reduce the risk of infection during PV is unknown. In contrast to arthrodesis procedures (99), the risk of infection from PV is extremely low (<1 percent). Therefore, elucidating the efficacy of prophylactic antibiotics would require a clinical trial with an extremely large population size for such a study to have sufficient statistical power. For immunocompromised patients, some clinicians routinely add antibiotics to the cement mixture (13).

It is also unknown what effect adding antibiotics to PMMA cement prepared for PV has on the cement's material properties. The addition of antibiotics to PMMA cement used in arthroplasty reportedly does not affect the cement's fatigue properties (100) and may increase its compressive strength (99).

Mechanical Tests

Cement Tests

Most mechanical tests for determining the material properties of acrylic bone cements are performed based on the American Society for Testing and Materials (ASTM) standard F451 (101) or similar test standards. To measure compressive material properties of acrylic cement, the cement components typically are weighed, mixed, and then poured into a mold consisting of cylindrical holes, each 6 mm in diameter and 12 mm high. The mold is then placed between two stainless steel plates, compressed, and subsequently placed in a saline (0.09%) bath maintained at 37°C for a given period of time. The cement specimens are sanded flush with the mold, pressed out of the mold, and inspected for defects. Specimens containing defects greater than 10 percent of their cross-section are culled from the group of test specimens. The specimens then are individually placed between loading platens on a materials testing machine and compressed to failure. Stress and strain data, obtained by dividing the load and deformation data by a specimen's cross-sectional area and initial length, respectively, are plotted for each specimen (Figure 6.9). Ultimate compressive stress is defined as peak (maximum) stress. Compressive modulus is defined as the slope of the linear (Hookean) portion of the stress-versus-strain curve. Compressive yield strength is determined using the 2% offset method, in which a line is drawn parallel to the Hookean portion of the stress-versus-strain curve but offset along the strain axis a distance equal to 2% of the specimen's initial height.

Compression is the loading mode most often used to test cements for PV. Although the cement undoubtedly experiences shear and tensile stresses in vivo, the dominant stress likely is compressive. It is unknown if cement fatigue is of clinical concern for the practice of PV. There are no clinical reports describing mechanical failure (fatigue or otherwise) of the cement. Furthermore, it is unknown if the stress magnitudes, in vivo, are sufficient to cause fatigue. It is unlikely that the stress magnitudes typically experienced by bone cement used with hip arthroplasty are similar to those experienced in the spine. For example,

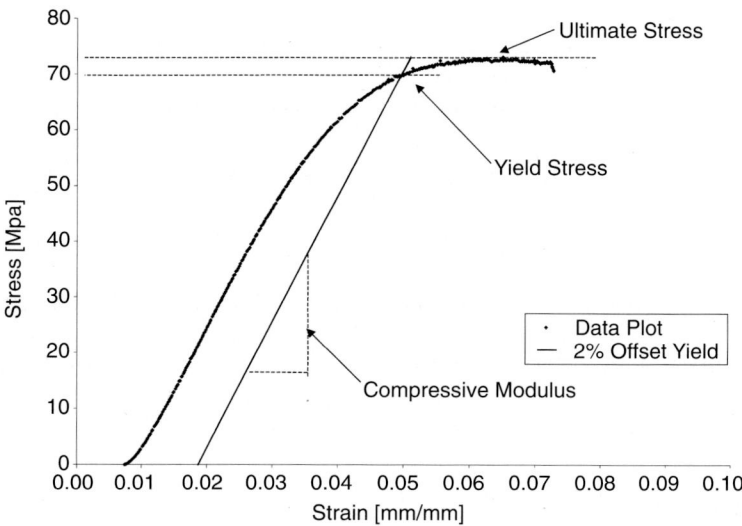

Figure 6.9. Typical compressive material behavior of cement specimens. (From J.M. Mathis, H. Deramond, and S.M. Belkoff [eds], Percutaneous Vertebroplasty. New York: Springer, 2002, with permission.)

the strength of one PMMA cement manufactured for use in vertebroplasty is 65 megapascals (MPa) (93), and an average cross-sectional area of a lumbar vertebral body endplate is 1,200 mm (2,102). An axial load on the spine of approximately 78 kilonewtons (kN) would be needed to generate enough stress to cause cement failure. For a 70-kg man, an axial load of 78 kN equates to 114 times body weight, which is well beyond the failure strength of a lumbar vertebra, even of normal density (102).

It is also unlikely that the cement used for PV would be exposed to enough cycles to cause fatigue. Most PV is performed on patients advanced in age (>70 years) whose remaining life span may not be long or active enough to elicit a fatigue response. Because of the relatively recent introduction of the practice of PV, no patients have follow-up of more than 20 years after treatment.

Vertebral Body Tests

As with tests conducted on isolated cement specimens, mechanical tests conducted on vertebral bodies to determine their prefracture (initial) and postrepair structural parameters have been almost exclusively compressive (46,47,62,75). Typically, impressions of the vertebral body endplates are made using a common epoxy to distribute contact stresses across the endplates during compression tests. The potted specimens are placed between loading platens on a materials testing

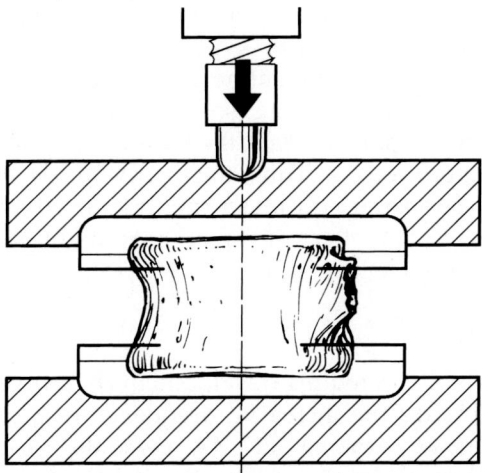

Figure 6.10. Compression test of an osteoporotic vertebral body. (From J.M. Mathis, H. Deramond, and S.M. Belkoff [eds], Percutaneous Vertebroplasty. New York: Springer, 2002, with permission.)

machine and compressed (Figure 6.10). In this manner, the initial stiffness and failure loads of the vertebral body are determined. The vertebral bodies then are repaired with the particular method under investigation and recompressed. Strength and stiffness values of the repaired specimens then are compared with the initial values to determine the biomechanical effect of the repair (Figure 6.11).

Although the spine is loaded predominantly in compression, the effects of bending and torsional loading should not be ignored. Wilson

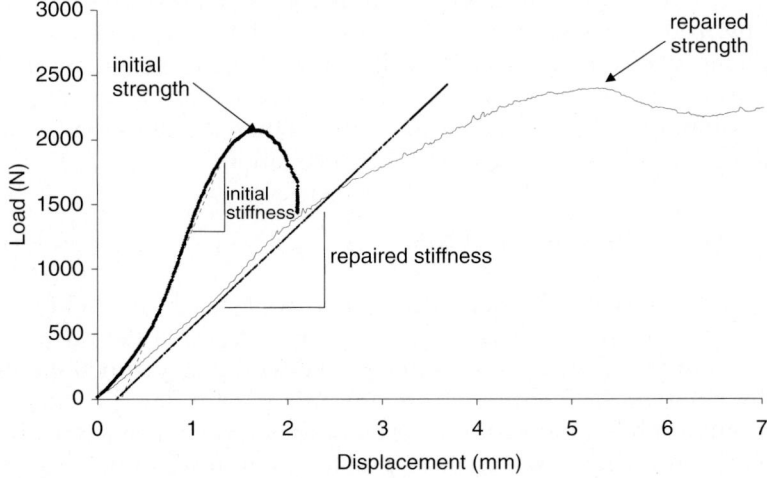

Figure 6.11. Mechanical behavior of an osteoporotic vertebral body during initial compression test and after repair. (From J.M. Mathis, H. Deramond, and S.M. Belkoff [eds], Percutaneous Vertebroplasty. New York: Springer, 2002, with permission.)

et al. (78) used a multisegment cadaver model to investigate potential altered kinematics as a result of kyphoplasty or PV. Although such models have the benefit of evaluating spine kinematics in a more clinically relevant manner than using isolated specimens, it is difficult in the multisegment model to create the simulated fractures needed to evaluate subsequent repairs. Thus, treatments in the study by Wilson et al. (78) were performed on intact (nonfractured) vertebral bodies, and it is unknown what effect the treatments might have on vertebral bodies mechanically weakened by VCFs.

Alternative Cements

Two factors have motivated the development of new types of cements and injection devices: the increasing frequency of the practice of PV and deficiencies in existing PMMA cements for use with PV (46,103–105). These cements are bioactive (106–109) or bioresorbable (103,105,110–113), are naturally radio-opaque (93,105), and have lower exothermic reactions (38,103,105) than PMMA cements.

Until recently (77,105), the use of calcium-phosphate cements in PV has been impeded substantially by their difficulty of injection (103). These more biocompatible cements may eliminate concerns about thermal necrosis and cytotoxicity and appear to result in mechanical stabilization of fractured vertebral bodies similar to that of PMMA (105). Yet, if thermal or chemical mechanisms are found to play an antitumoral role, then the non-PMMA cements may not be as effective for use in patients with tumors. Bioresorbable cements may be most appealing for use in prophylactic augmentation because injected vertebral bodies would be mechanically augmented immediately, whereas the cement would provide an osteoconductive material for subsequent bone repair and remodeling. The subsequent risk of fracture after the cement is remodeled or resorbed is unknown. Bioresorbable cements also may have application with PV for treating burst fractures in young healthy patients (104). Despite the allure of using such cements, some caution is warranted because the calcium may initiate coagulation and clot formation, thus placing the patient at risk for cardiac arrest (114). Many questions regarding the clinical use of these cements remain and need to be resolved through careful investigation.

Summary and Conclusions

The practice of PV has experienced explosive growth in recent years and, with it, many questions regarding the efficacy of the procedure and its optimal practice. Percutaneous vertebroplasty functions primarily to stabilize fractures, thus preventing pain and providing a stable environment for healing. The amount of cement needed to affect stabilization is unknown, but it is probably 4 to 6 mL rather than the volume needed to fill the vertebral body completely (>10 mL), as previously thought necessary. Altering the cement composition by adding antibiotics, opacifying agents, and more monomer alters the material properties of the cement, but with the availability of cements approved by the Conformitè Europèene or the FDA, such alterations are of more academic than clinical interest. The primary concerns relative to cement selection are whether or not the cement can be injected easily and visualized properly under fluoroscopy.

References

1. Alleyne CH, Jr, Rodts GE, Jr, Haid RW. Corpectomy and stabilization with methylmethacrylate in patients with metastatic disease of the spine: a technical note. J Spinal Disord 1995; 8(6):439–443.
2. Cortet B, Cotten A, Deprez X, et al. [Value of vertebroplasty combined with surgical decompression in the treatment of aggressive spinal angioma. Apropos of 3 cases.] Rev Rhum Ed Fr 1994; 61(1):16–22.
3. Cybulski GR. Methods of surgical stabilization for metastatic disease of the spine. Neurosurgery 1989; 25(2):240–252.
4. Harrington KD. Anterior decompression and stabilization of the spine as a treatment for vertebral collapse and spinal cord compression from metastatic malignancy. Clin Orthop 1988; 233:177–197.
5. Harrington KD, Sim FH, Enis JE, et al. Methylmethacrylate as an adjunct in internal fixation of pathological fractures. Experience with three hundred and seventy-five cases. J Bone Joint Surg 1976; 58A(8):1047–1055.
6. Mavian GZ, Okulski CJ. Double fixation of metastatic lesions of the lumbar and cervical vertebral bodies utilizing methylmethacrylate compound: report of a case and review of a series of cases. J Am Osteopath Assoc 1986; 86(3):153–157.
7. O'Donnell RJ, Springfield DS, Motwani HK, et al. Recurrence of giant-cell tumors of the long bones after curettage and packing with cement. J Bone Joint Surg 1994; 76A(12):1827–1833.
8. Persson BM, Ekelund L, Lovdahl R, et al. Favourable results of acrylic cementation for giant cell tumors. Acta Orthop Scand 1984; 55(2):209–214.
9. Sundaresan N, Galicich JH, Lane JM, et al. Treatment of neoplastic epidural cord compression by vertebral body resection and stabilization. J Neurosurg 1985; 63(5):676–684.
10. Knight G. Paraspinal acrylic inlays in the treatment of cervical and lumbar spondylosis and other conditions. Lancet 1959; 2:147–149.
11. Galibert P, Deramond H, Rosat P, et al. [Preliminary note on the treatment of vertebral angioma by percutaneous acrylic vertebroplasty.] Neurochirurgie 1987; 33(2):166–168.
12. Lapras C, Mottolese C, Deruty R, et al. [Percutaneous injection of methylmethacrylate in osteoporosis and severe vertebral osteolysis (Galibert's technic).] Ann Chir 1989; 43(5):371–376.
13. Jensen ME, Evans AJ, Mathis JM, et al. Percutaneous polymethylmethacrylate vertebroplasty in the treatment of osteoporotic vertebral body compression fractures: technical aspects. Am J Neuroradiol 1997; 18(10):1897–1904.
14. Cyteval C, Sarrabere MPB, Roux JO, et al. Acute osteoporotic vertebral collapse: open study on percutaneous injection of acrylic surgical cement in 20 patients. Am J Roentgenol 1999; 173(6):1685–1690.
15. McGraw JK, Lippert JA, Minkus KD, et al. Prospective evaluation of pain relief in 100 patients undergoing percutaneous vertebroplasty: results and follow-up. J Vasc Intervent Radiol 2002; 13(9 Pt 1):883–886.
16. Evans AJ, Jensen ME, Kip KE, et al. Vertebral compression fractures: pain reduction and improvement in functional mobility after percutaneous

polymethylmethacrylate vertebroplasty—retrospective report of 245 cases. Radiology 2003; 226(2):366–372.
17. Grados F, Depriester C, Cayrolle G, et al. Long-term observations of vertebral osteoporotic fractures treated by percutaneous vertebroplasty. Rheumatology 2000; 39:1410–1414.
18. Peh WCG, Gilula LA, Peck DD. Percutaneous vertebroplasty for severe osteoporotic vertebral body compression fractures. Radiology 2002; 223(1):121–126.
19. Peh WCG, Gelbart MS, Gilula LA, et al. Percutaneous vertebroplasty: treatment of painful vertebral compression fractures with intraosseous vacuum phenomena. Am J Roentgenol 2003; 180(5):1411–1417.
20. Weill A, Chiras J, Simon JM, et al. Spinal metastases: indications for and results of percutaneous injection of acrylic surgical cement. Radiology 1996; 199(1):241–247.
21. Cotten A, Duquesnoy B. Vertebroplasty: current data and future potential. Rev Rhum Engl Ed 1997; 64(11):645–649.
22. Alvarez L, Perez-Higueras A, Quinones D, et al. Vertebroplasty in the treatment of vertebral tumors: postprocedural outcome and quality of life. Eur Spine J 2003; 12(4):356–360.
23. Fourney DR, Schomer DF, Nader R, et al. Percutaneous vertebroplasty and kyphoplasty for painful vertebral body fractures in cancer patients. J Neurosurg 2003; 98(Suppl 1):21–30.
24. Bostrom MPG, Lane JM. Future directions. Augmentation of osteoporotic vertebral bodies. Spine 1997; 22(Suppl 24):38S–42S.
25. Deramond H, Depriester C, Galibert P, et al. Percutaneous vertebroplasty with polymethylmethacrylate. Technique, indications, and results. Radiol Clin North Am 1998; 36(3):533–546.
26. Srikumaran U, Wong W, Belkoff SM, McCarthy EF: Histopathologic analysis of human vertebral bodies after kyphoplasty. J Bone Joint Surg 2005; 87(8):1838–1843.
27. Togawa D, Bauer TW, Lieberman IH, et al. Histologic evaluation of human vertebral bodies after vertebral augmentation with polymethyl methacrylate. Spine 2003; 28(14):1521–1527.
28. Verlaan JJ, Oner FC, Slootweg PJ, et al. Histologic changes after vertebroplasty. J Bone Joint Surg 2004; 86A(6):1230–1238.
29. Lewis G. Properties of acrylic bone cement: state of the art review. J Biomed Mater Res 1997; 38(2):155–182.
30. Hasenwinkel JM, Lautenschlager EP, Wixson RL, et al. A novel high-viscosity, two-solution acrylic bone cement: effect of chemical composition on properties. J Biomed Mater Res 1999; 47(1):36–45.
31. Leeson MC, Lippitt SB. Thermal aspects of the use of polymethylmethacrylate in large metaphyseal defects in bone. A clinical review and laboratory study. Clin Orthop 1993; 295:239–245.
32. Mjoberg B, Pettersson H, Rosenqvist R, et al. Bone cement, thermal injury and the radiolucent zone. Acta Orthop Scand 1984; 55(6):597–600.
33. Eriksson RA, Albrektsson T, Magnusson B. Assessment of bone viability after heat trauma. A histological, histochemical and vital microscopic study in the rabbit. Scand J Plast Reconstr Surg 1984; 18(3):261–268.
34. Rouiller C, Majno G. Morphologische und chemische Untersuchung an Knochen nach Hitzeeinwirkung. Beitr Pathol Anat Allg Pathol 1953; 113:100–120.
35. Li S, Chien S, Branemark PI. Heat shock–induced necrosis and apoptosis in osteoblasts. J Orthop Res 1999; 17(6):891–899.
36. Jefferiss CD, Lee AJC, Ling RSM. Thermal aspects of self-curing polymethylmethacrylate. J Bone Joint Surg 1975; 57B(4):511–518.

37. De Vrind HH, Wondergem J, Haveman J. Hyperthermia-induced damage to rat sciatic nerve assessed in vivo with functional methods and with electrophysiology. J Neurosci Methods 1992; 45(3):165–174.
38. Deramond H, Wright NT, Belkoff SM. Temperature elevation caused by bone cement polymerization during vertebroplasty. Bone 1999; 25(Suppl 2):17S–21S.
39. Belkoff SM, Molloy S. Temperature measurement during polymerization of polymethylmethacrylate cement used for vertebroplasty. Spine 2003; 28(14):1555–1559.
40. Verlaan JJ, Oner FC, Verbout AJ, et al. Temperature elevation after vertebroplasty with polymethylmethacrylate in the goat spine. J Biomed Mater Res 2003; 67B(1):581–585.
41. Dahl OE, Garvik LJ, Lyberg T. Toxic effects of methylmethacrylate monomer on leukocytes and endothelial cells in vitro [published erratum appears in Acta Orthop Scand 1995 Aug; 66(4):387]. Acta Orthop Scand 1994; 65(2):147–153.
42. Svartling N, Pfaffli P, Tarkkanen L. Blood levels and half-life of methylmethacrylate after tourniquet release during knee arthroplasty. Arch Orthop Trauma Surg 1986; 105(1):36–39.
43. Wenda K, Scheuermann H, Weitzel E, et al. Pharmacokinetics of methylmethacrylate monomer during total hip replacement in man. Arch Orthop Trauma Surg 1988; 107(5):316–321.
44. San Millan Ruiz D, Burkhardt K, Jean B, et al. Pathology findings with acrylic implants. Bone 1999; 25(Suppl 2):85S–90S.
45. Belkoff SM, Deramond H, Jasper LE, et al. Biomechanical evaluation of a hydroxyapatite cement for use with vertebroplasty. Presented at the 11th Interdisciplinary Research Conference on Biomaterials (Groupe de Recherches Interdisciplinaire sur les Biomateriaux Osteo-articulaires Injectables, GRIBOI), March 8, 2001.
46. Belkoff SM, Mathis JM, Erbe EM, et al. Biomechanical evaluation of a new bone cement for use in vertebroplasty. Spine 2000; 25(9):1061–1064.
47. Tohmeh AG, Mathis JM, Fenton DC, et al. Biomechanical efficacy of unipedicular versus bipedicular vertebroplasty for the management of osteoporotic compression fractures. Spine 1999; 24(17):1772–1776.
48. Garfin SR, Blair B, Eismont FJ, et al. Thoracic and upper lumbar spine injuries. In Skeletal Trauma: Fractures, Dislocations, Ligamentous Injuries, 2nd Ed. BD Browner, JB Jupiter, AM Levine, et al (eds). Philadelphia: WB Saunders Co, 1998:947–1034.
49. Mow VC, Hayes WC. Basic Orthopaedic Biomechanics. New York: Raven Press, 1991.
50. WHO Study Group. Assessment of fracture risk and its application to screening for postmenopausal osteoporosis. Report of a WHO Study Group. WHO Tech Rep Ser 1994; 843:1–129.
51. Ross PD, Davis JW, Epstein RS, et al. Pre-existing fractures and bone mass predict vertebral fracture incidence in women. Ann Intern Med 1991; 114(11):919–923.
52. Eastell R, Cedel SL, Wahner HW, et al. Classification of vertebral fractures. J Bone Miner Res 1991; 6(3):207–215.
53. Riggs BL, Melton LJ, III. The worldwide problem of osteoporosis: insights afforded by epidemiology. Bone 1995; 17(Suppl 2):505S–511S.
54. Lyritis GP, Mayasis B, Tsakalakos N, et al. The natural history of the osteoporotic vertebral fracture. Clin Rheumatol 1989; 8(Suppl 2):66–69.
55. Gaughen JR, Jr, Jensen ME, Schweickert PA, et al. The therapeutic benefit of repeat percutaneous vertebroplasty at previously treated vertebral levels. Am J Neuroradiol 2002; 23(10):1657–1661.

56. Gilula L. Is insufficient use of polymethylmethacrylate a cause for vertebroplasty failure necessitating repeat vertebroplasty [letter]? Am J Neuroradiol 2003; 24(10):2120–2121.
57. Cotten A, Boutry N, Cortet B, et al. Percutaneous vertebroplasty: state of the art. RadioGraphics 1998; 18(2):311–323.
58. Molloy S, Mathis JM, Belkoff SM. The effect of vertebral body percentage fill on mechanical behavior during percutaneous vertebroplasty. Spine 2003; 28(14):1549–1554.
59. Barr JD, Barr MS, Lemley TJ, et al. Percutaneous vertebroplasty for pain relief and spinal stabilization. Spine 2000; 25(8):923–928.
60. Cotten A, Dewatre F, Cortet B, et al. Percutaneous vertebroplasty for osteolytic metastases and myeloma: effects of the percentage of lesion filling and the leakage of methyl methacrylate at clinical follow-up. Radiology 1996; 200(2):525–530.
61. Kallmes DF, Jensen ME, Marx WF. Response to letter "Is insufficient use of polymethylmethacrylate a cause for vertebroplasty failure necessitating repeat vertebroplasty?" [letter]. Am J Neuroradiol 2003; 24(10):2121–2122.
62. Belkoff SM, Mathis JM, Jasper LE, et al. The biomechanics of vertebroplasty: the effect of cement volume on mechanical behavior. Spine 2001; 26(14):1537–1541.
63. Liebschner MAK, Rosenberg WS, Keaveny TM. Effects of bone cement volume and distribution on vertebral stiffness after vertebroplasty. Spine 2001; 26(14):1547–1554.
64. Terjesen T, Apalset K. The influence of different degrees of stiffness of fixation plates on experimental bone healing. J Orthop Res 1988; 6(2):293–299.
65. Mathis JM. Percutaneous vertebroplasty: complication avoidance and technique optimization. Am J Neuroradiol 2003; 24(8):1697–1706.
66. Baroud G, Nemes J, Heini P, et al. Load shift of the intervertebral disc after a vertebroplasty: a finite-element study. Eur Spine J 2003; 12(4):421–426.
67. Ananthakrishnan D, Berven S, Deviren V, et al. The effect on anterior column loading due to different vertebral augmentation techniques. Clin Biomech (Bristol, Avon) 2005; 20(1):25–31.
68. Higgins KB, Harten RD, Langrana NA, et al. Biomechanical effects of unipedicular vertebroplasty on intact vertebrae. Spine 2003; 28(14):1540–1547; disc, 1548.
69. Dean JR, Ison KT, Gishen P. The strengthening effect of percutaneous vertebroplasty. Clin Radiol 2000; 55(6):471–476.
70. Lyles KW, Gold DT, Shipp KM, et al. Association of osteoporotic vertebral compression fractures with impaired functional status. Am J Med 1993; 94(6):595–601.
71. Silverman SL. The clinical consequences of vertebral compression fracture. Bone 1992; 13(Suppl 2):S27–S31.
72. Schlaich C, Minne HW, Bruckner T, et al. Reduced pulmonary function in patients with spinal osteoporotic fractures. Osteoporos Int 1998; 8(3):261–267.
73. Leech JA, Dulberg C, Kellie S, et al. Relationship of lung function to severity of osteoporosis in women. Am Rev Respir Dis 1990; 141(1):68–71.
74. Leidig-Bruckner G, Minne HW, Schlaich C, et al. Clinical grading of spinal osteoporosis: quality of life components and spinal deformity in women with chronic low back pain and women with vertebral osteoporosis. J Bone Miner Res 1997; 12(4):663–675.

75. Belkoff SM, Mathis JM, Fenton DC, et al. An ex vivo biomechanical evaluation of an inflatable bone tamp used in the treatment of compression fracture. Spine 2001; 26(2):151–156.
76. Belkoff SM, Mathis JM, Deramond H, et al. An ex vivo biomechanical evaluation of a hydroxyapatite cement for use with kyphoplasty. Am J Neuroradiol 2001; 22(June/July):1212–1216.
77. Belkoff SM, Mathis JM, Jasper LE, et al. An ex vivo biomechanical evaluation of a hydroxyapatite cement for use with vertebroplasty. Spine 2001; 26(14):1542–1546.
78. Wilson DR, Myers ER, Mathis JM, et al. Effect of augmentation on the mechanics of vertebral wedge fractures. Spine 2000; 25(2):158–165.
79. Hiwatashi A, Moritani T, Numaguchi Y, et al. Increase in vertebral body height after vertebroplasty. Am J Neuroradiol 2003; 24(2):185–189.
80. Lieberman IH, Dudeney S, Reinhardt MK, et al. Initial outcome and efficacy of "kyphoplasty" in the treatment of painful osteoporotic vertebral compression fractures. Spine 2001; 26(14):1631–1638.
81. Phillips FM, Todd WF, Lieberman I, et al. An in vivo comparison of the potential for extravertebral cement leak after vertebroplasty and kyphoplasty. Spine 2002; 27(19):2173–2178.
82. Baroud G, Bohner M, Heini P, et al. Injection biomechanics of bone cements used in vertebroplasty. Biomed Mater Eng 2004; 14(4):487–504.
83. Tomita S, Molloy S, Abe M, et al. Ex vivo measurement of intravertebral pressure during vertebroplasty. Spine 2004; 29(7):723–725.
84. Kim SH, Kang HS, Choi JA, et al. Risk factors of new compression fractures in adjacent vertebrae after percutaneous vertebroplasty. Acta Radiol 2004; 45(4):440–445.
85. Uppin AA, Hirsch JA, Centenera LV, et al. Occurrence of new vertebral body fracture after percutaneous vertebroplasty in patients with osteoporosis. Radiology 2003; 226(1):119–124.
86. Magerl F, Aebi M, Gertzbein SD, et al. A comprehensive classification of thoracic and lumbar injuries. Eur Spine J 1994; 3(4):184–201.
87. Lin EP, Ekholm S, Hiwatashi A, et al. Vertebroplasty: cement leakage into the disc increases the risk of new fracture of adjacent vertebral body. Am J Neuroradiol 2004; 25(2):175–180.
88. Berlemann U, Ferguson SJ, Nolte LP, et al. Adjacent vertebral failure after vertebroplasty. A biomechanical investigation. J Bone Joint Surg 2002; 84B(5):748–752.
89. Mathis JM, Deramond H, Belkoff SM. Percutaneous Vertebroplasty. New York: Springer, 2002.
90. Deramond H, Depriester C, Toussaint P, et al. Percutaneous vertebroplasty. Semin Musculoskel Radiol 1997; 1(2):285–295.
91. Belkoff SM, Sanders JC. The effect of the monomer-to-powder ratio on the material properties of acrylic bone cement. J Biomed Mater Res 2002; 63(4):396–399.
92. Jasper LE, Deramond H, Mathis JM, et al. The effect of monomer-to-powder ratio on the material properties of Cranioplastic. Bone 1999; 25(Suppl 2):27S–29S.
93. Jasper LE, Deramond H, Mathis JM, et al. Material properties of various cements for use with vertebroplasty. J Mater Sci Mater Med 2002; 13:1–5.
94. Svartling N, Pfaffli P, Tarkkanen L. Methylmethacrylate blood levels in patients with femoral neck fracture. Arch Orthop Trauma Surg 1985; 104(4):242–246.

95. Jasper L, Deramond H, Mathis JM, et al. Evaluation of PMMA cements altered for use in vertebroplasty. Presented at the 10th Interdisciplinary Research Conference on Injectible Biomaterials, Amiens (France), March 14–15, 2000.
96. Padovani B, Kasriel O, Brunner P, et al. Pulmonary embolism caused by acrylic cement: a rare complication of percutaneous vertebroplasty. Am J Neuroradiol 1999; 20(3):375–377.
97. Wilkes RA, MacKinnon JG, Thomas WG. Neurological deterioration after cement injection into a vertebral body. J Bone Joint Surg 1994; 76B(1):155.
98. Perrin C, Jullien V, Padovani B, et al. [Percutaneous vertebroplasty complicated by pulmonary embolus of acrylic cement.] Rev Mal Respir 1999; 16(2):215–217.
99. Saha S, Pal S. Mechanical properties of bone cement: a review. J Biomed Mater Res 1984; 18(4):435–462.
100. Riser WH. Introduction. Vet Pathol 1975; 12:235–238.
101. American Society for Testing and Materials. Standard specification for acrylic bone cement. In Annual Book of ASTM Standards. West Conshohocken, PA: American Society for Testing and Materials, 1997: 47–53.
102. Singer K, Edmondston S, Day R, et al. Prediction of thoracic and lumbar vertebral body compressive strength: correlations with bone mineral density and vertebral region. Bone 1995; 17(2):167–174.
103. Schildhauer TA, Bennett AP, Wright TM, et al. Intravertebral body reconstruction with an injectable in situ–setting carbonated apatite: biomechanical evaluation of a minimally invasive technique. J Orthop Res 1999; 17(1):67–72.
104. Mermelstein LE, McLain RF, Yerby SA. Reinforcement of thoracolumbar burst fractures with calcium phosphate cement. A biomechanical study. Spine 1998; 23(6):664–670.
105. Bai B, Jazrawi LM, Kummer FJ, et al. The use of an injectable, biodegradable calcium phosphate bone substitute for the prophylactic augmentation of osteoporotic vertebrae and the management of vertebral compression fractures. Spine 1999; 24(15):1521–1526.
106. Kim SB, Kim YJ, Yoon TL, et al. The characteristics of a hydroxyapatite-chitosan-PMMA bone cement. Biomaterials 2004; 25(26):5715–5723.
107. Lim TH, Brebach GT, Renner SM, et al. Biomechanical evaluation of an injectable calcium phosphate cement for vertebroplasty. Spine 2002; 27(12):1297–1302.
108. Zhao F, Lu WW, Luk KDK, et al. Surface treatment of injectable strontium-containing bioactive bone cement for vertebroplasty. J Biomed Mater Res B Appl Biomater 2004; 69(1):79–86.
109. Mendez JA, Fernandez M, Gonzalez-Corchon A, et al. Injectable self-curing bioactive acrylic-glass composites charged with specific anti-inflammatory/analgesic agent. Biomaterials 2004; 25(12):2381–2392.
110. Fujita H, Nakamura T, Tamura J, et al. Bioactive bone cement: effect of the amount of glass-ceramic powder on bone-bonding strength. J Biomed Mater Res 1998; 40(1):145–152.
111. Tomita S, Kin A, Yazu M, et al. Biomechanical evaluation of kyphoplasty and vertebroplasty with calcium phosphate cement in a simulated osteoporotic compression fracture. J Orthop Sci 2003; 8:192–197.
112. Barralet JE, Grover LM, Gbureck U. Ionic modification of calcium phosphate cement viscosity. Part II: hypodermic injection and strength improvement of brushite cement. Biomaterials 2004; 25(11):2197–2203.

113. Gbureck U, Barralet JE, Spatz K, et al. Ionic modification of calcium phosphate cement viscosity. Part I: hypodermic injection and strength improvement of apatite cement. Biomaterials 2004; 25(11):2187–2195.
114. Bernards CM, Chapman J, Mirza S. Lethality of embolized norian bone cement varies with the time between mixing and embolization [abstr]. Trans Orthop Res Soc 2005; 29:254.

7

Percutaneous Vertebroplasty: Procedure Technique

John M. Mathis

This chapter presents the general technique used to perform a percutaneous vertebroplasty (PV) and presumes that the reader has appropriate knowledge of issues discussed in earlier chapters such as pertinent spinal anatomy, patient selection and evaluation, biomechanics of PV, and bone cement selection. If more information about these subjects is needed, see the preceding chapters.

Informed Consent

Written permission for the procedure is recommended following a complete discussion of the risks and complications of the procedure with the patients and/or their representatives. Now that Food and Drug Administration (FDA)—approved bone cement for percutaneous vertebroplasty and balloon kyphoplasty (KP) is available (Spineplex, Stryker-Howmedica, Kalamazoo, MI), there is no good reason to use nonapproved cements except as part of an investigational review board (IRB)—approved investigation (with an FDA-approved device exemption). The discussion of risks and complications should include potential side effects that are known to be possible with these procedures. These include bleeding and infection (both rare), temporary pain exacerbation, cement leaks (resulting in neural or pulmonary compromise), and death (which has been reported due to severe cement allergy or pulmonary compromise).

There are clinical and anatomic situations that help the operator categorize a patient's risk as low or high. Examples of low-risk patients are those with no known comorbidities and who have simple anatomic fractures (such as a mild, single-level fracture in the low thoracic or lumbar region). High-risk patients have complex anatomic situations such as a vertebra partially destroyed by a tumor or a tumor extending into the epidural space. In these situations, neural compression, due to cement leak or additional extrusion of tumor, make clinical complications more likely. Other high-risk situations would include patients with preexisting pulmonary compromise. These patients may have otherwise simple fractures that still can pose a significant risk as small amounts of marrow fat or cement embolized to the lungs may produce respiratory failure. Remember, all PV and KP procedures result in hydraulic displacement of marrow elements that end up in the lung (even without cement emboli). In severe chronic obstructive pulmonary disease (COPD) this can result in substantial pulmonary compromise, respiratory failure, and even death.

Patients in the high-risk category should be informed of this situation during consent discussions. Even when the expected risk is low, potentially severe complications should be discussed and understood.

Image Guidance

Since the first PV procedure (1), fluoroscopy has been the preferred method of image guidance for performing PV, although computed tomography (CT) has infrequently been used as a primary or adjunctive tool (2,3). Because this procedure was initiated and popularized by interventional neuroradiologists, biplane fluoroscopic equipment was commonly available and often used (Figure 7.1A). This equipment allows multiplanar, real-time visualization for cannula introduction and cement injection and permits rapid alternation between imaging planes without complex equipment moves or projection realignment. However, this type of radiographic equipment is expensive and not as commonly available in interventional suites or operating rooms unless they are used for neurointerventional procedures.

It takes longer to acquire two-plane guidance and monitoring information with a single-plane than with a biplane system. However, it is feasible and safe to use a single-plane fluoroscopic system as long as the operating physician recognizes the necessity of orthogonal projection visualization during the PV (or KP) to ensure a safe procedure. With a single-plane system for PV, the C arm moves will mean a slower procedure compared with biplane. A temporary biplane configuration can be made using two mobile C arms together (or a mobile C arm with a fixed plane angiographic instillation) (Figure 7.1B). Set-up time is longer, but the resulting biplane configuration will result in a more rapid procedure with less attention by the operator to continually move the imaging plane to obtain pictures in multiple projections.

Gangi et al. (3) introduced the concept of using a combination of CT and fluoroscopy for PV. This method gained a brief period of popularity in the United States when the study by Barr et al. (2) was published. They subsequently abandoned CT for routine PV. Although the contrast resolution with CT is superior to that with fluoroscopy, the CT method does not include the ability to monitor needle placement and cement injection in real time. This may be acceptable for needle placement, particularly if a small-gauge guide needle is first placed to ensure accurate and safe location before introducing a large-bore, trocar–cannula system. However, it is certainly not optimum for monitoring the injection of cement. For this reason, Gangi et al. (3) and Barr et al. (2) used fluoroscopy in the CT suite during cement introduction

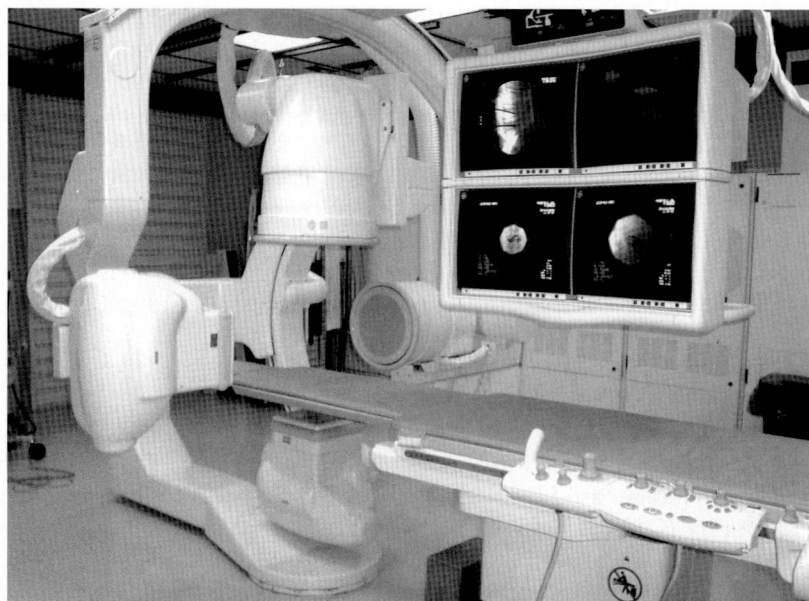

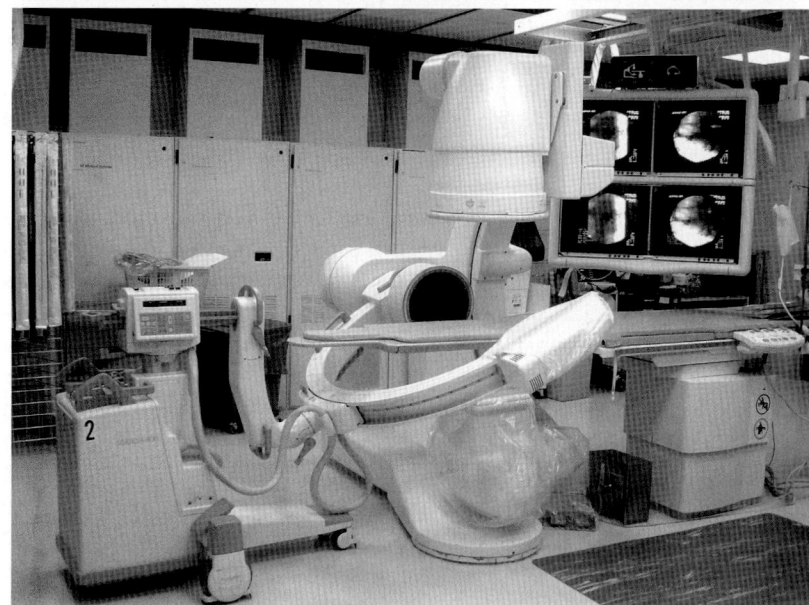

Figure 7.1. **(A)** Typical biplane configuration with independent imaging planes capable of producing images in two projections without complex equipment movements. **(B)** This shows a temporary biplane arrangement with a mobile C arm moved into position along with a fixed single-plane fluoroscopic system. Although not necessary routinely, this type of configuration may be advantageous when starting PV or KP to make the imaging acquisitions faster. **(C)** Combined CT and mobile fluoroscopy setup. In this arrangement, fluoroscopy may be constrained to lateral images only based on the size and configuration of the CT table. (A, from J.M. Mathis [ed], Image-Guided Spine Interventions. New York: Springer, 2004, with permission.)

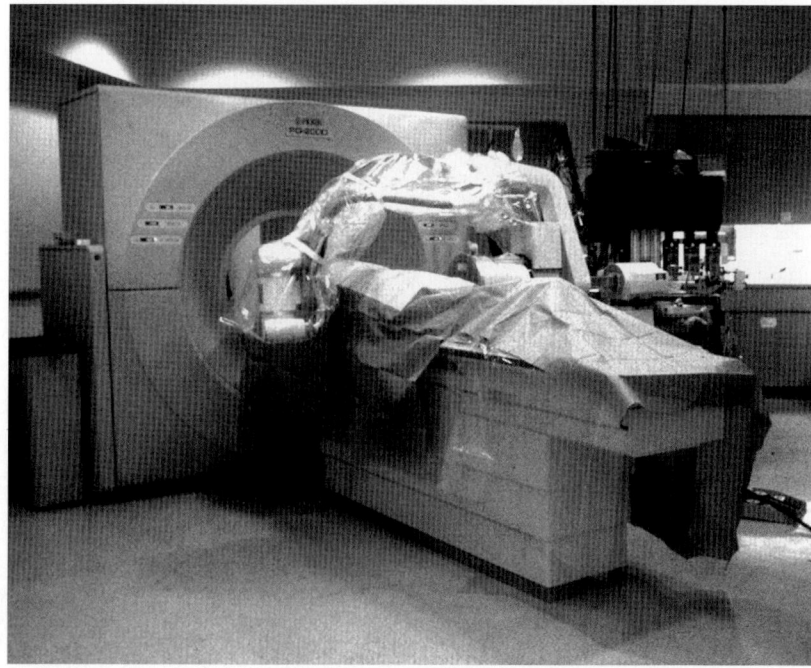

Figure 7.1. *Continued*

(Figure 7.1C). Computed tomography does not afford one the opportunity to watch the cement as it is being injected or to alter the injection volume in real time if a leak occurs. Also, unless a large section is scanned with each observation, it is possible to have leaks outside the scan plane that may be missed by looking only locally in the middle of the injected body. Barr et al. (2) used general anesthesia with their CT-guided cases because of the need to minimize patient motion. This was successful but added a small additional risk to the procedure and considerable complexity and cost. For all of these reasons, CT has not found a primary role in image guidance for PV; it is reserved for extremely difficult cases.

Examples of situations where CT is preferred over fluoroscopy include the treatment of cervical or high thoracic vertebra (where the approach is anterior and fluoroscopy is inadequate to see critical structures such as carotid or vertebral arteries), destroyed vertebra where there is a risk of tumor displacement into the spinal canal during cement introduction, and in the treatment of sacral insufficiency fractures. Here one must modify the cement injection technique. Computed tomography scans are made frequently after injections of small aliquots of cement. In this situation, cement leaks should be detected before they are large and clinical symptoms avoided (Figure 7.2). These techniques are discussed more fully in Chapter 11.

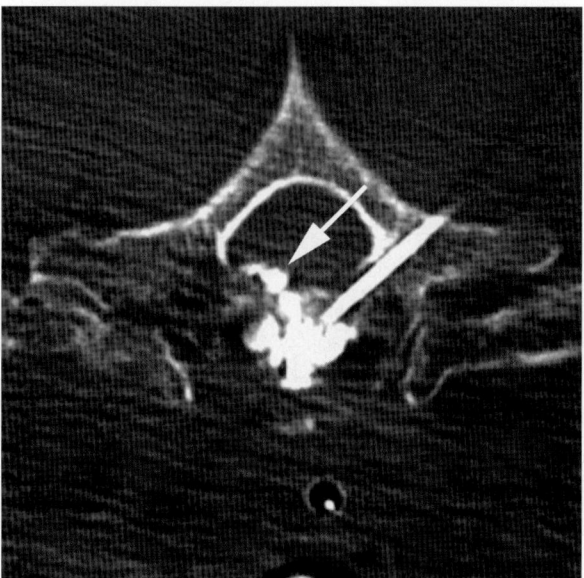

Figure 7.2. A CT image taken during PV showing cement filling of a T1 vertebra (invaded by tumor) with a small (asymptomatic) cement leak into the spinal canal (white arrow). Cement injection was terminated, and the patient had a good result from the PV.

Laboratory Evaluations

Coagulation test results should be normal, and the patient should not be taking coumadin. Coumadin may be discontinued and replaced with enoxaparin sodium (Lovenox, Rhône-Poulenc Rorer Pharmaceuticals, Inc, Collegeville, PA), taken once or twice a day on an outpatient basis. Coumadin may also be stopped and replaced with heparin, but this medication must be administered intravenously, requiring hospital admission. Both enoxaparin sodium and heparin can be reversed with protamine sulfate before PV and restarted postprocedure. Aspirin use is not a contraindication to the procedure.

Percutaneous vertebroplasty is not recommended for patients with signs of active infection, but elevated white blood cell counts clearly associated with medical conditions such as myeloma or secondary to steroid use are not contraindications.

Antibiotics

For PV, as for other surgical procedures that implant devices into the body, intravenous antibiotics are routinely given, usually 30 minutes before starting the procedure. The most common antibiotic used in this application is cephazolin (1g) (4). If an alternative must be used because of allergy, ciprofloxacin (500mg orally, two times daily) may be substituted and continued for 24 hours after the completion of the procedure. Optimally, an oral antibiotic should be started 12 hours before a PV procedure.

Antibiotics are added to the cement only in the situation of immunocompromise. This is due to the very low risk of infection after PV with only minimal evidence that any benefit occurs from antibiotics in the cement (and then only in the situation of immunocompromise). Additionally, there is a mechanical change in the cement that is produced by the addition of the antibiotic. This should be avoided unless definitely necessary.

Anesthesia

During PV, it is common to use both local anesthetics and conscious sedation to make the patient comfortable and relaxed. Patients who request not to receive intravenous (IV) sedation or who cannot have it for safety reasons still can be treated with only mild discomfort if appropriate attention is given to local anesthetic placement. To reduce the sting and discomfort associated with locally administered anesthetics (lidocaine, etc.), one may buffer the anesthetic by the addition of a mixture of 1 mL of bicarbonate to 9 mL of lidocaine. This mixture reduces, but does not eliminate, the anesthetic sting. I commonly use a lidocaine mixture that contains both bicarbonate and Ringer's lactate, and this essentially eliminates the sting of the local anesthetic. At my institution, this mixture is prepared on a daily basis for all procedures requiring local anesthetics. The excess is discarded at the end of each day. This preparation has a low concentration of lidocaine (0.5%) and allows the use of a more generous volume locally with less risk of toxicity (Table 7.1).

Whatever the chosen local anesthetic preparation, the skin, subcutaneous tissues along the expected needle tract, and periosteum of the bone at the bone entry site must be thoroughly infiltrated. Once this is accomplished, the patient will experience only mild discomfort while the bone needle is being placed, regardless of whether conscious sedation is used. Local anesthesia alone may be insufficient if a mallet is used for needle introduction. In this case, IV procedural sedation is required for patient comfort.

Intravenous procedural sedation has become a common adjunctive method for pain and anxiety control in awake patients who undergo minimally invasive procedures. I use a combination of IV midazolam

Table 7.1. Modified Local Anesthetic Solutions.

Solution	Lidocaine (4%)	Lactated Ringer's	Bicarbonate	Epinephrine
1	4 mL	24 mL	2 mL	0
2	4 mL	24 mL	2 mL	0.15 mL (1:1,000)

Solution 1 makes a "sting-free" local anesthetic with 0.5% lidocaine. Solution 2 is "sting free" with 0.5% lidocaine and 1:200,000 epinephrine. These should be mixed daily and discarded at the end of the day. The total volume of each mix is 30 mL.

(Versed, Roche, Manati, PR) and fentanyl (Sublimase, Abbott Labs, Chicago). To decrease anxiety and diminish the discomfort associated with positioning, it may be helpful to begin these medications before placing the patient on the operative table. Dosages are chosen according to patient size and medical condition. The final amount is determined with titration while observing the patient's response.

General anesthesia is rarely needed for PV, but it is used occasionally for patients in extreme pain who cannot tolerate the prone position used in PV or for patients with psychological disability that would preclude a conscious procedure. It is not needed for routine PV (or KP) and should be avoided when possible because it adds a small additional risk and considerable cost to the procedure. As described previously, Barr et al. (2) used general anesthesia routinely with CT-guided procedures to ensure minimum patient motion.

Needle Introduction and Placement

The original choice of a device for percutaneous cement introduction was based on device availability. The size of these devices was empirically chosen to allow the viscous polymethylmethacrylate (PMMA) cement to be injected. Originally 10- to 11-gauge trocar–cannula systems were used. Needle systems have now been specifically developed for cement introduction into collapsed vertebra (Figure 7.3A). It is becoming progressively common to see smaller gauge needles used routinely (13–15 gauge). All will work with the least resistance during injection found with the larger bore systems. The smaller systems are necessary in small pedicles or in the cervical spine. A 13-gauge cannula can be placed through any adult pedicle from the thoracic through lumbar spine without fear of it being too large. (I now use 13-gauge systems for all levels and have stopped stocking 11-gauge devices for routine use.) Regardless of size, the diamond tip configuration (Figure 7.3B) offers the maximal ease of needle introduction into bone. Bevel tip needles have been described as useful for changing the tip direction according to which way the bevel is oriented. This is certainly true with small needles (i.e., 21–25 gauges), but I doubt that 13-gauge and larger needles are significantly directable by soft, osteoporotic bone. The bevel tip is certainly harder to introduce into bone as it tends to slip off any surface that is not flat.

Bone biopsy can be accomplished easily with the trocar removed (Figure 7.3C). This does require removing the cannula to get the biopsy specimen out. Biopsy devices are made that fit both the 13- and 11-gauge systems (Figure 7.3D) and allow biopsy and subsequent PV without removing the cannula.

Several introductory routes for needle delivery are possible, including (1) transpedicular, (2) parapedicular (transcostovertebral), (3) posterolateral (lumbar only), and (4) anterolateral (cervical or high thoracic). These are discussed in detail in Chapter 2. The classic route for most PV procedures is transpedicular (Figure 7.4); see also Figure 2.8A. It offers the following advantages:

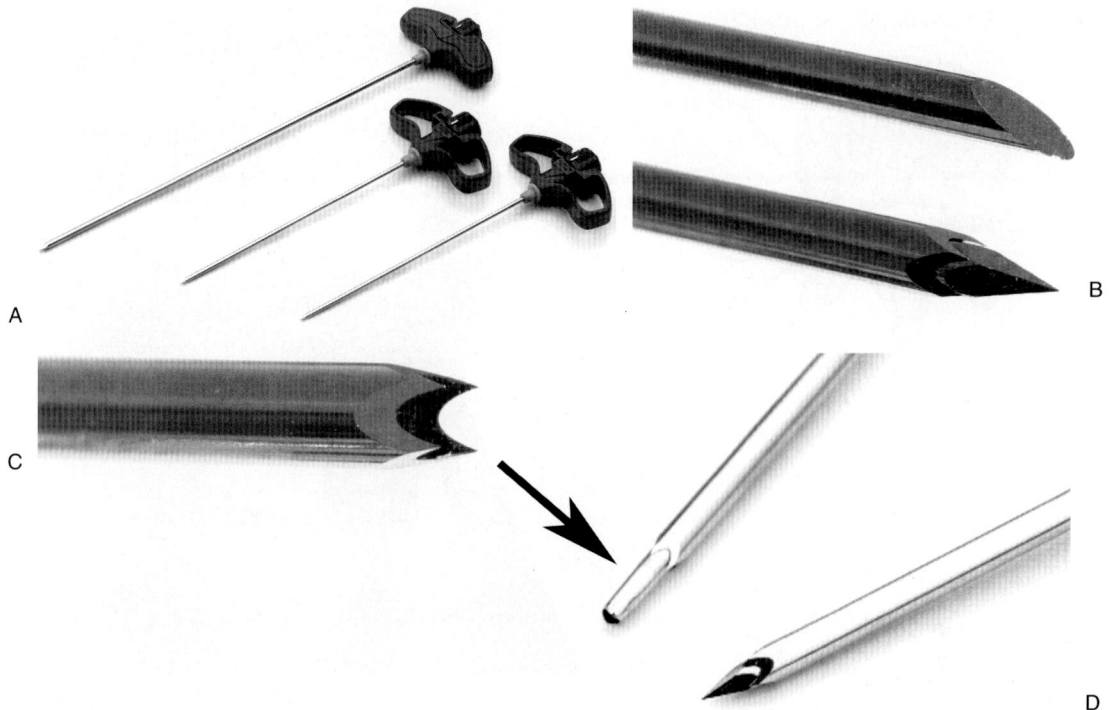

Figure 7.3. **(A)** Needle systems for PV developed by Stryker Medical Instruments for cement delivery. These needles have a fixed handle for ease of introduction into bone. They are made in various lengths and sizes, with 13 and 11 gauge being most common. **(B)** Close-up views of the needle points showing a match-ground diamond point with a very sharp tip that engages the bone surface to prevent slipping during the start of needle placement. The flat facets of the point cut bone with a back and forth motion of the hand during needle introduction. **(C)** Close-up view of the Stryker cannula with the trocar removed. This can be used to obtain a bone biopsy specimen but will require removal to retrieve the specimen. **(D)** Close-up view of the Stryker biopsy device (black arrow) inserted through the cannula. This allows a biopsy specimen to be extracted through the cannula. The trocar is then reinserted and the trocar–cannula placed in final position for PV. (Courtesy of Stryker Medical Instruments, Kalamazoo, MI.)

- It provides the operating physician with a definite anatomic landmark for needle targeting.
- It is very effective for PV and for biopsy of lesions inside the vertebral body.
- It is inherently safe, with no other adjacent anatomic structures that might be damaged with the needle (e.g., nerve root, lung) as long as an intrapedicular location is maintained.
- It provides a safe entry point that allows easy compression of overlying soft tissues, postprocedure, to minimize bleeding.

In the upper thoracic region and in small patients, the size of the pedicle may be too narrow for an 11-gauge needle. In this situation, a 13-gauge needle should be used.

The parapedicular or transcostovertebral approach (Figure 7.5; see also Figure 2.8B,C) was devised to allow access when the transpedicular route is not desirable or possible (e.g., small pedicle). As the needle

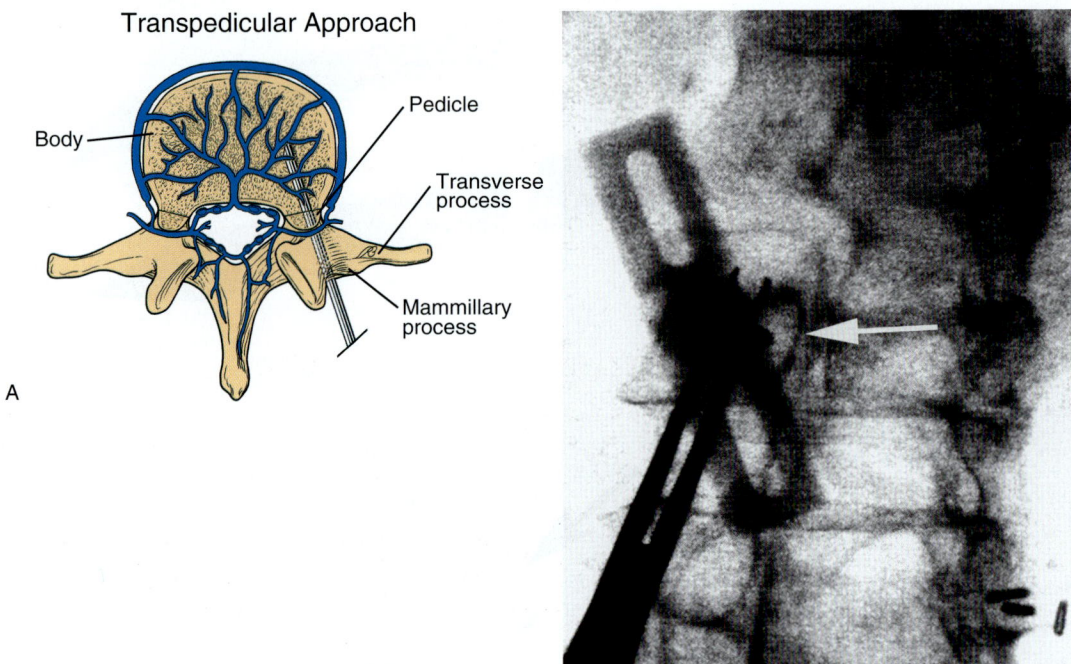

Figure 7.4. (A) Drawing of the transpedicular approach with a needle traversing the pedicle. The pedicle provides a bone channel that allows access from the skin surface to the vertebral body and that bypasses critical areas like the spinal canal. **(B)** Oblique fluoroscopic image of a needle being introduced via the transpedicular approach. The pedicle (white arrow) is seen as an oval target through which the needle can be safely placed.

passes along the lateral aspect of the pedicle, rather than through it, a small pedicle does not preclude using an 11-gauge needle for cement introduction. Also, this approach angles the needle tip more toward the center of the vertebral body than does the transpedicular approach. At least in theory, this angle may allow easier filling of the vertebra with a single injection (this may not be the case if an early cement leak occurs). A parapedicular approach has a higher chance of creating a pneumothorax than does the transpedicular route. A second potential problem with the parapedicular route is that the needle enters the body only through its lateral wall. This approach may increase the risk of paraspinous hematoma after needle removal. Because the osteotomy site occurs laterally along the side of the vertebra with a parapedicular approach, one cannot apply local pressure after needle removal as can be done with the transpedicular route.

In the cervical spine, a transpedicular route is very difficult, so an anterolateral approach may be used as an alternative. Needle introduction must avoid the carotid–jugular complex, the vertebral artery, and the esophagus. To accomplish this, the operating physician (as in cervical discography) can select a right-sided approach (opposite the esophagus) and manually push the carotid out of the path of the needle (Figure 7.6; see also Figure 2.3). Alternatively, CT can be used to visualize the carotid, and a safe trajectory that will miss the vascular structures can then be chosen. A small guide needle can be inserted to ensure accurate placement outside the carotid complex. I prefer the guide needle alternative because it gives positive guidance and confirmation without excessive fluoroscopy to my hands during needle introduction. However, because osteoporotic fractures in this area are rare, the cervical spine only occasionally undergoes PV. Neoplastic disease usually produces the uncommon need for PV intervention in the cervical spine (additional information on this approach can be found in the case series on "cervical approach"; see Case 6 in Section II).

Once the needle route is chosen, IV procedural sedation and local anesthesia are administered. A small dermatotomy incision is made with a No. 11 scalpel blade. The trocar and cannula system are introduced through the skin incision and subcutaneous tissue to the periosteum of the bone. This introduction can be facilitated with a sterile clamp to guide the needle during fluoroscopy (Figure 7.7), thus avoiding radiation to the operating physician's hands. In osteoporotic bone, penetrating the bone cortex and advancing the needle into the body is usually very easy. In a patient with neoplastic disease, the bone may still be very dense and strong (except where it has been destroyed by a tumor), and, in this situation, the use of a mallet to advance the needle is a technique clearly superior to that of manual advancement.

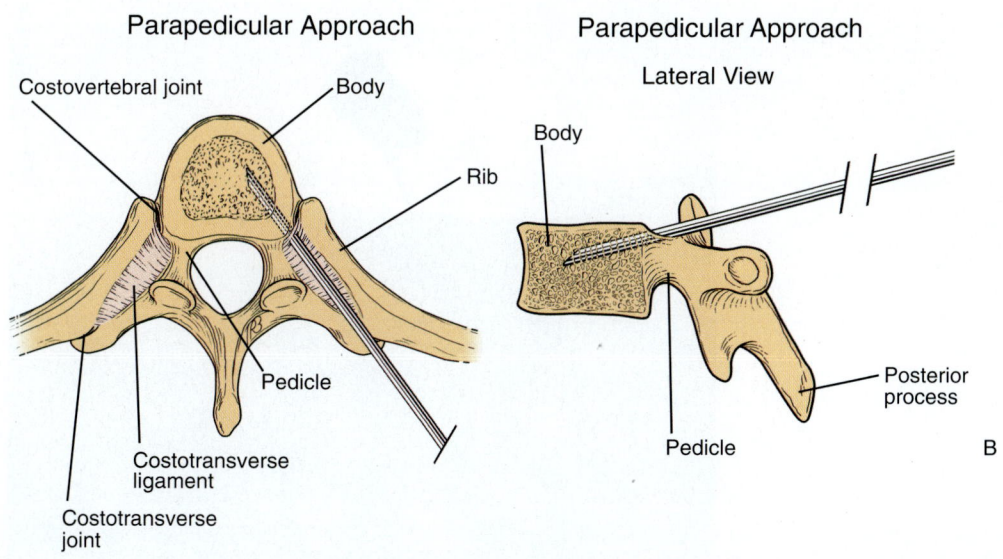

Figure 7.5. (A,B) Drawings that show needle position for a parapedicular approach from two views. The needle position is lateral to the pedicle and approaches the vertebra from above the transverse process. This avoids the exiting nerve root that courses under the pedicle. The needle entry site is along the lateral aspect of the vertebra. This location does not allow access for local pressure after needle removal, making the chance for bleeding higher than with the transpedicular approach.

Anterior Cervical Approach

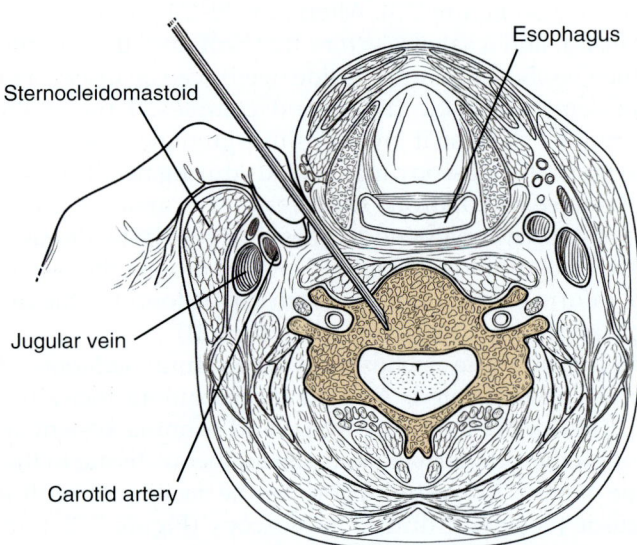

Figure 7.6. Drawing showing manual displacement of the carotid–jugular complex and guide needle insertion. This allows access to the vertebra and spares injury to the neck vessels. Needle position can be confirmed with CT.

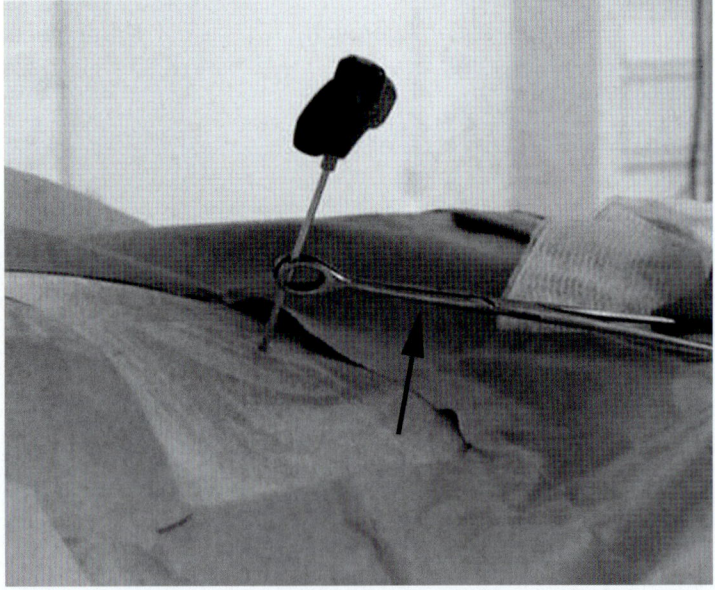

Figure 7.7. This picture shows a long clamp (black arrow) used to hold and position the needle during fluoroscopy to minimize radiation to the operator's hands. Once the needle is positioned in this manner, the fluoroscope is turned off and manual needle introduction proceeds.

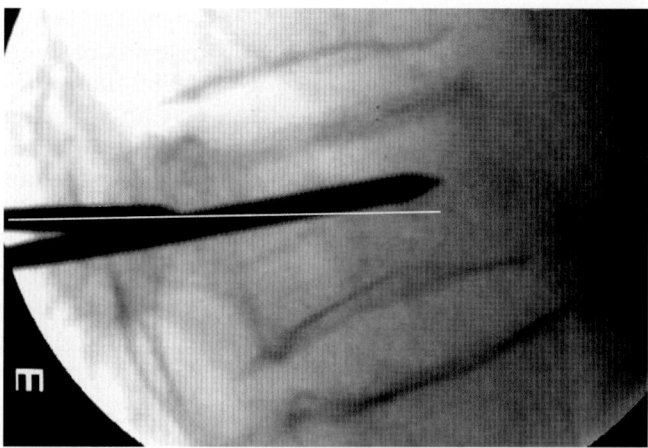

Figure 7.8. Lateral image showing one needle in place with the tip at the junction of the anterior and middle third of the vertebra. This position allows good safety for cement injection away from the large venous confluence in the posterior of the vertebra. The second needle is just beginning to be introduced. The white line shows its trajectory based on its angle of entry. This preliminary evaluation of trajectory allows the operator to predict the ultimate needle tract and make adjustments as the needle is being introduced.

Regardless of whether a transpedicular or parapedicular route has been chosen, the tip of the needle should be ultimately positioned beyond the vertebral midpoint as viewed from the lateral projection. I usually try to obtain an even more anterior position by placing the needle tip at the junction of the anterior and middle thirds (Figure 7.8).

Two needles are routinely placed, usually via the transpedicular approach (Figure 7.9). This takes minimally longer than a single-needle

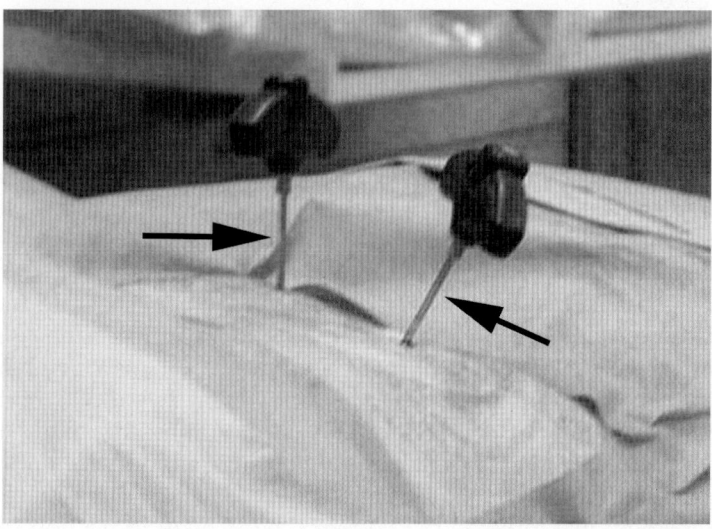

Figure 7.9. Two needles in place (black arrows) for a single-level PV via a transpedicular approach. Both needles are placed prior to cement mixing.

placement and affords a large margin of safety for being able to dependably complete a vertebral fill with a single mix of cement while minimizing cement leaks and maximizing vertebral filling. There is no question that a single-needle placement can give an adequate fill in a large number of cases. However, the single-needle method fails to produce uniform fills more often than the double-needle technique and may cause the operator to accept a larger cement leak during filling (when a leak is seen during injection through the first needle, the operator can finish filling through the second needle and minimize the initial cement leak). Larger leaks occur with one needle because the operator will almost always try to finish a PV through the single existing needle rather than placing a second needle and remixing cement. I teach and routinely use the two-needle technique.

Venography

Venography was never used much in Europe and was introduced in the United States in an attempt to discover potential leak sites using radiographic contrast and prior to injecting cement. However, this worked poorly because the viscosities of contrast and bone cement are very different. The predictive value of where the cement would go by using contrast was low. Occasionally, contrast would pool in a cavity or the disc space and even impede visualization during cement injection (Figure 7.10). Finally, venography increased the radiation burden to the patient and physician, added exposure of contrast to the procedure risks, and was usually very uncomfortable for the patient during the injection. For all these reasons, I discontinued using venography in 1996 and have found no disadvantage or safety loss without its use (5). Other long-term proponents of venography have belatedly stopped its use in routine PV as they found no safety benefit after reviewing their prior cases (6).

Cement Injection

Cement is prepared only after all needles are placed. Spineplex (Figure 7.11A; Stryker-Howmedica), which is now FDA approved for PV and KP, is prepared per the manufacturer's directions using a sterile, vacuum mixing device (Figure 7.11B,C). It is then injected using small syringes (typically 1 cc) or devices made specifically for injection (Figure 7.11C). This allows easy control of the cement introduction. Either the cement injection should be monitored in real time or small quantities (i.e., 0.1–0.2 mL) injected and the result visualized before additional cement is introduced. The latter approach allows monitoring while minimizing the operator's radiographic exposure (as it allows one to step back from the syringe or injection device and minimize exposure during visualization).

Any cement leak outside the vertebral body is an indication to stop the injection. When a rapidly polymerizing cement (e.g., Spineplex) is used, this may be necessary only for a minute or two while the injected

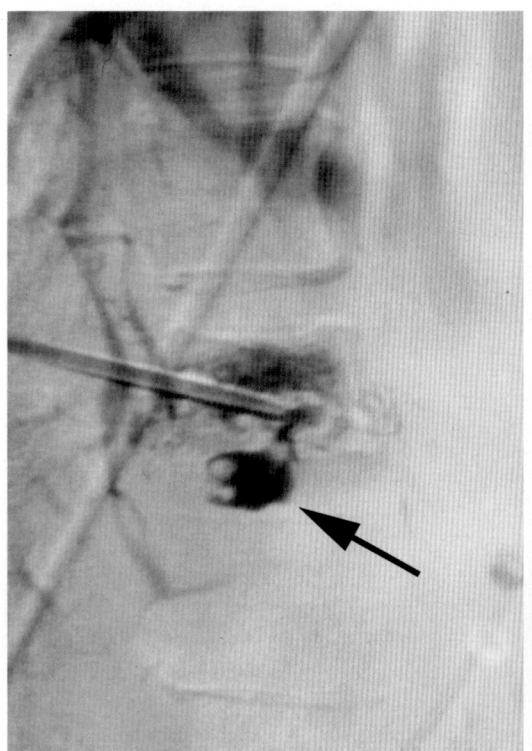

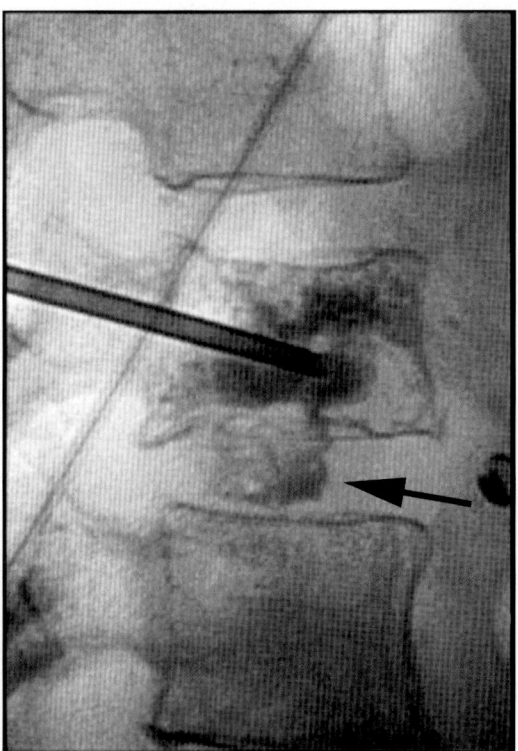

Figure 7.10. (A) Digital subtraction venogram showing contrast leaking into the disc space (black arrow) through an endplate fracture. This finding would predict a cement leak into the disc through the same hole. **(B)** As cement is injected we see that the contrast that has pooled in the disc space from the venogram slowly goes away (black arrow). Nevertheless, its presence makes it hard to distinguish between residual contrast and potential leak of cement into this area. **(C)** The final image shows good filling of the vertebra with cement and progressive resolution of the contrast in the disc (black arrow). There was no cement leak into the disc, and therefore the contrast leak was not predictive of where the cement would go. Also, the contrast obscures detection of early cement leak in this situation.

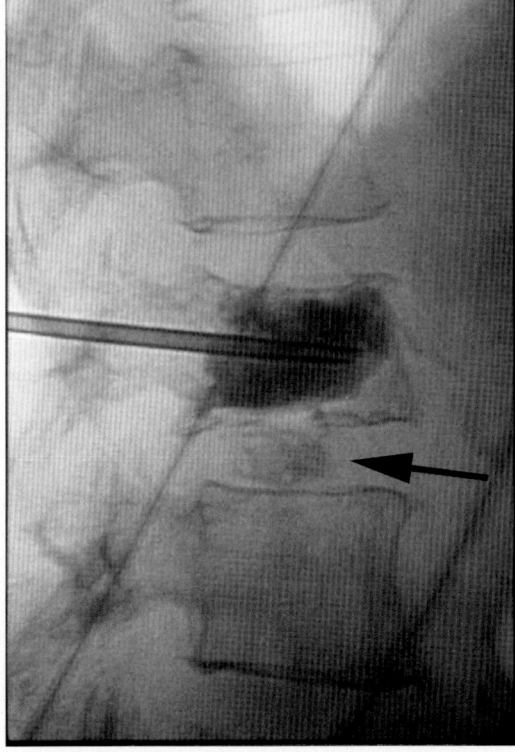

126   J.M. Mathis

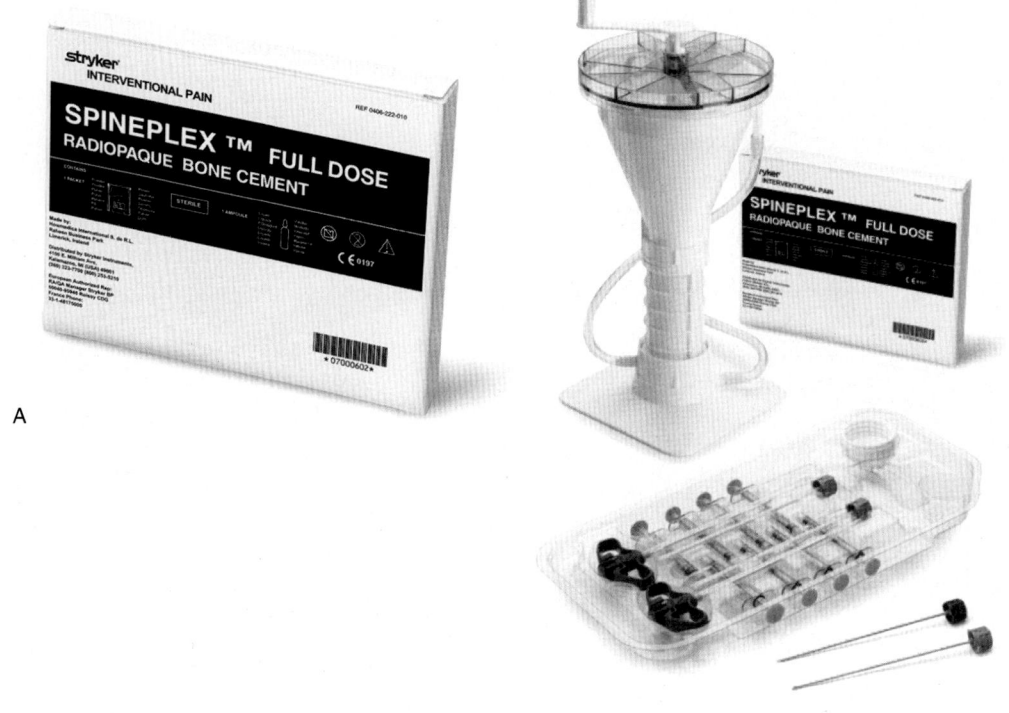

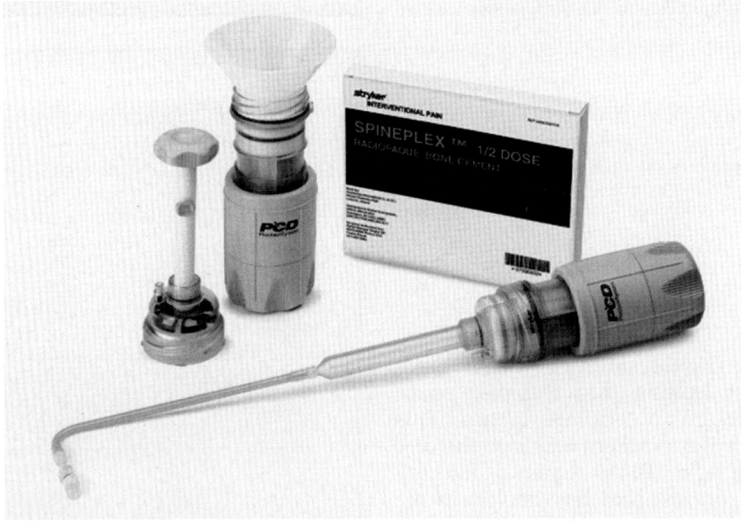

Figure 7.11. (A) Spineplex is a polymethylmethacrylate specially prepared and FDA approved for PV and KP. It contains 30% barium sulfate by weight, which allows easy visualization of the cement during injection. Mixture of the co-polymer (powder) and monomer (liquid) is adjusted to give adequate room temperature working times for PV and KP. **(B)** This picture shows the "full dose" vacuum mixing device that is supplied in a kit for PV containing two bone needles and multiple syringes for injection. **(C)** The vacuum mixing and injection device shown provides a closed system for mixing and cement delivery. It provides a mechanical advantage during cement injection to facilitate an easier delivery of cement. (Courtesy of Stryker-Howmedica, Kalamazoo, MI.)

cement partially polymerizes and becomes more viscous. Restarting the injection may then redirect flow into other areas of the vertebra away from areas already filled by cement. If leakage is still seen, it is advisable to terminate the cement injection through this needle and move to a second or alternate needle. This will usually allow completion of the vertebral fill without further leakage. The original leak will be occluded by the prior cement injected as it will now have hardened. One should work through a single needle at a time. This avoids contamination of both needles at once and preserves a route (the second needle) for subsequent injection if a leak is encountered early. Injection of thick cement is considered safer than using a very liquid consistency. Cement can still be introduced after the injection devices are no longer able to deliver it. The trocar is useful to push additional thick cement from the cannula into the vertebra. The 5-inch, 13-gauge cannula holds 0.5 mL of cement, and the 5-inch, 11-gauge cannula holds 0.9 mL. Reintroducing the trocar will push this amount of cement (respectively) into the vertebra. This is done only if this additional amount of cement is desired. The cannula can be removed safely without reintroduction of the trocar when the cement is hardened beyond when it can be injected. Simply twisting the needle through several revolutions will break the cement at the tip of the cannula and will prevent leaving a trail of cement in the soft tissues. However, removing the cannula before the cement sufficiently hardens can allow cement to track backward from the bone into the soft tissues and may create local pain (Figure 7.12).

The amount of cement needed to produce pain relief has not been accurately documented in available clinical reports. As we believe pain relief is related to fracture stabilization, the amount of cement needed to restore the initial vertebral body's mechanical integrity should give

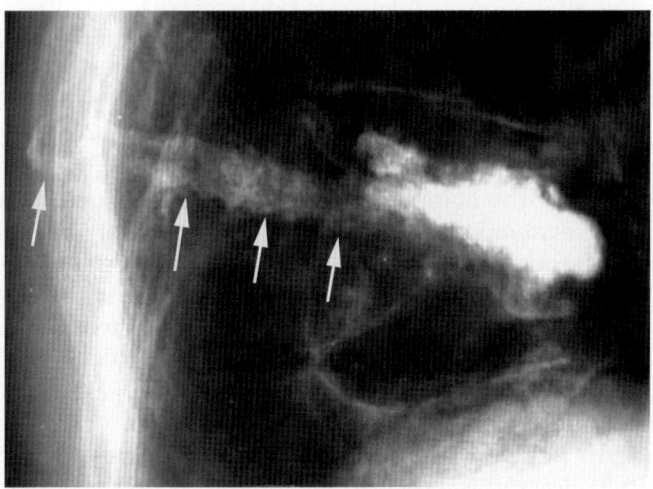

Figure 7.12. Lateral radiograph showing cement that was too liquid when injected that tracked backward along the needle path, leaving cement in the soft tissues (white arrows). This can happen easily when using cements with long work times (i.e., Cranioplastic, Vertebroplastic, or Secore).

an approximation of the quantity needed also to relieve pain clinically. In an in vitro study, we showed that the initial prefracture strength and stiffness of a vertebra could be restored by injecting 2.5–4 mL of Simplex P in a thoracic vertebra, while 6–8 mL provided similar augmentation in the lumbar region (7). A reasonable guideline for the quantity of cement to be injected is the amount that is needed to fill 50%–70% of the residual volume of the compressed vertebra (Figure 7.13). These amounts should not be taken as an absolute but rather as a guide. This indicates that relatively small amounts of cement are needed to restore vertebral biomechanical strength and that these amounts vary with the vertebral level in the spine, an individual's body size, and the degree of vertebral collapse.

We have also demonstrated that significant strength restoration is provided to the vertebral body with a unipedicular injection when cement filling crosses the midline of the vertebral body (8). This would suggest that unipedicular fills that achieve adequate cement injection volumes and distribution are likely to be successful at achieving pain relief. This fact notwithstanding, there is a higher likelihood of achieving more uniform fills, with smaller leaks, while using two needles rather than one.

Postprocedure Care

After adequate vertebral filling has been achieved, the needles are removed. Occasionally, venous bleeding is experienced at the needle entry site. Hemostasis is easily achieved with local pressure for 3–5 minutes. The entry site is dressed with betadine ointment and a sterile bandage. The patient is maintained recumbent for 1–2 hours after the procedure and monitored for changes in neurologic function or for signs of any other clinical change or side effects (Table 7.2).

Any sign of adverse affect should trigger a search of the explanatory cause using appropriate imaging modalities (usually CT). It is well known that 1%–2% of patients will have a transient period of benign increase in local pain following PV. However, this is a diagnosis of exclusion, and increased pain should prompt extended monitoring (or hospitalization if the pain is severe and requires aggressive therapy) and imaging evaluation to exclude other causes for the pain (such as cement extravasation). Pain alone will usually be adequately treated with analgesics, nonsteroidal anti-inflammatory drugs (such as Toradol), or local steroid injections adjacent to affected nerve roots or into the epidural space. Large cement leaks or neurologic dysfunction should prompt an immediate surgical consultation.

Percutaneous vertebroplasty is easily performed on an outpatient basis with the patient discharged after 2 hours of uneventful recovery. (Table 7.2). Follow-up is indicated to monitor the results of therapy and should be incorporated into a quality management program. Complications and results should be maintained by the facility as well as for each individual provider. Additional information and recommendations about the credentialing and quality management for PV can be

Figure 7.13. Lateral **(A)** and anteroposterior **(B)** radiographs following a bilateral transpedicular PV reveals 70% or greater filling (white arrow in A) with no evidence of leak. It is important to fill the anterior 2/3–3/4 of the vertebral body. In the anteroposterior view, cement should cross the midline to reinforce both halves of the vertebra (white arrows). **(C)** Anteroposterior radiograph of a unipedicular PV shows distribution of cement into both halves of the vertebra.

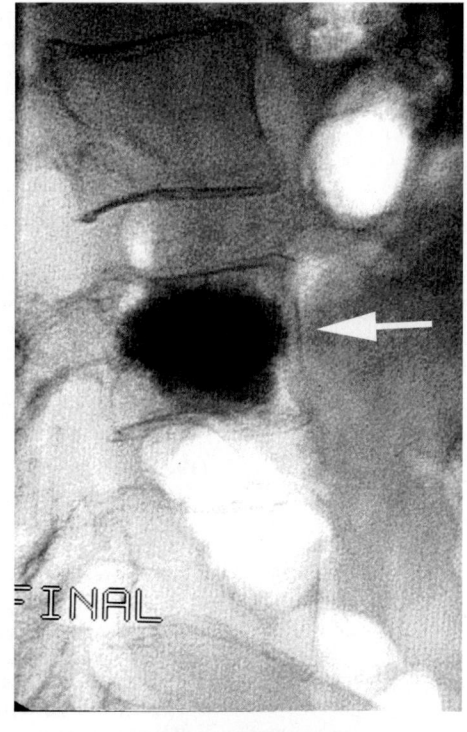

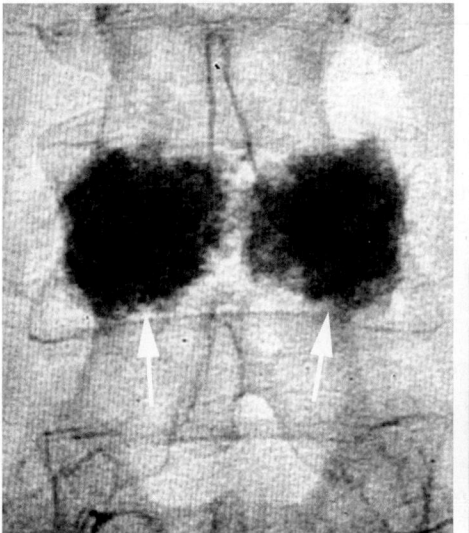

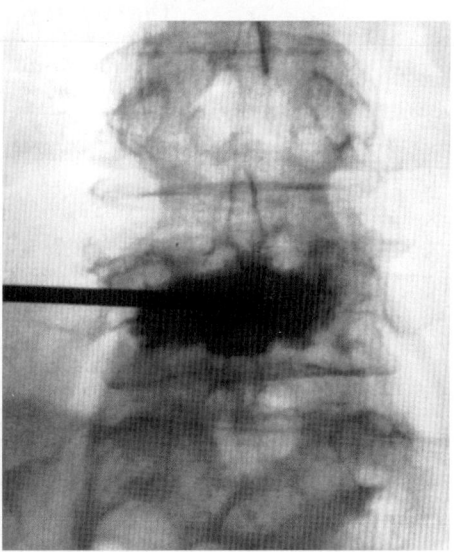

Table 7.2. Sample Postprocedure Orders and Discharge Instructions.

Postprocedure
- Bed rest 1 hour postprocedure (may roll side to side)
- May sit up after 1 hour with assistance
- Vital signs and neurologic examinations (focused on the lower extremities) every 15 minutes for the first hour, then every 30 minutes for the second hour
- Record pain level (visual analog scale, 1 to 10) at end of procedure and at 2 hours postprocedure (before discharge). Compare with baseline values and notify physician if pain increases above baseline
- May have liquids by mouth if no nausea
- Discontinue oxygen (if used) after procedure (if saturation is normal)
- Discontinue intravenous drips after 1 hour if recovery is otherwise uneventful
- Discharge patient home with adult companion after 2 hours if recovery is uneventful

Discharge
- Return home; bed rest or minimal activity for next 24 hours
- May resume regular diet and medications
- Keep operative site covered for 24 hours. Bandages may then be removed and site washed with a damp cloth. Do not soak
- Notify physician/facility if you have increasing pain, redness, swelling, or drainage from the operative site
- Notify physician/facility if you have difficulty with walking, changes in sensation in your hips or legs, new pain, or problems with bowel or bladder function
- The area of your procedure will be tender to the touch for 24 to 48 hours. This is to be expected
- If you continue to have pain similar to that before your procedure, you may continue to take prescribed pain medications as needed

found in the standards of practice published by the American College of Radiology or Society of Interventional Radiology (see Chapter 14).

Results

Relatively few prospective trials are available looking at the results of PV. Zoarski et al. (9) presented a small prospective (nonrandomized) evaluation of the effectiveness of PV for relieving pain. This report utilized the MODEMS method to establish that 22 of 23 patients improved after PV and remained satisfied during the 15–18 month follow-up period. McGraw et al. (10) prospectively treated and evaluated 100 patients with PV looking at pain scores before and after the procedure. They found a statistically significant improvement in pain following PV (10). Additionally, numerous retrospective series are available and uniformly report good pain relief and reduced requirements for analgesics following PV (2,11–14). This is especially true of pain related to compression fractures produced by osteoporosis where significant pain relief of between 80% and 90% has been observed. This pain relief is persistent with rare reports of additional compression of vertebra previously treated with PV (15). Additional fractures at other levels remain a possibility and primary source of morbidity. Once osteoporotic compression fracture occurs, every effort to minimize future bone loss medically should be made. Also, modifications in lifestyle should be attempted to minimize mechanical stress on the spine and thereby lessen the risk of additional fractures.

Complications

Complications were initially considered and reported as low. Unfortunately, complications are higher for inexperienced physicians and for those who attempt the procedure without adequate image guidance or appropriate materials. Adequate training needs to be completed before attempting the procedure. Recommendations can be obtained from the American College of Radiology Standards of Practice on Percutaneous Vertebroplasty or the Society of Interventional Radiology (see Chapter 14). A complete discussion of known and potential complications and methods for complication avoidance is given in Chapter 13.

In osteoporotic induced vertebral fractures, clinical reports of complications are around 1% (11–14). Many of these are transient and include short-term increase in local pain after cement introduction (nonradicular and not associated with neurologic deficit). This is usually easily treated with nonsteroidal anti-inflammatory drugs and resolves within 2–24 hours. Uncommonly, cement leaking from the vertebra adjacent to a nerve root may produce radicular pain. Analgesics combined with local steroid and anesthetic injections usually provide adequate relief. A trial of this type of therapy is warranted as long as there are no associated motor deficits. The discovery of a motor deficit (or bowel or bladder dysfunction) should initiate an immediate surgical consult. This type of severe complication will almost always be associated with large volume leaks that result in neurologic compression. Severe complications are rare in the hands of experienced operators.

Cement leaks have also been implicated in producing pulmonary embolus (11). These are usually not symptomatic but rarely have produced the clinical symptoms accompanying pulmonary infarct. With a right-to-left shunt this can result in cerebral infarct (16). Patients should be categorized into low or high pulmonary risk on the basis of existing pulmonary function. Those with severe respiratory disability should have limited procedures to minimize adverse effects of even small embolic events.

Infection has been rare with PV, with only a single case reported in the literature (15).

The complication rate found when treating compression fractures resulting from malignant tumors is considerably higher than complications found in osteoporosis (13,17–20). This occurs because there are frequently areas of destroyed bone involving the vertebral cortex creating more of a propensity for cement to leak into the surrounding tissues or vessels. Cement leaks resulting in symptomatic complications occur in up to 5% of patients in this setting. These difficult cases should be undertaken only by experienced individuals.

Death is a known complication of PV. Nussbaum et al. (21) reported death in 1/50,000 cases of both PV and KP. These may be related to severe allergic reactions to the bone cement or to pulmonary compromise created by cement or fat emboli. The risk of this extreme complication increases with the number of levels performed during each session. Mathis et al. (4) reported the first multilevel PV therapy treating seven vertebrae in a 35-year-old with multiple fractures associated with steroid use for lupus. This patient's therapy occurred in three treatment sessions. Because the introduction of cement is a hydraulic event with as much marrow pushed out of the trabecular space as cement injected, there is concern about fat emboli in large-volume cement injections. I recommend treating no more than three vertebrae in any one session. Additionally, there are no data that support the prophylactic use of PV to treat vertebrae that are believed to be at risk of fracture. Except for prophylactic use, there is little conceivable reason to perform PV on large numbers of vertebrae at one time.

Any deviation from an expected good result (such as increased pain or neurologic compromise) should initiate an immediate imaging search with CT to look for a cause of the clinical change. Unremitting or progressive symptoms may require surgical or aggressive medical intervention, and outpatients should be hospitalized and monitored.

Conclusions

Percutaneous vertebroplasty has been shown to be very effective at relieving the pain associated with compression fractures of vertebra caused by both primary (age-related) and secondary (steroid-induced) osteoporosis. It also has substantial benefit in neoplastic-induced vertebral compression fracture pain but with a higher chance of associated complication. Percutaneous vertebroplasty is rapidly becoming the standard of care for compression fracture pain not responding to conservative medical therapy. However, this simple procedure must be treated with respect, as its application, without appropriate preparation and physician knowledge, can quickly produce increased pain, permanent neurologic injury, and even death.

References

1. Galibert P, Deramond H, Rosat P, Le Gars D [Preliminary note on the treatment of vertebral angioma by percutaneous acrylic vertebroplasty.] Neurochirurgie 1987; 33:166–168.
2. Barr JD, Barr MS, Lemley TJ, McCann RM. Percutaneous vertebroplasty for pain relief and spine stabilization. Spine 2000; 25:923–928.
3. Gangi A, Kastler BA, Dietemann JL. Percutaneous vertebroplasty guided by a combination of CT and fluoroscopy. Am J Neuroradiol 1994; 15:83–86.
4. Mathis JM, Petri M, Naff N. Percutaneous vertebroplasty treatment of steroid-induced osteoporotic compression fractures. Arthritis Rheum 1998; 41:171–175.

5. Wong W, Mathis JM. Commentary: is intraosseous venography a significant safety measure in performance of vertebroplasty? J Vasc Intervent Radiol 2002; 13:137–138.
6. Gaughen JR, Jensen ME, Schweickert PA, et al. Relevance of antecedent venography in percutaneous vertebroplasty for the treatment of osteoporotic compression fractures. Am J Neuroradiol 2002; 23:594–600.
7. Belkoff SM, Mathis JM, Jasper LE, et al. The biomechanics of vertebroplasty: the effect of cement volume on mechanical behavior. Spine 2001; 26:1537–1541.
8. Tohmeh AG, Mathis JM, Fenton DC, Levine AM, Belkoff SM. Biomechanical efficacy of unipedicular versus bipedicular vertebroplasty for the management of osteoporotic compression fractures. Spine 1999; 24:1772–1776.
9. Zoarski GH, Snow P, Olan WJ, et al. Percutaneous vertebroplasty for osteoporotic compression fracture: quantitative prospective evaluation of long-term outcomes. J Vasc Intervent Radiol 2002; 13:139–148.
10. McGraw JK, Lippert JA, Minkus KD, et al. Prospective evaluation of pain relief in 100 patients undergoing percutaneous vertebroplasty: results and follow-up. J Vasc Intervent Radiol 2002; 13:883–886.
11. Jensen ME, Evans AJ, Mathis JM, Kallmes DF, Cloft HJ, Dion JE. Percutaneous polymethylmethacrylate vertebroplasty in the treatment of osteoporotic vertebral body compression fractures: technical aspects. Am J Neuroradiol 1997; 18:1897–1904.
12. Mathis JM, Barr JD, Belkoff SM, et al. Percutaneous vertebroplasty: a developing standard of care for vertebral compression fractures. Am J Neuroradiol 2001; 22:373–381.
13. Chiras J, Depriester C, Weill A, Sola-Martinez MT, Deramond H [Percutaneous vertebral surgery. Technics and indications.] J Neuroradiol 1997; 24:45–59.
14. Cyteval C, Sarrabere MP, Roux JO, Thomas E, Jorgensen C, Blotman F, Sany, Taourel P. Acute osteoporotic vertebral collapse: open study on percutaneous injection of acrylic surgical cement in 20 patients. Am J Roentgenol 1999; 173:1685–1690.
15. Mathis JM. Percutaneous vertebroplasty: complication avoidance and technique optimization. Am J Neuroradiol 2003; 24:1697–1706.
16. Scroop R, Eskridge J, Britz GW. Paradoxical cerebral arterial embolization of cement during intraoperative vertebroplasty: case report. Am J Neuroradiol 2002; 23:868–870.
17. Cotten A, Dewatre F, Cortet B, Assaker R, Leblond D, Duquesnoy B, Chastanet P, Clarisse J. Percutaneous vertebroplasty for osteolytic metastases and myeloma: effects of the percentage of lesion filling and the leakage of methyl methacrylate at clinical follow-up. Radiology 1996; 200:525–530.
18. Deramond H, Depriester C, Toussaint P [Vertebroplasty and percutaneous interventional radiology in bone metastases: techniques, indications, contra-indications.] Bull Cancer Radiother 1996; 83:277–282.
19. Deramond H, Depriester C, Toussaint P, Galibert P. Percutaneous vertebroplasty. Semin Musculoskel Radiol 1997; 1:285–295.
20. Weill A, Chiras J, Simon J, et al. Spinal metastases: indications for and results of percutaneous injection of acrylic surgical cement. Radiology 1996; 199:241–247.
21. Nussbaum DA, Gaulloud P, Murphy K. A review of complications associated with vertebroplasty and kyphoplasty as reported to the FDA medical device related web site. J Vasc Intervent Radiol 2004; 15:1185–1192.

8
Balloon Kyphoplasty and Lordoplasty

Paul F. Heini, René Orler, and Bronek Boszczyck

The expected increase in the elderly population over the next decades will present major challenges for the health care systems in Western countries. Maladies of the musculoskeletal system represent the second or third most important burden of disease, and osteoporosis and osteoporotic fractures are the leading causes of disability among the elderly (1). The fracture incidence increases exponentially as patient age increases (2,3). The spine is the most commonly affected site of osteoporotic fractures. At the age of 75 years, about 25% of all women have at least one fractured vertebra. By the age of 80 years this percentage grows to 50% (4).

Differentiated Indications for Vertebroplasty, Kyphoplasty, and Lordoplasty

Percutaneous vertebroplasty (PV) initially was not evaluated for associated height restoration after fracture. Prone patient positioning creates hyperextension and can allow some height gain with PV alone (Figure 8.1). At times, this is equivalent to that obtained with kyphoplasty. Kyphoplasty (KP) was developed to restore the VB height and to address the kyphotic deformity that may be associated with some vertebral body compression fractures (5,6). Height restoration and reduction of cement leakage are the main points that theoretically distinguish KP from PV (7,8). However, the kyphosis reduction achieved by KP appears limited; the average kyphotic angle correction is reportedly 8.5° (Table 8.1) (9,10). The excessive cost and the more complex procedure of KP relative to PV place in question its clinical usefulness. Kyphoplasty is reported to have the potential benefit of allowing injection of a more viscous cement than does PV, which could minimize extravasation (10). However, the incidence of leakage from KP does not differ from that of standard PV (10). Indications for KP are restricted to (1) selected patients in whom height loss is related to a spinal stenosis and height restoration can relieve the symptoms and (2) patients with traumatic fractures in whom repositioning of the endplate is

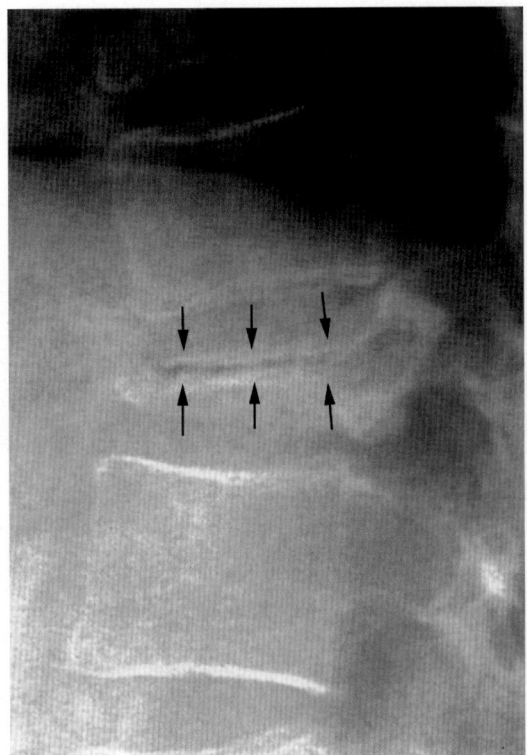 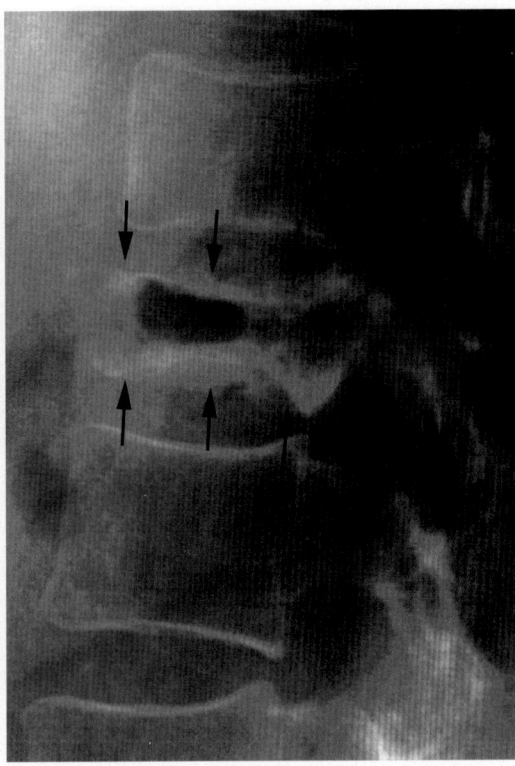

Figure 8.1. (A) Standing lateral radiograph shows marked collapse of the vertebra with minimal residual height (black arrows). **(B)** With patient prone there are distraction forces placed on the spine simply from positioning. This shows considerable height gain (black arrows) with positioning alone.

attempted (Figure 8.2) and for whom the cavity formation might help in difficult indications for tumorous lesions (7,9,11,12).

An alternative to KP for VB height restoration and kyphosis reduction is lordoplasty. Analogous to the established principle of the "fixateur interne," an indirect reduction maneuver is performed (13). Cannulae are placed into the pedicles of the vertebral bodies above and below the fractured level, and cement is injected into the cannulae. The cement is allowed to cure, after which the cannulae are used as levers to reduce the collapsed VB, and cement is injected into the collapsed level and allowed to cure (9). This procedure may be combined with KP to overcome a weakness of KP, namely, the partial loss of the initial reduction after the balloons are deflated. Lordoplasty may be indicated

Table 8.1. Comparison of Kyphosis Correction with Lordoplasty and Kyphoplasty.

Parameter	Kyphoplasty (27 Patients)	Lordoplasty (31 Patients)
Minimum follow-up	1 year	1 year
Average kyphosis correction	8.5° (47%)	12.4° (68%)
Average cost of procedure	$4,000.00	$400.00

Source: Data from Berlemann et al. (15), with permission.

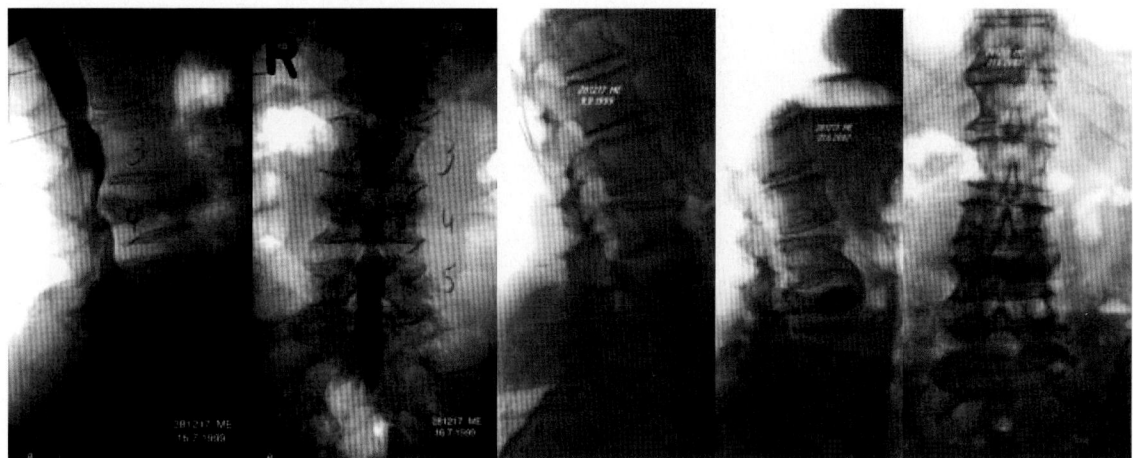

Figure 8.2. The potential of height restoration with kyphoplasty. From left to right: Spinal stenosis secondary to a fracture at L4 (left images) in an 82-year-old woman. A kyphoplasty procedure was performed and anterior height of L4 was restored, which relieved the leg pain, and the patient regained her mobility (middle image). Three years after the procedure, an autofusion between L3 and L4 was apparent (right images).

if a substantial kyphotic deformity is present that has a potential for reduction.

Surgical Technique

General Principles

The following items are valid for PV and KP.

Positioning

The patient is placed in a prone position resting on padding, such as a beanbag, that allows adjustment and provides maximal comfort. While under general anesthesia, the patient can be placed in hyperextension to reduce the compressed vertebra (Figure 8.3).

Monitoring and Anesthesia

Percutaneous vertebroplasty, but not lordoplasty, can be performed under local anesthesia with monitored anesthesia care (MAC). Because local anesthesia of the puncture site and of the periosteum may not provide sufficient analgesia lordoplasty can require additional analgesics. [Editor's note: In the United States, radiologists often perform KP successfully without general anesthesia.]

With the patient in the prone position, maintenance of a patent airway and sufficient spontaneous ventilation is mandatory. For most patients, standard monitoring (electrocardiogram, noninvasive blood pressure, and pulse oximetry) with additional end-expiratory carbon dioxide monitoring via a nasal cannula is sufficient. Oxygen is administered by face mask at 6–10 L/min. Because PV does not cause serious postoperative pain, an infusion of the short-acting opioid fentanyl is the method of choice for intraoperative analgesia during MAC.

Bradycardia, hypotension, and loss of consciousness can be signs of intravascular embolism of fat or polymethylmethacrylate. During cement injection, measurement of blood pressure should be performed at short intervals (every 2 minutes).

Lordoplasty and KP are performed under general anesthesia with tracheal intubation at the authors' institution.

Visualization and Imaging
Free access to the C arm in the posteroanterior and lateral projection at the level of pathology is mandatory. A high-quality C arm with a wide distance between tube and camera is essential, and a biplanar installation is advantageous. The area to be treated is identified before it is draped and cleaned. If fluoroscopy is to be used, the levels to be treated must be clearly visible in both projections. Visualization of the upper thoracic spine (T2–T5) often is difficult, and imaging with computed tomography (CT) may be necessary (Figure 8.4).

After the patient is draped, the vertebrae to be augmented are identified with the C arm, which is adjusted in the posteroanterior view so that the view is parallel to the endplates; in this position, the pedicles are well visualized. The authors prefer to have a strict posteroanterior view, although it is possible to use the so-called bulls-eye view. The principle for the orientation of wire insertion is shown in Figure 8.5. Computed tomography guidance for cannula placement is reported to be helpful, but monitoring of the cement application can be performed in real time only with fluoroscopy (14) or fluoro-CT.

Kyphoplasty

Percutaneous Transpedicular Kyphoplasty
All individual surgical steps are performed bilaterally. The skin is opened by means of a small, transverse, stab incision craniolateral to the pedicle entry site. A bone needle is placed at the junction between the transverse process and cranial articular process (Figure 8.5). The

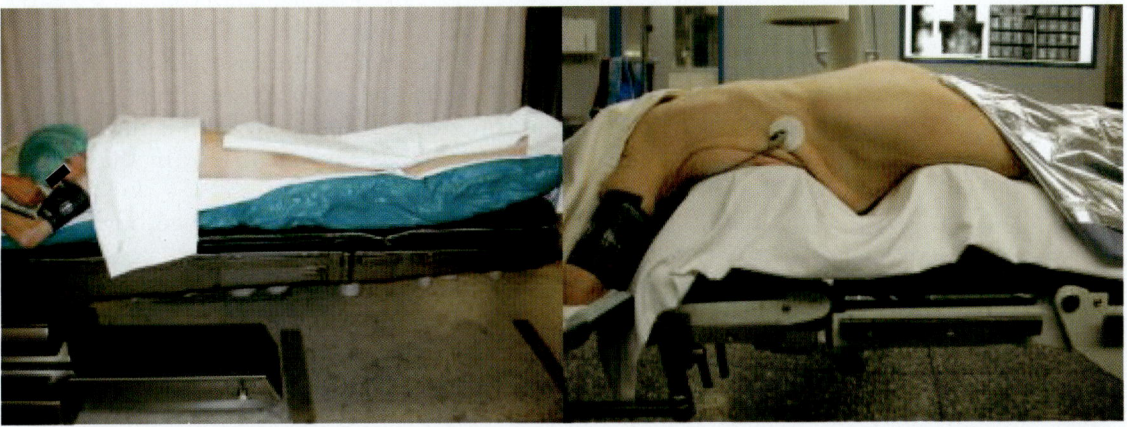

Figure 8.3. Patient positioning. If local anesthesia is an option, the patient may be positioned on a beanbag (left). When general anesthesia is used, positioning the patient in hyperextension can promote spontaneous reduction of the fractured vertebra (right).

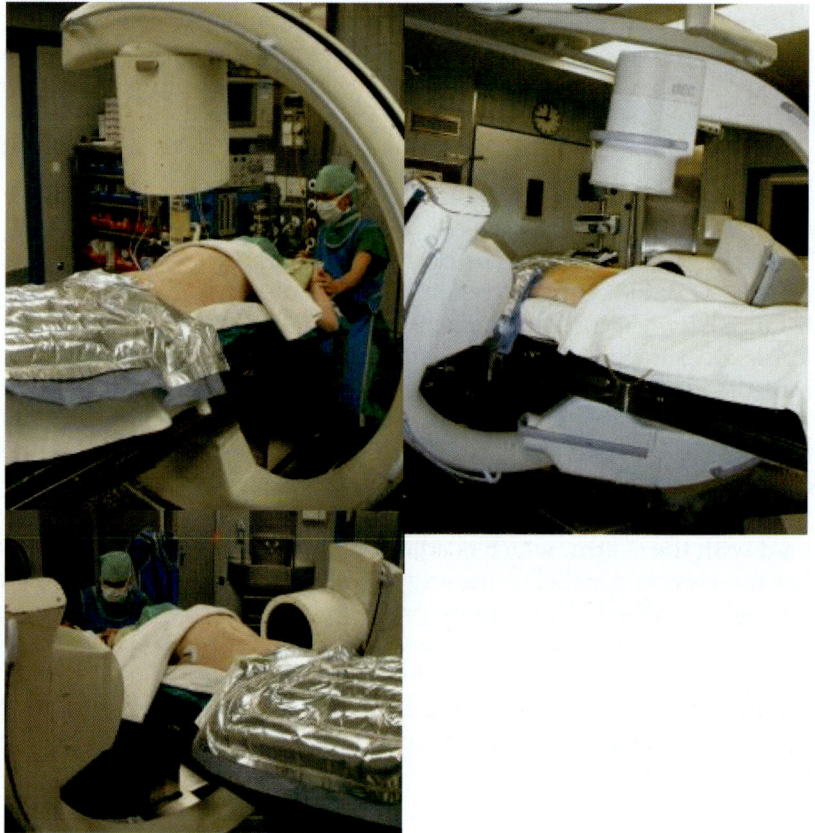

Figure 8.4. A high-quality C arm is essential, and free access for the c arm in the posteroanterior (upper left) and lateral (lower left) projections at the area of interest is mandatory. The area to be treated is examined before draping, and the levels to be treated are marked. Upper right image shows that installation of two image intensifiers (to control the anteroposterior and lateral planes) will obviate the need to switch projections during the filling procedure.

bone needle is driven into the pedicle with light mallet blows, and the passage though the pedicle is monitored fluoroscopically in both planes. Spinal canal violation is avoided by strictly ensuring that the medial pedicle cortex (in the anteroposterior projection) is not crossed before the posterior vertebral wall has been reached (in the lateral projection).

The initial trajectory of the bone needle must be based on fracture type (i.e., whether it is osteoporotic or traumatic). The final needle position for osteoporotic fractures is in the middle of the VB's cancellous bone. The target for traumatic fractures is the fracture zone because, unlike osteoporotic bone, healthy cancellous bone will not yield to the pressure of balloon inflation.

The next step involves feeding a Kirschner wire through the bone needle to serve as a guide for the working cannula, which is driven into the VB over the wire. Once the Kirschner wire and the trocar of the cannula have been removed, the working cannula remains in the posterior third of the VB. All subsequent steps in the VB must carefully avoid perforating the cortex, which would provide points of minimal resistance through which cement could leak during injection. If required, a biopsy specimen of the VB can be taken at this point.

Channels, made on each side with a hand drill, are convergent toward the midline, and deflated KP balloons are placed into each channel (Figure 8.6). The size of the balloon is chosen relative to the size of the VB (15 mm long with a filling volume of 4 mL or 20 mm long with a filling volume of 6 mL). Each end of the balloon is fitted with radio-opaque markers, thus allowing the final position of the balloons to be verified in both planes fluoroscopically. With a manual pressure-injection system, pressures of up to 28 bars (~400 psi) can be generated in the balloons. However, a pressure of approximately 7 bars (~100 psi) usually is sufficient if the balloon's position is correct. The gradual, pressure-controlled inflation of the balloons displaces the damaged cancellous bone and, ideally, lifts the adjacent endplate. Once the fracture has been reduced or a sufficiently large cavity has been created, the balloons are deflated and removed.

The cavity (defect zone) that remains in the VB is filled with augmentation material (usually polymethylmethacrylate) through the cannulae. To prevent epidural or paravertebral leaks, the augmentation material should be highly viscous and introduced gradually with low pressure. The cavity-filling volume, known from the volume reached by the KP balloons, is slightly exceeded to achieve interdigitation with the cancellous bone.

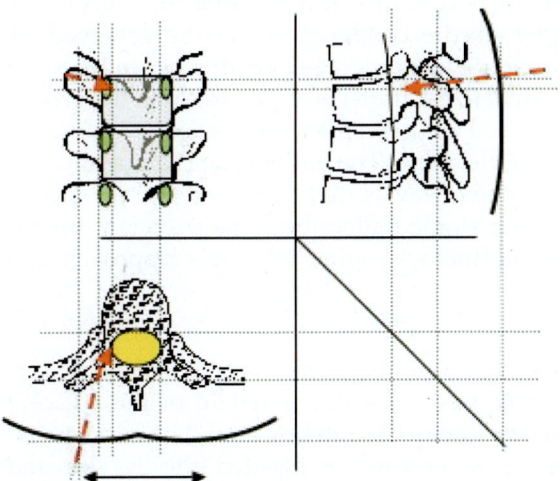 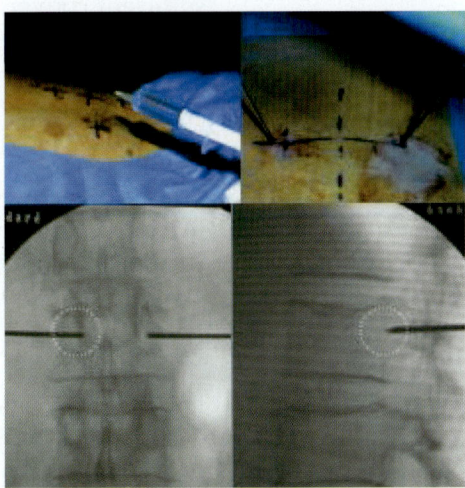

Figure 8.5. Left: The insertion of the guide wire is planned based on the anteroposterior and lateral views. Right (upper left to lower right): Local anesthesia is administered, and guide wires are advanced under c arm control. The surgeon needs to combine the anteroposterior and lateral views to aim the guide wire accurately into the vertebral body. Depending on the size of the pedicle, the guide wire is inserted transpedicularly (for large pedicles) or parapedicularly (for small pedicles). As soon as the tip reaches the medial border of the outlines of the pedicle, its depth should reach the posterior border of the vertebra.

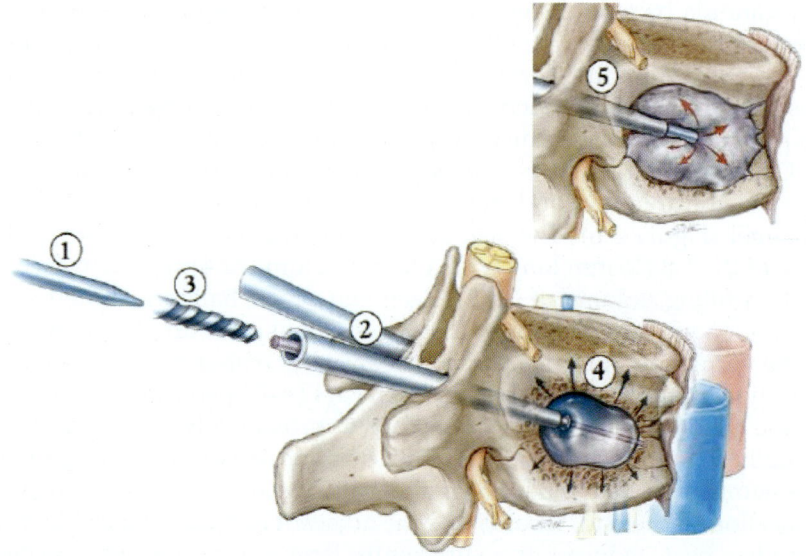

Figure 8.6. The five steps of kyphoplasty: 1, placement of a guide wire; 2, insertion of a working cannula; 3, reaming working channels beyond the cannula tips; 4, balloon insertion, inflation, deflation, and removal; 5, injection of void filler.

Percutaneous Extrapedicular Kyphoplasty
The pedicles of the midthoracic spine are slender and usually oriented more toward the sagittal plane than their lumbar counterparts. With a transpedicular approach, therefore, it often is not possible to achieve sufficient convergence of the needle tips into the anterior third of the vertebral body. A stronger needle convergence can be achieved by means of the so-called extrapedicular access. In this procedure, the bone needle is inserted cranial to the transverse process, into the groove between the neck of the rib and the lateral pedicle cortex. This position results in a more medial needle angle. The balloons and augmentation material are inserted in the same way as that described for transpedicular access. Introduction of a single balloon may be sufficient for the smaller vertebrae of the midthoracic spine with this approach and medial needle angle.

Lordoplasty

Lordoplasty consists of three steps: (1) reinforcement of the adjacent vertebrae, (2) reduction of the fractured vertebra, and (3) reinforcement of the fractured vertebra. Local anesthetic is injected into the skin and the subcutaneous tissue down to the periosteum at the guide wire insertion site. At each site, 3 to 5 mL of anesthetic is administered. To avoid repeated changes from the posteroanterior to the lateral view, all vertebrae to be reinforced are injected with local anesthetic. With the C arm control, a stab incision in the skin is made approximately 6 cm lateral of the midline, and the guide wire is advanced along the angle of the pedicle. When the tip of the wire reaches the bony surface, it should be located in the cranial and lateral corner of the pedicle. The wire is guided convergently and directed caudally. To penetrate the surface of the bone, some gentle blows with a hammer may be necessary. The direction of the guide wire is adjusted as required and advanced continuously under C arm control. As soon as the tip of the wire reaches the medial border of the pedicle, the position of the wire needs to be verified in the lateral projection (Figure 8.7).

Before changing the projection, the wires are inserted at all levels where cement injection is planned. Once the wires are inserted preliminarily, a picture of their position is stored in the image intensifier, and the c arm then is switched to the lateral position. In the lateral projection, the tips of the wires must be at least at the level of the posterior wall of the spinal canal; if they are not, they need to be relocated by switching back to the posteroanterior view. [Editor's note: Needle or wire insertion also can be monitored accurately in the anteroposterior oblique projection by looking directly down the axis of the needle or wire.] The guide wire then is advanced cautiously with gentle hammer blows and, if necessary, redirected to reach the posterior third of the VB. The filling cannulae are inserted over the guide wires with rotating movements. This procedure can be painful, and the anesthesiologist should be informed so that appropriate analgesia can be given. Preferentially, the procedure is performed with the patient under general anesthesia and positioned in hyperextension (see Figure 8.3).

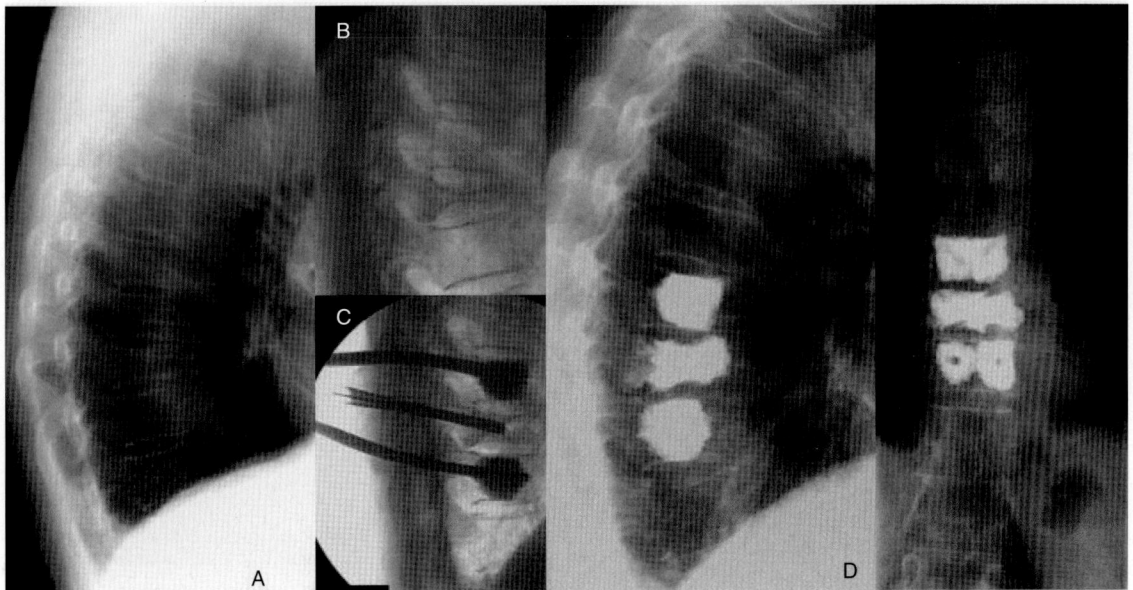

Figure 8.7. Female patient with localized pain and a compression fracture at T9. **(A)** Radiograph obtained at initial presentation. **(B)** A follow-up radiograph taken 5 weeks later depicts a nearly complete collapse of the vertebral body. **(C)** Lordoplasty procedure restored height to the collapsed VB. **(D)** The follow-up lateral and anteroposterior radiographs show a well-maintained alignment of the spine.

The tip of the cannula should be advanced until the anterior half of the vertebral body is reached (Figure 8.8). The guide wire must not be pushed forward during cannula insertion. After insertion of the cannula, the guide wire is removed, and a blunt trocar is used to clear the tip of the cannula. Anterior VB perforation must be avoided.

Once the cannulae are placed, the VBs immediately caudal and cranial to the fractured VB are reinforced with cement. The trocars are reinserted in these cannulae to prevent cannular kinking during the lordoplasty reduction. The clinician needs to keep in mind that approximately 1 mL of cement resides in each cannula and is injected when the trocar is reinserted. With the trocars in place, each cannula then is advanced carefully approximately 5 to 10 mm, placing it into the injected bolus of cement.

After the cement has cured, the reduction maneuver is performed: Analogous to the technique used with the "fixateur interne," the cannulae are used as a lever for height restoration (13). The kyphotic

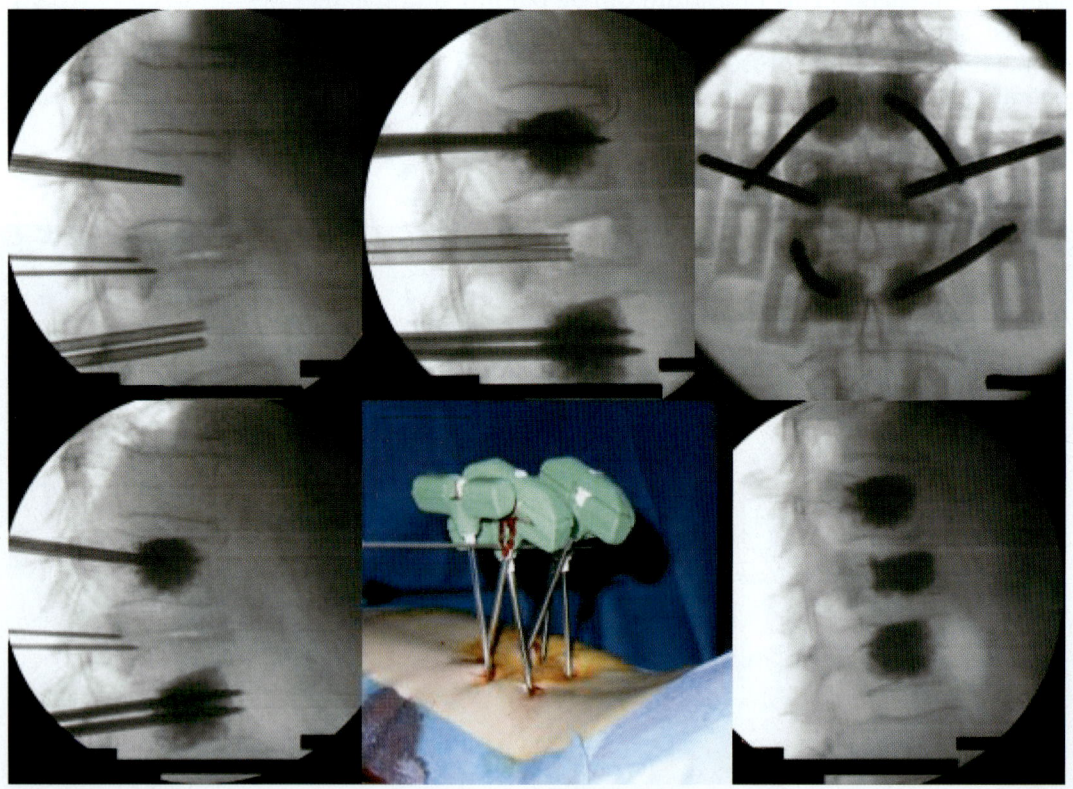

Figure 8.8. Lordoplasty: The filling cannulae are inserted with rotating movements over the previously placed guide wires (top left). The VBs are then reinforced with cement (bottom left). After the cement has cured, the reduction maneuver is performed (top middle). The reduction is temporarily secured by connecting the cannulae with a bar or using fixation clamps (bottom middle). The fractured VB is reinforced according to the standard PV (top right). After the cement has cured, the cannulae are rotated about their long axis, breaking their bond with the cement, and they can be removed (bottom right).

deformity will be corrected by ligamentotaxis. The reduction is temporarily secured by connecting the cannulae with a bar or using fixation clamps.

The fractured VB is reinforced according to the standard VP technique described previously. Only after the cement has cured are the connections between the cranial and caudal cannulae released. The cannulae then are rotated about their long axis, breaking their bond with the cement, and they can be removed. This technique can be combined with KP. After the reduction maneuver is applied, the balloons are inflated to provide a direct reduction force. After deflation, the defect is filled with polymethylmethacrylate. This technique overcomes one of the limitations of the KP procedure: It avoids the reduction loss seen after balloon deflation. If there is only moderate osteoporosis, the lordoplasty may be used without the need of reinforcing the vertebrae cranial and caudal to the fractured level. Table 8.1 compares the results achieved in a prospective series of 31 patients (minimal follow up, 1 year) treated with lordoplasty with those achieved in a series of patients treated with KP (15).

References

1. Ryan PJ, Blake G, Herd R, et al. A clinical profile of back pain and disability in patients with spinal osteoporosis. Bone 1994; 15(1):27–30.
2. Cooper C, Campion G, Melton LJ, III. Hip fractures in the elderly: a worldwide projection. Osteoporos Int 1992; 2(6):285–289.
3. European Prospective Osteoporosis Study (EPOS) Group. Incidence of vertebral fracture in Europe: results from the European Prospective Osteoporosis Study (EPOS). J Bone Miner Res 2002; 17(4):716–724.
4. Melton LJ, III, Kan SH, Frye MA, et al. Epidemiology of vertebral fractures in women. Am J Epidemiol 1989; 129(5):1000–1011.
5. Garfin SR, Yuan HA, Reiley MA. New technologies in spine: kyphoplasty and vertebroplasty for the treatment of painful osteoporotic compression fractures. Spine 2001; 26(14):1511–1515.
6. Wong W, Reiley MA, Garfin S. Vertebroplasty/kyphoplasty. J Women's Imag 2001; 2(3):117–124.
7. Myers ME. Vertebroplasty and kyphoplasty: is one of these procedures the best choice for all patients [letter]? Am J Neuroradiol 2004; 25(7):1297.
8. Phillips FM, Wetzel TF, Lieberman I, et al. An in vivo comparison of the potential for extravertebral cement leak after vertebroplasty and kyphoplasty. Spine 2002; 27(19):2173–2178.
9. Heini PF, Orler R. Kyphoplasty for treatment of osteoporotic vertebral fractures. Eur Spine J 2004; 13(3):184–192.
10. Lieberman IH, Dudeney S, Reinhardt MK, et al. Initial outcome and efficacy of "kyphoplasty" in the treatment of painful osteoporotic vertebral compression fractures. Spine 2001; 26(14):1631–1638.
11. Groen RJM, du Toit DF, Phillips FM, et al. Anatomical and pathological considerations in percutaneous vertebroplasty and kyphoplasty: a reappraisal of the vertebral venous system. Spine 2004; 29(13):1465–1471.
12. Mathis JM, Ortiz AO, Zoarski GH. Vertebroplasty versus kyphoplasty: a comparison and contrast. Am J Neuroradiol 2004; 25(5):840–845.
13. Dick W. The "fixateur interne" as a versatile implant for spine surgery. Spine 1987; 12:882–900.

14. Gangi A, Kastler BA, Dietemann JL. Percutaneous vertebroplasty guided by a combination of CT and fluoroscopy. Am J Neuroradiol 1994; 15(1):83–86.
15. Berlemann U, Franz T, Orler R, et al. Kyphoplasty for treatment of osteoporotic vertebral fractures: a prospective non-randomized study. Eur Spine J 2004; 13(6):496–501.

9

Vertebroplasty Versus Kyphoplasty: A Comparison and Contrast*

John M. Mathis, A. Orlando Ortiz, and Gregg H. Zoarski

The phrase *vertebroplasty versus kyphoplasty* evokes images of competitive procedures and battling groups of entrenched physicians. Our involvement in the development and introduction of percutaneous vertebroplasty (PV) and kyphoplasty (KP) in the United States has given us a unique perspective on the safety and efficacy of both procedures. We believe that both procedures offer potential benefit with acceptable safety when used by skilled physicians. However, they are not the same; they have some distinct differences, including cost and possibly even complication rates. The real hurdles are to further assess and develop the appropriate indications, advantages, and shortcomings of each procedure. We must then select the appropriate method of therapy to maximally benefit our patients. Finally, all practitioners must venture beyond the dogma of their respective subspecialties and understand the full spectrum of tools and techniques that are available to treat vertebral compression fractures. This chapter reviews the published data regarding KP and PV and put these data in perspective with regard to the marketing comments so often encountered when dealing with sales personnel or physicians who use only one tool.

History

The history of the development of each procedure explains how a competitive environment has arisen among many of the physicians who use either PV or KP. Percutaneous vertebroplasty was introduced in France in 1984 by the interventional neuroradiologist Hervé Deramond and his colleagues (1). It was found useful for the treatment of pain associated with vertebral compression fractures (VCFs) resulting from benign and malignant tumors, as well as osteoporotic compression fractures (1,2). The technique began to be used by interventional neuroradiologists in the United States in 1993, with the first U.S. case series reported in 1997 (3). Percutaneous vertebroplasty has experienced a

---

* Modified with permission from Am J Neurol Radiol 2004; 25:840–845.

rapid rise in popularity in the radiologic community and with patients. There are approved reimbursement codes (CPTs) for PV with many third-party payers (including Medicare) who recognize and reimburse for the procedure.

Since the introduction of PV, many papers have documented the positive biomechanical effects of PV and the pain relief resulting from this treatment for VCFs (1–18). A review of this literature shows that all reports reveal favorable results of pain relief and restoration of activities of daily living following PV. (However, no prospective, randomized series comparing PV with alternative therapy has been accomplished.) Clinical complications are rare in the hands of experienced operators. Some reports do list a higher risk of complications for patients with malignant disease, which includes myeloma and osteolytic metastases (myeloma is thought to be less risky than osteolytic malignancy).

The idea of attempting to treat a VCF with an inflatable balloon tamp (and thereby restore the vertebral body height and minimize the associated kyphotic deformity) was conceived by an orthopedic surgeon, Dr. Mark Reiley, in the early 1990s. The initial biomechanical investigations of the Kyphx inflatable balloon tamp (Kyphon Corporation, Sunnyvale, CA) were performed as a combined effort by this orthopedic surgeon and an interventional neuroradiologist (J.M.M.) familiar with PV (19–21). The device was given 510k approval by the FDA as a "bone tamp." A randomized clinical trial that compared "kyphoplasty" with conservative medical management was attempted, but patient entry was slow, and this initiative was ultimately abandoned in favor of a clinical registry tabulating the results of patients treated with KP. Like PV, KP has not been tested in a comparison trial against conservative therapy. There are only a few peer-reviewed studies available with which to judge the safety and efficacy of KP (22,23). Case reports and opinion papers are also found (24–28).

In one study, pain relief with KP was found to be similar to that observed with PV, and the perioperative complication rate was 10% (although no complications related to the procedure were claimed by the authors) (22). The complications that occurred included a perioperative myocardial infarction and two patients who experienced rib fractures during the procedure. An 8.5% asymptomatic cement leak rate was observed. Height restoration was enthusiastically reported by the authors, but analysis of their data reveals that the average height gained per vertebra treated was 3mm at the center of the vertebral endplate. This leaves open for debate the effectiveness of the KP procedure for predictably restoring significant vertebral height in vertebral compression fractures.

Another early series of 15 patients, who underwent 24 uncomplicated KP procedures for osteoporotic vertebral compression fractures that were present for an average duration of 14 weeks, reported immediate pain relief in all of the patients (23). The mean height restoration as measured on lateral radiographs was 1.5mm in the posterior vertebral body, 4.7mm in the midvertebral body, and 3.7mm in the anterior vertebral body. In a larger series of 226 consecutive KP procedures, similar results, with respect to height restoration, were reported (24). A 1% complication rate in this series included one case of epidural hematoma that required surgical decompression, one case of spinal cord injury, and one case with transient adult respiratory distress syndrome. A multicenter registry of 1,439 patients with 2,194 treated fractures with KP showed an efficacy of 90% with respect to pain relief and a major complication rate of 0.2% per fracture (25).

Only one report is available for KP as a treatment of pathologic VCFs. In a series of 18 patients with multiple myeloma who underwent 55 uncomplicated kyphoplasty procedures, significant pain relief was achieved in all patients (26). Height restoration was only reported in 39 treated levels and was listed as 34%.

The initial reports and editorials concerning KP were generated primarily in the orthopaedic literature and reflected an unqualified, positive opinion. Some of this literature seemed simply to echo marketing statements that were, as yet, unproved by clinical or laboratory investigation. The procedure, however, was not as well received in the radiologic community. This initial difference of opinion has not been substantially altered over time. Kyphoplasty has flourished in the surgical community as this physician group has been the direct beneficiaries of extensive marketing and educational support. They tend to see KP as a potential "high dollar" replacement for PV. There has been growing competition for patients between the two groups that favor one or the other of these two procedures. Unfortunately, the competitive environment between radiologists and surgeons has been compounded due to limited access by Kyphon to KP training courses for radiologists.

Substantial differences exist in the costs of PV and KP. The KP kit (without bone cement) is ~$3,400, while a PV kit (with bone cement) is less than $400. Although not a requirement of the procedure, KP is often performed in the operating room with general anesthesia. The patients are commonly kept overnight in the hospital for observation. Percutaneous vertebroplasty is usually performed with intravenous sedation only and a brief period of observation followed by discharge home after the procedure. All of these differences combine to make KP cost 10–20 times more than PV. This cost difference is acceptable only if there are proven, substantial positive benefits for the more expensive procedure. Kyphoplasty marketing claims that these benefits include improved safety due to fewer symptomatic cement leaks and substantial height restoration with kyphosis reduction that might improve pulmonary and gastrointestinal function. Actual published data are sparse that address these claims directly, but an attempt here is made to compare and contrast results based on published information.

Jargon Versus Reality

It seems that the majority of physicians would agree that both PV and KP have similar success rates for relieving the pain associated with VCFs. This would seem logical because KP relies on the same vertebral stabilization principle used in PV, which is the introduction of bone cement into a structurally compromised vertebra. Kyphoplasty is even sometimes referred to as "balloon-assisted vertebroplasty" (29). Biomechanical data comparing the mechanical stabilization by PV and KP show similar results (19).

Beyond these basics, reality seems to be blurred by marketing jargon. Manufacturers and champions of any device always describe their individual advantages. This has been no less true of KP proponents who routinely point out the reduced likelihood for cement leaks with this procedure compared with PV (30). This is alleged to occur because the injection of cement in PV is purportedly under "high pressure," while KP fills a void created by the bone tamp and is therefore "low pressure." For years this marketing-driven claim went unchallenged, and it was often repeated by physicians even though no scientific data existed that actually measured or compared the injection pressures with these devices. Recently, independent groups of investigators demonstrated quantitatively that under usual operating conditions, intraosseus "high-pressure" was *not* observed with any (PV or KP) of these percutaneous vertebral fracture reduction procedures (31,32). In fact, the variables that seemed to influence intravertebral pressures were the rate of injection and the size of the cannula. Higher intravertebral pressures were recorded with higher injection rates and larger bore systems and when a metal trocar was used to drive cement through the cannula (31).

Lieberman et al. (22) reported a cement leak rate during KP of 8.6%. Fortunately, as with PV, the vast majority of cement leaks are asymptomatic. Reports of KP have noted very high cement leak incidences with PV but have usually failed to distinguish between symptomatic and asymptomatic leaks. When this is done, little difference seems to be present in the two procedures. Symptomatic cement leaks have occurred with both procedures (33) (Figures 9.1 and 9.2). Concern for patient safety prompted the FDA in April of 2003 (34) to issue a warning regarding the use of polymethylmethacrylate (PMMA) in both PV and KP.

Even in vitro the capability of KP to reliably produce height restoration in fractures and compressed vertebral bodies remains controversial (Figure 9.3). Biomechanical evaluations by Belkoff et al. (20) reported "significant" height restoration with KP than with PV. However, their investigation only looked at vertebrae that had a maximum height loss of 25%. Percutaneous vertebroplasty was noted to yield height recovery but less than KP in this study. The height gained by KP was on the order of 3 mm. Unfortunately, no in vitro investigations are available that determine if this effect can be achieved, without destroying the vertebra, when compression is more severe than 25%. Indeed, the data of Lieberman et al. (22), which shows an average height restoration of approximately 3 mm per vertebra treated, suggest that KP may have a limited effect at height restoration for many patients. Alternatively, this limited clinical result could be due to indiscriminate patient selection. Patients in the Lieberman et al. (22) series, whose average symptom duration was 5.9 months, were treated

Figure 9.1. Computed tomography scan of a thoracic vertebra following kyphoplasty. There was a lateral blowout fracture of the vertebra caused by balloon inflation and a large cement leak (white arrow) into the mediastinum. The patient had severe pain requiring hospitalization and protracted analgesic therapy for weeks following therapy. (From Mathis [33], with permission.)

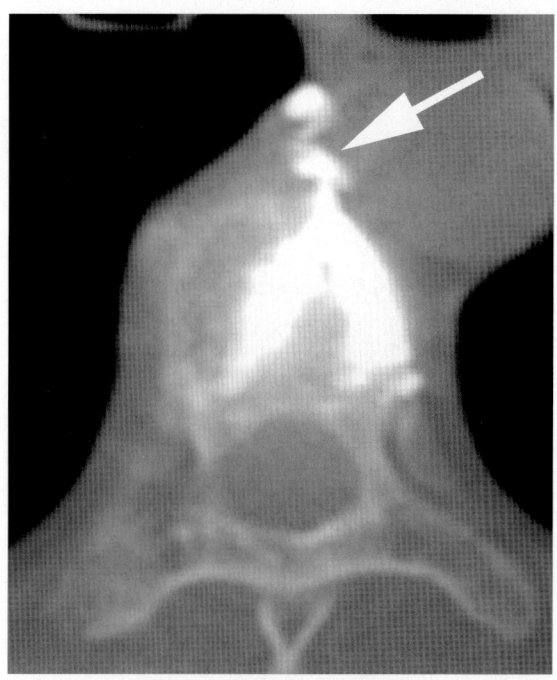

Figure 9.2. Radiograph following PV and KP showing small, asymptomatic cement leaks at both levels. The PV level (above) had a small cement leak into an adjacent vein (white arrows). The KP level (below) had small cement leaks into both adjacent disc levels (white arrowheads).

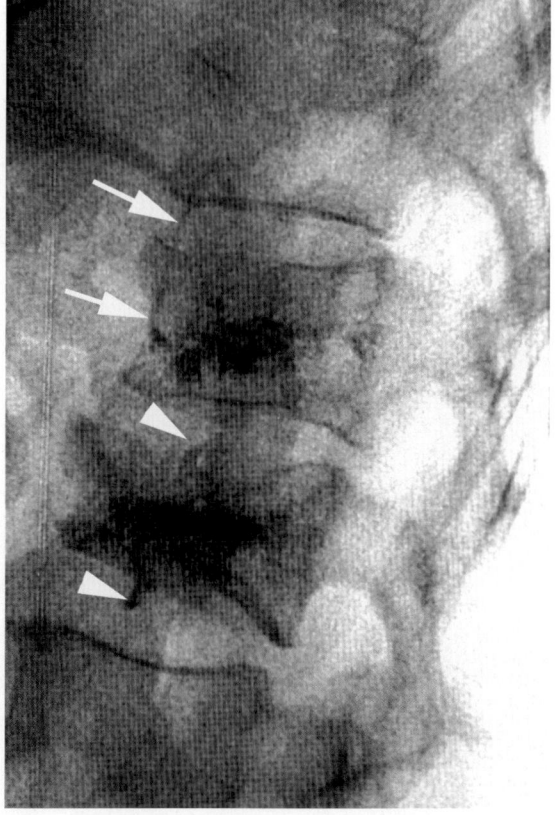

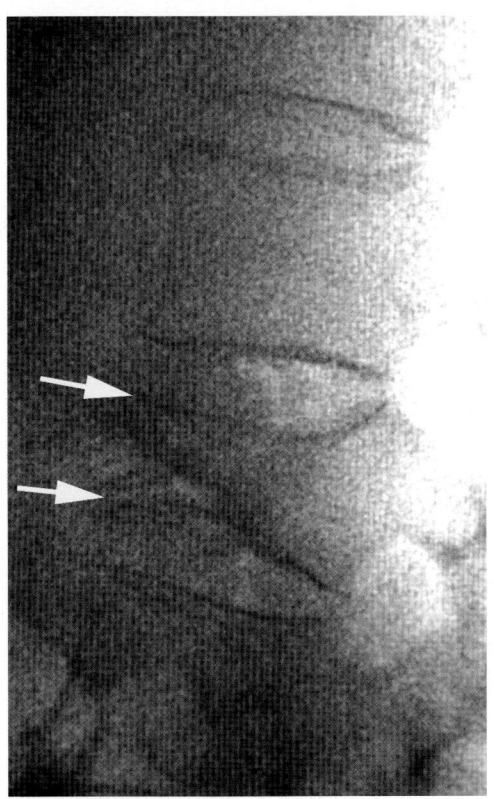

Figure 9.3. (A) Compression fracture with anterior cleft prior to KP. Endplates are marked with white arrows. The height is estimated at 50% of the height of the adjacent level above. **(B)** Fluoroscopic image showing balloon inflation during KP. **(C)** After cement injection the height gain is approximately 4 mm or 25% of a vertebral height (when compared with the adjacent level above). There was essentially no kyphosis to start with, and this vertebra had a cleft originally and therefore would be expected to be a good candidate for height restoration with either KP or PV. (White bars indicated upper and lower vertebral margins.)

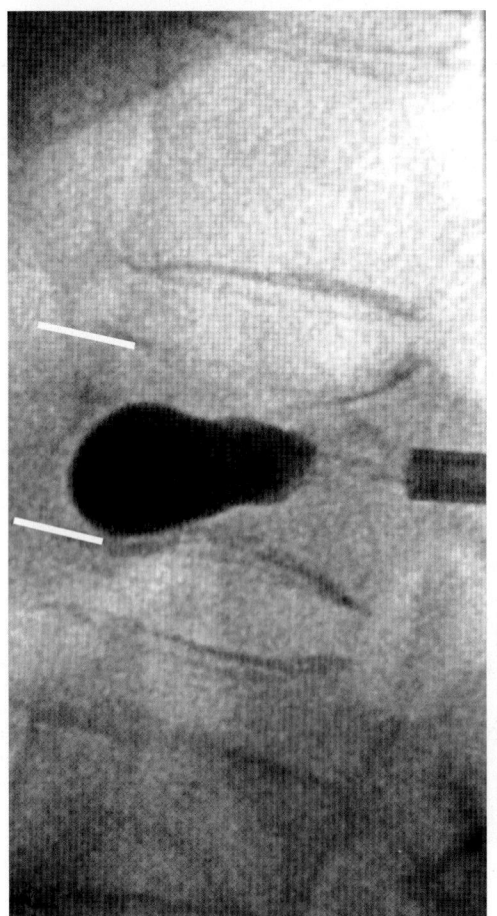
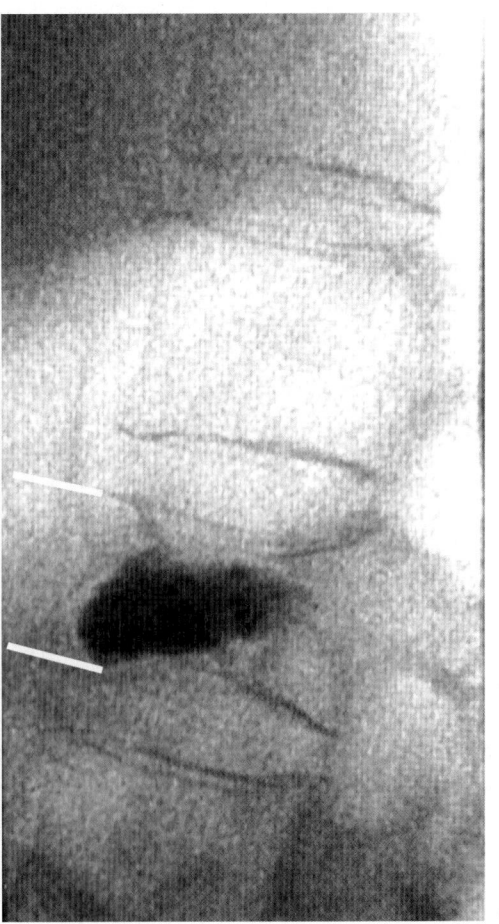

relatively late after fracture, and many of these patients could have experienced partial fracture healing prior to KP. Although these reports are anecdotal, it does seem that VCFs treated closer to their date of incidence tend to experience more height restoration (22). While the average height restoration in a clinical setting ranges from 2.5 to 3.5mm (35), no clinical trials are available that help us select those patients who will predictably get maximum height restoration with KP. Pain relief seems less sensitive to "time since fracture." Pain relief in the series of Lieberman et al. (22) was not adversely affected by treatment delay or the amount of height restoration achieved and was similar to that seen with PV.

Vertebral height restoration reported in some KP studies has been linked to correction of associated kyphotic deformity of the spine (23,36). Theodorou and coworkers (23) reported an average kyphosis correction of 62.4% ± 16.7%; however, patients who are pain free following VP or KP usually experience less muscle spasm and tend to stand straighter with the elimination of spine pain. Mathis (33) demonstrated this effect in a PV case with 50% kyphosis reduction after PV alone (Figure 9.4). Teng et al. (37) reported kyphosis improvement

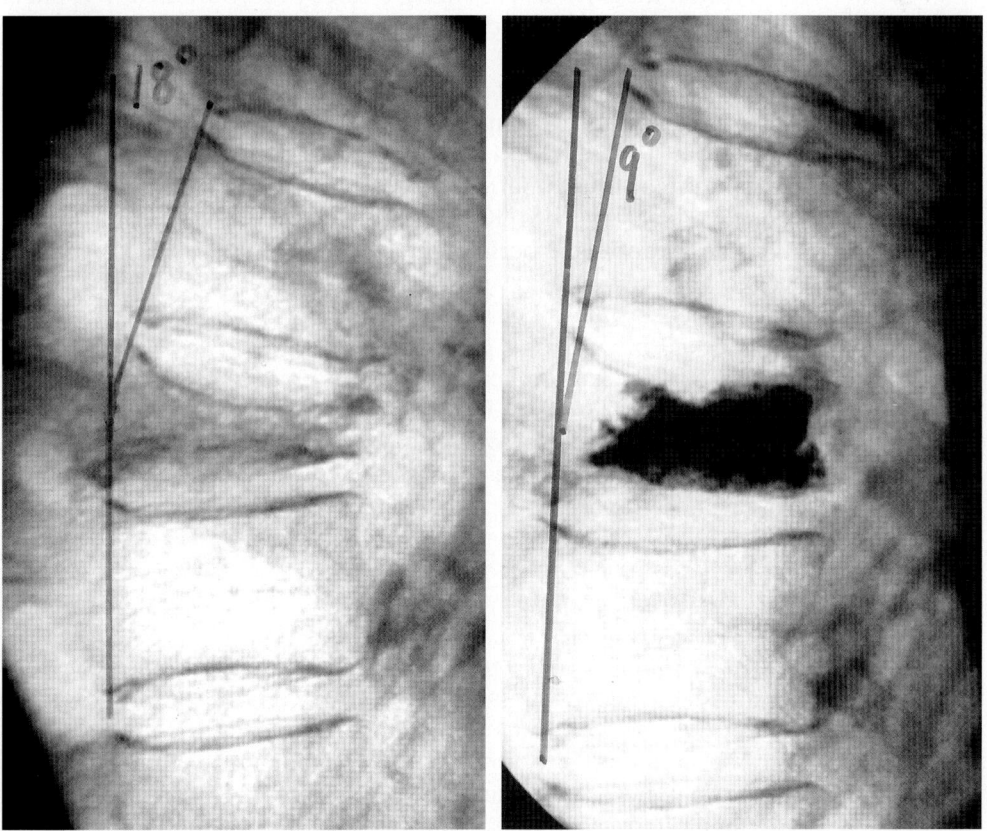

Figure 9.4. (A) Radiograph of a compression fracture and 18° of kyphosis. **(B)** Following PV there is modest height gain estimated at 3–4mm and a reduction in kyphosis to 9°. (From Mathis [33], with permission.)

following PV in 45 of 53 patients, with 49% having a kyphotic angle reduction of 5° or more. Studies on the secondary benefits of kyphosis correction, such as improved pulmonary function, are not yet available. Obviously, this is another place where the corrections of both PV and KP need to be compared with control to determine the relative difference between the therapies.

What has often been neglected in the controversy regarding height restoration with KP is that PV can, in selected patients, also restore vertebral body height (Figure 9.4). Hiwatashi et al. (38) have shown that vertebral body height can be augmented by an average of 2.2 mm with PV simply by hyperextending the affected spinal segment. Similarly, McKiernan et al. (39) demonstrated dynamic fracture mobility in 35% of 65 VCFs that they treated with PV. When they used PV alone, they found that the "average anterior vertebral height increased 106% compared with initial fracture height (absolute increase, 8.41 ± 0.4 mm)" in patients with these mobile fractures. Their kyphotic angle reduction was 40% (39). If some height restoration can be expected from PV alone, then the meager height recovery found in a series like that of Lieberman et al. (22) may be partially measuring the effect due to prone positioning rather than that due to the balloon inflation.

Kyphon touts KP as providing a safer procedure than PV. There are no direct comparison studies to prove or disprove this claim. However, using data accumulated by the FDA (on their Web site devoted to medical devices and related complications), Nussbaum et al. (40) found that the permanent complication rates for KP were approximately 20–30 times higher on a per basis case than those reported for PV. Although not from a perfect source, the finding disputes the claim for improved safety with KP. Without question, both procedures are capable of producing permanent neurologic injury. This is usually associated with cement leaks into the spinal canal (Figure 9.5). These large cement leaks should be avoidable if good imaging equipment is used by prudent physicians.

Death is a rare complication and was equal in KP and PV, occurring in about 1/50,000 cases. Death may occur in either procedure related to severe cement allergy or cardiopulmonary failure created by the procedure (usually in those with severe chronic obstructive pulmonary disease).

Authors' Opinions

Without doubt, both PV and KP need additional trials that conclusively establish the effectiveness of each compared with conservative medical therapy and to each other. Attempts to perform these types of studies have been stymied by poor patient enrollment in the control arm of each trial. This occurs due to the positive public awareness about these augmentation techniques and the dramatic benefit that previously treated patients have experienced. Few patients are willing to accept the chance of undergoing a sham procedure when the available treatments seem reliably safe and effective. A randomized comparison of

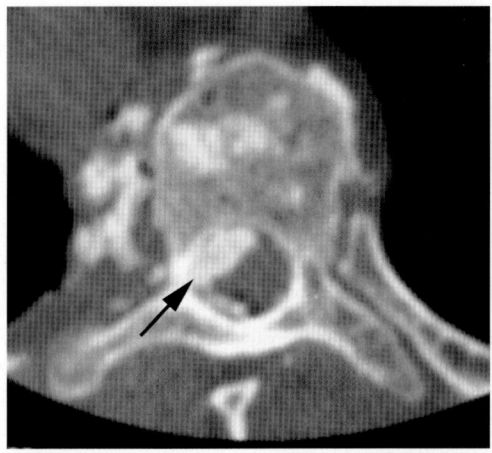 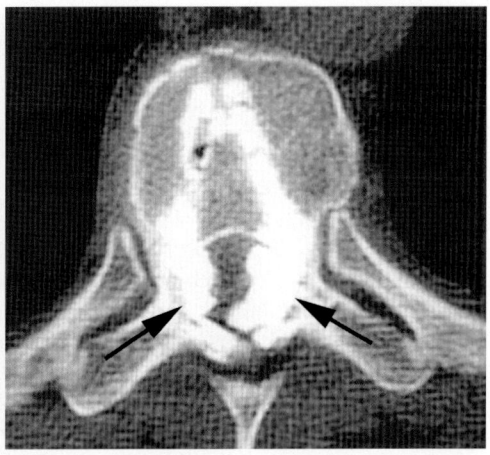

Figure 9.5. **(A)** Computed tomography image postvertebroplasty that shows a large cement leak into the spinal canal (black arrow) that resulted in permanent neurologic injury. **(B)** Computed tomography following kyphoplasty demonstrating a large cement leak into the spinal canal (black arrows). The complications resulted in cord compression and permanent paralysis.

PV and KP would also help establish patient selection criteria and individual procedure advantages, allowing physicians to better utilize these procedures to the patients' benefit. Until these data are available, we will likely continue to hear considerable jargon and relentless marketing claims about the relative safety and therapeutic advantages of each procedure.

The authors believe that both procedures relieve pain and can be performed with acceptable complication rates by prudent, well-trained physicians. We do note the large differential in cost of the procedures. If KP is going to be worthwhile, it should reliably produce significantly more height restoration than does PV. In our practices, we employ KP differently but agree to its use when we think that height restoration (beyond that usually achieved by PV) is feasible and would be beneficial. Our implementation of KP is driven by the "time since fracture" and is markedly different within our own ranks. One extreme requires fractures of 3 weeks or less (J.M.M.), and another tack includes fractures of less than 3 months (O.O.). Even with these guidelines, we are unable to ensure large height restoration in all patients.

At present, we recommend that both procedures be available in the treatment armamentarium of all operators, thus allowing the physician, not the marketplace, to determine patient selection criteria.

All VCFs are not the same, and certain fracture subtypes may be more amenable to one or the other procedure. Regardless of which procedure is chosen, safety depends on operator experience, excellent imaging equipment, and adequate cement opacification. Complications that have occurred with either procedure most often have been a result of poor operator judgment or experience or of inadequate anatomic and cement visualization. Time and accumulated data will tell whether the promise of reliable height restoration with KP is realistic. Until then, careful use of either procedure should successfully relieve the pain associated with vertebral compression injury.

References

1. Galibert P, Deramond H, Rosat P. [Preliminary note on the treatment of vertebral angioma by percutaneous acrylic vertebroplasty.] Neurochirurgie 1987; 33:166–168.
2. Bascoulergue Y, Duquesnel J, Leclercq R. Percutaneous injection of methyl methacrylate in the vertebral body for the treatment of various diseases: percutaneous vertebroplasty [abstr]. Radiology 1988; 169:372.
3. Jensen ME, Evans AJ, Mathis JM, Kallmes DF, Cloft HJ, Dion JE. Percutaneous polymethylmethacrylate vertebroplasty in the treatment of osteoporotic vertebral compression fractures: technical aspects. Am J Neuroradiol 1997; 18:1897–1904.
4. Mathis JM, Barr JD, Belkoff SM, et al: Percutaneous vertebroplasty: a developing standard of care for vertebral compression fractures. Am J Neuroradiol 2001; 22:373–381.
5. Mathis JM, Eckel TS, Belkoff SM, Deramond H. Percutaneous vertebroplasty: a therapeutic option for pain associated with vertebral compression fracture. J Back Musculoskel Rehab 1999; 13:11–17.
6. Mathis JM, Petri M, Naff N. Percutaneous vertebroplasty treatment of steroid-induced osteoporotic compression fractures. Arthritis Rheum 1998; 41:171–175.
7. Belkoff SM, Mahoney M, Fenton DC, Mathis JM. An in vitro biomechanical evaluation of bone cements used in percutaneous vertebroplasty. Bone 1999; 25:23s–26s.
8. Belkoff SM, Mathis JM, Erbe EM, Fenton DC. Biomechanical evaluation of a new bone cement for use in vertebroplasty. Spine 2000; 25:1061–1064.
9. Tohmeh AG, Mathis JM, Fenton DC, Levine AM, Belkoff SM. Biomechanical efficacy of unipedicular versus bipedicular vertebroplasty for the management of osteoporotic compression fractures. Spine 1999; 24:1772–1776.
10. Belkoff SM, Mathis JM, Jasper LE, Deramond H. The biomechanics of vertebroplasty: the effect of cement volume on mechanical behavior. Spine 2001; 26:1537–1541.
11. Jasper LE, Deramond H, Mathis JM, Belkoff SM. The effect of monomer-to-powder ratio on the material properties of Cranioplastic. Bone 1999; 25:27s–29s.
12. Jasper LE, Deramond H, Mathis JM, Belkoff SM. Material properties of various cements for the use with vertebroplasty. J Mater Sci Mater Med 200; 14:1–5.
13. Belkoff SM, Mathis JM, Jasper LE, Deramond H. An ex vivo biomechanical evaluation of a hydroxyapatite cement for use with vertebroplasty. Spine 2001; 26:1542–1546.
14. Cotton A, Dewatre F, Cortet B. Percutaneous vertebroplasty for osteolytic metastases and myeloma. Radiology 1996; 200:525–530.
15. Weill A, Chiras J, Simon JM. Spinal metastases: indications for and results of percutaneous injection of acrylic surgical cement. Radiology 1996; 199:241–247.

16. Cyteval C, Sarrabere MP, Roux JO, Thomas E, Jorgensen C, Blotman F. Acute osteoporotic vertebral collapse: open study on percutaneous injection of acrylic surgical cement in 20 patients. Am J Roentgenol 1999; 173:1685–1690.
17. Barr JD, Barr MS, Lemley TJ, McCann RM. Percutaneous vertebroplasty for pain relief and spinal stabilization. Spine 2000; 25:923–928.
18. Zoarski GH, Snow P, Olan WJ, Stallmeyer MJ, Dick BW, Hebel JR, De Deyne M. Percutaneous vertebroplasty for osteoporotic compression fractures: quantitative prospective evaluation of long-term outcomes. J Vasc Intervent Radiol 2002; 13:139–148.
19. Wilson DR, Myers ER, Mathis JM, Scribner RM, Conta JA, Reiley MA, Talmadge K. Effect of augmentation on the mechanics of vertebral wedge fractures. Spine 2000; 25:158–165.
20. Belkoff SM, Mathis JM, Fenton DC, Scribner RM, Reiley ME, Talmadge K. An ex vivo biomechanical evaluation of an inflatable bone tamp used in the treatment of compression fractures. Spine 2001; 26:151–156.
21. Belkoff SM, Mathis JM, Deramond H, Jasper LE. An ex vivo biomechanical evaluation of a hydroxyapatite cement for use with kyphoplasty. Am J Neuroradiol 2001; 22:1212–1216.
22. Lieberman IH, Dudeney S, Reinhardt MK, Bell G. Initial outcome and efficacy of "kyphoplasty" in the treatment of painful osteoporotic vertebral compression fractures. Spine 2001; 26:1631–1638.
23. Theodorou DJ, Theodorou SJ, Duncan TD, et al: Percutaneous balloon kyphoplasty for the correction of spinal deformity in painful vertebral body compression fractures. J Clin Imaging 2002; 26:1–5.
24. Lane JM, Girardi F, Parvaianen H, et al: Preliminary outcomes of the first 226 consecutive kyphoplasties for the fixation of painful osteoporotic vertebral compression fractures [abstr]. Osteoporosis Int (Suppl) 2000; 11:S206.
25. Garfin S, Lin G, Lieberman I, et al: Retrospective analysis of the outcomes of balloon kyphoplasty to treat vertebral body compression fracture (VCF) refractory to medical management. Eur Spine J 2001; 10(Suppl):S7.
26. Dudeney S, Lieberman IH, Reinhardt MK, et al. Kyphoplasty in the treatment of osteolytic vertebral compression fractures as a result of multiple myeloma. J Clin Oncol 2002; 20:2382–2387.
27. Ledlie JT, Renfro M. Balloon kyphoplasty: one-year outcomes in vertebral body height restoration, chronic pain, and activity levels. J Neurosurg 2003; 98(Suppl 1):36–42.
28. Watts NB, Harris ST, Genant HK: Treatment of painful osteoporotic vertebral fractures with percutaneous vertebroplasty or kyphoplasty. Osteoporos Int 2001; 12:429–437.
29. Olan WJ. Kyphoplasty: balloon-assisted vertebroplasty. ASNR Spine Symposium. Vancouver, BC, May 11–12, 2002:115–117.
30. Phillips FM, Wetze FT, Lieberman I, Campbell-Hupp M. An in vivo comparison of the potential for extravertebral cement leak after vertebroplasty and kyphoplasty. Spine 2002; 27:2173–2179.
31. Agris JM, Zoarski GH, Stallmeyer MJB, Ortiz O. Intravertebral pressure during vertebroplasty: a study comparing multiple delivery systems. Presented at the Annual Meeting of the American Society of Spine Radiology; February 19–23, 2003, Scottsdale, AZ.
32. Tomita S, Malloy S, Abe M, Belkoff SM. Ex vivo measurement of intramedullary pressure during vertebroplasty. Spine 2004; 29:723–725.
33. Mathis JM. Percutaneous vertebroplasty: complication avoidance and technique optimization. Am J Neuroradiol 2003; 24:1697–1706.

34. FDA Public Health Web Notification: Complications related to the use of bone cement in treating compression fractures of the spine. 4/2003; http://www.fda.gov/cdrh/safety/bonecement.html.
35. Wong WH, Olan WJ, Belkoff SM: Balloon kyphoplasty. In Percutaneous Vertebroplasty. JM Mathis, H Deramond, SM Belkoff (eds). New York: Springer, 2002:109–124.
36. Garfin SR, Yuan HA, Reiley MA: Kyphoplasty and vertebroplasty for the treatment of painful osteoporotic compression fractures. Spine 2001; 26:1511–1515.
37. Teng MMH, Wei CJ, Wei LC, et al. Kyphosis correction and height restoration effects of percutaneous vertebroplasty. Am J Neuroradiol 2003; 24:1893–1900.
38. Hiwatashi A, Moritani T, Numaguchi Y, Westesson PL. Vertebral height restoration following percutaneous vertebroplasty. Am J Neuroradiol 2003; 24:185–189.
39. McKiernan F, Jensen R, Faciszewski T. The dynamic mobility of vertebral compression fractures. J Bone Miner Res. 2003; 18:24–29.
40. Nussbaum DA, Gailloud P, Murphy K. A review of complications associated with vertebroplasty and kyphoplasty as reported to the FDA medical device related web site. J Vasc Intervent Radiol 2004; 15:1185–1192.

10
Tumors

Hervé Deramond, Jacques Chiras, and Anne Cotten

Osteolytic metastases and myeloma are the most frequent malignant destructive lesions involving the spine. Affected patients often experience severe back pain and disability related to the vertebral fractures induced by these destructive lesions. The aim of percutaneous vertebroplasty (PV) in these disease processes is to produce pain relief and reinforcement by the injection of acrylic cement. This treatment may be used adjunctively with radiation therapy and chemotherapy.

Percutaneous vertebroplasty is rarely indicated for benign tumors. Spinal osteoid osteoma and aneurismal bone cysts do not need structural reinforcement and therefore are not an indication for PV, although they can be treated by other percutaneous methods (1,2). Fibrous dysplasias, eosinophilic granulomas, and vertebral hemangiomas (VHs) are osteolytic lesions weakening bone, and PV can be used for their treatment (3–5). The most frequent indication for PV in the treatment of benign tumors is VH. This chapter describes the role of PV in the treatment of metastatic lesions, myelomas, and VHs.

Percutaneous Vertebroplasty and Metastatic Lesions

Pathology and Patient Demographics

Patients with cancer eventually present with bone metastases in 27% of the cases (6). The vertebral bodies are the most frequent site of bone metastatic disease (7). The incidence of metastatic lesion to the spine depends on the primary cancer: 80% of patients with prostate cancer, 50% of patients with breast cancer, and 30% of patients with lung, thyroid, or renal cell cancer (8). Breast (30%), prostate (10%), and lung (25%) cancers are the three main etiologies of metastases to the spine (7,8).

The 1-year survival rate after diagnosis of spinal metastases is high for patients with prostate (83%) or breast (78%) cancer (hormonal-dependent cancers) but low for patients with lung cancer (22%) (9). Survival rates for patients with renal cell or thyroid cancer depend on the histologic classification of the tumor cells (9). The detection of spinal metastasis from the time of primary lesion diagnosis is shortest for patients with lung cancer (3.6–6.1 months) and longest for patients with breast cancer (29.4–33.5 months) (10). About 7.5% of patients present with spinal metastases before the diagnosis of the primary lesion (10). The thoracic spine is the most common site of disease (70%), followed by the lumbar spine (20%), and cervical spine (10%). These data are important to consider when counseling patients for therapy.

Indications and Contraindications

The primary indication for PV is proven metastatic disease to the spine of a patient who is experiencing severe, focal, and mechanical back pain that limits normal activities and requires narcotic medications. Usually there will be a vertebral compression fracture (VCF) associated with the osteolytic metastatic lesion, although the amount of compression may be small.

Inherent in the process of malignant involvement of the spine is destruction of portions of the vertebral body. The greater the destruction, the more chance there is for vertebral collapse and pain. In addition, these lesions present problems for the physician considering PV, because destruction of the cortex of the vertebra, although not a contraindication, increases the possibility of cement leakage. In several studies, 40% of patients treated with PV had partial destruction of the posterior wall (Figure 10.1) (11–13). However, if there is extension of the tumor through the posterior wall (Figure 10.2), PV should be considered only after a multidisciplinary discussion, and a surgical team should be available in case spinal cord decompression is needed. Shimony et al. (14) demonstrated that PV could be performed safely

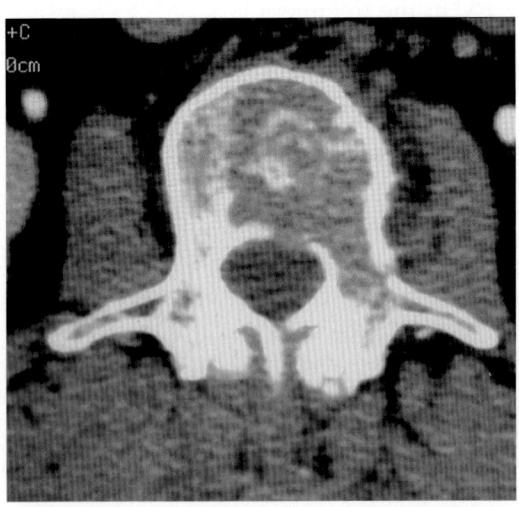 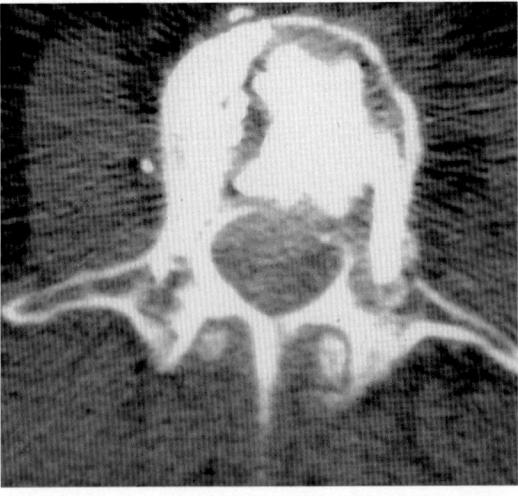

A B

Figure 10.1. Partial destruction of the posterior wall. Axial CT scans before **(A)** and after **(B)** injection of cement. Note the injection of both the "normal" part and the osteolytic part of the vertebral body. (From J.M. Mathis, H. Deramond, and S.M. Belkoff [eds], Percutaneous Vertebroplasty. New York: Springer, 2002, with permission.)

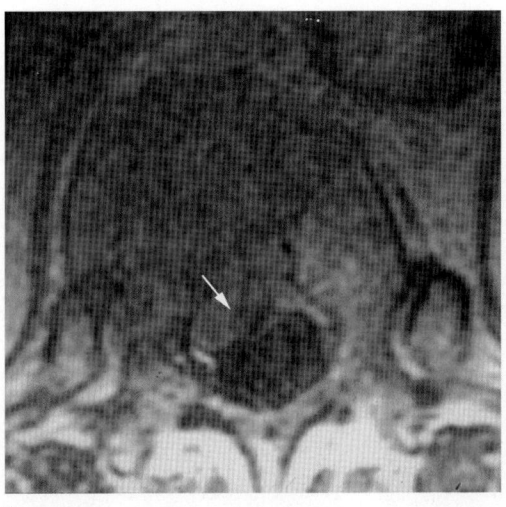 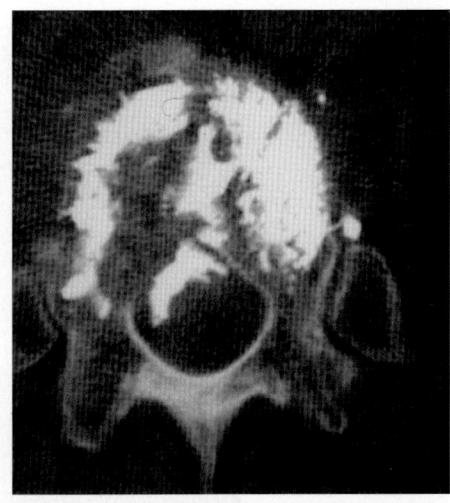

Figure 10.2. Partial destruction of the posterior wall with anterior epidural involvement by the tumor (white arrow in A). **(A)** Axial MR image before PV. **(B)** Axial CT scan after PV. Note the cement in the epidural component of the tumor; there were no neurologic complications. Both the "normal" and the osteolytic parts of the vertebral body were injected. (From J.M. Mathis, H. Deramond, and S.M. Belkoff [eds], Percutaneous Vertebroplasty. New York: Springer, 2002, with permission.)

and effectively with conscious sedation for patients with epidural involvement without neurologic symptoms. Conscious sedation provides an extra measure of safety because patients are able to tell if any pain, especially radicular pain, develops during the injection of polymethylmethacrylate (PMMA) (14). Clinical signs of compression of nerve roots or cord are contraindications to PV because there is a distinct risk of increasing compression with the injection of cement.

In general, PV is not indicated for asymptomatic lesions of the spine. One should first consider other therapies (radiotherapy, chemotherapy, thermoablation, etc.). Percutaneous vertebroplasty can be performed if other therapies have been exhausted and/or if there is a high risk of vertebral collapse (Figure 10.3).

The presence of multiple spinal lesions with diffuse back pain is not an indication for PV. Percutaneous vertebroplasty for focal pain with multiple lesions is appropriate, but the treatment of several lesions may be required to give adequate pain relief (Figure 10.4). The decision of which vertebra to treat depends on the correlation between the imaging examination and physical findings. Physical examination can be performed by using fluoroscopy to determine which level is symptomatic. No more than three vertebrae should be treated at one session.

Although lesions in the thoracic and lumbar spine are often treated with PV, those in the cervical region can be treated operatively without major surgical exposure. However, based on the situation, patient's condition, and age, PV may be useful for treating cervical metastatic lesions (Figure 10.5). As in all levels of the spine, metastatic lesions are associated with a high risk of epidural invasion or spinal cord damage in the presence of posterior wall compromise.

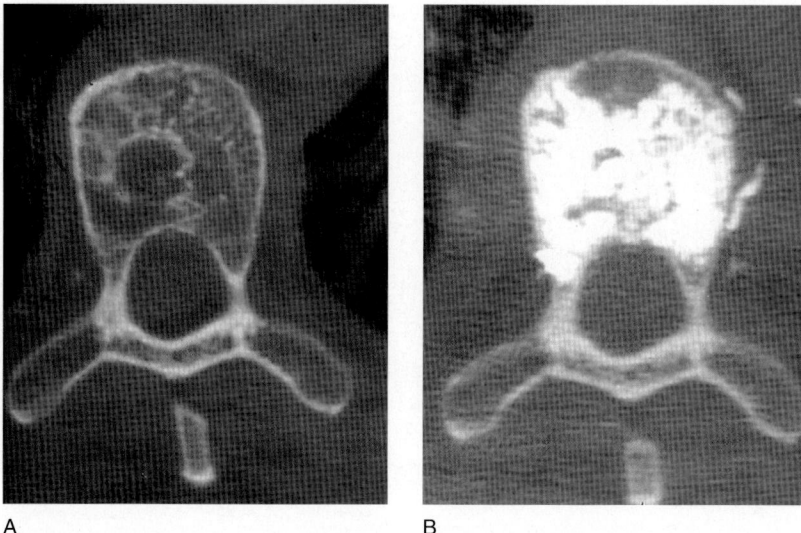

Figure 10.3. Patient with asymptomatic breast osteolysis of T8. **(A)** Axial CT before PV. **(B)** Axial CT after PV, which was performed because the extensive tumor placed the vertebral body at high risk for collapse. (From J.M. Mathis, H. Deramond, and S.M. Belkoff [eds], Percutaneous Vertebroplasty. New York: Springer, 2002, with permission.)

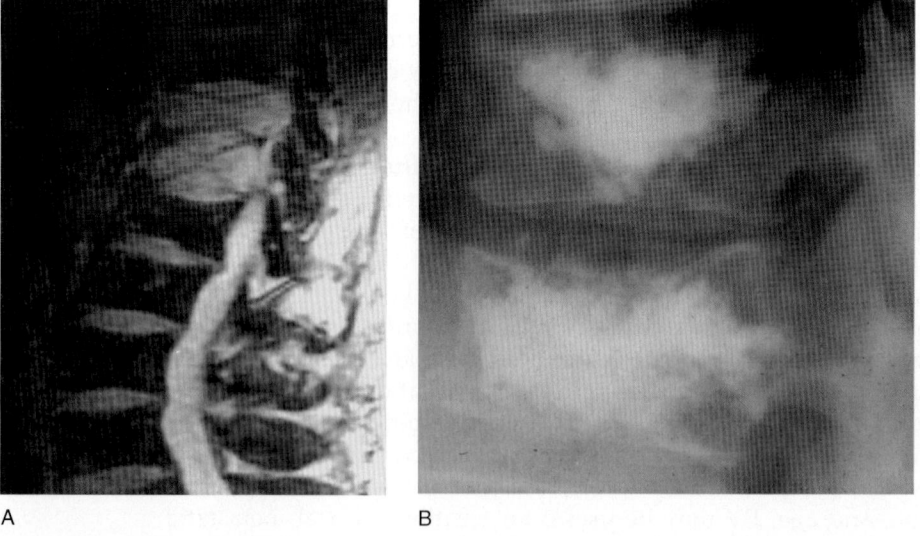

Figure 10.4. This patient presented with severe and focal back pain related to two metastatic lesions of T11–T12. MR image **(A)** and lateral view **(B)** after PV at two levels. (From J.M. Mathis, H. Deramond, and S.M. Belkoff [eds], Percutaneous Vertebroplasty. New York: Springer, 2002, with permission.)

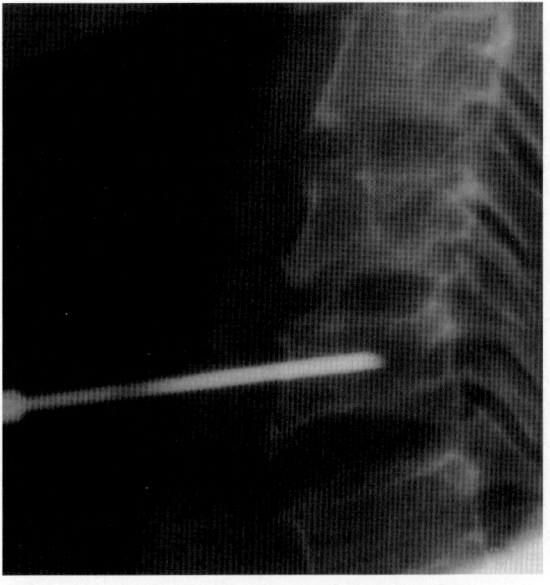 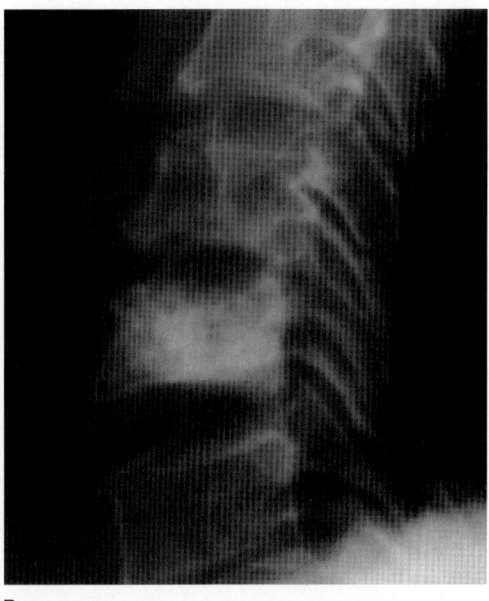

Figure 10.5. This patient presented with severe cervical pain related to a C5 lung cancer metastatic lesion. Lateral views before **(A)** and after **(B)** the injection of cement. (From J.M. Mathis, H. Deramond, and S.M. Belkoff [eds], Percutaneous Vertebroplasty. New York: Springer, 2002, with permission.)

Contraindications to PV with spinal metastatic lesions include (1) complete collapse of the vertebra (generally there needs to be 25% to 30% of the original height remaining to allow successful PV [12]); (2) pure osteoblastic lesions (a mixed sclerotic and destructive lesion with focal pain and collapse is a good indication for PV) (Figure 10.6); (3) nerve root or spinal cord compression related to epidural or foraminal extension of the tumor; (4) diffuse (nonfocal) back pain and failure to localize symptomatic level(s); (5) general infectious disorders; and (6) coagulation disorders (platelets below 100,000, prothrombin time greater than 3 above the upper limits of normal, and partial thromboplastin time more than 1.5 times normal).

Patient Selection and Evaluation

Generally, patients are referred for three main reasons: known cancer and back pain related to a spinal metastasis, known cancer and a recently diagnosed but asymptomatic spinal lesion, or back pain and suspicious lesions but no known diagnosis. Patient evaluation should consider all available clinical information, and clinical examination should identify the focal pain that correlates to the lesion considered for PV. Back pain usually increases when the patient is standing and decreases when the patient is recumbent. The patient's pain should be severe, altering activities of daily living or requiring substantial use of analgesics. This pain should be documented with measurement instruments such as visual analog scale and a quality-of-life questionnaire.

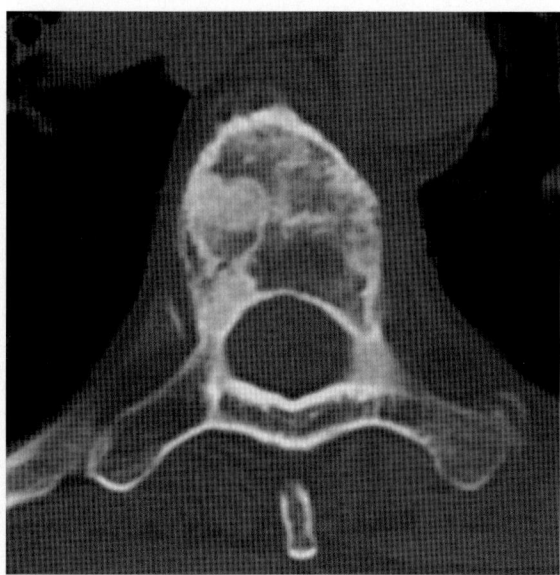

Figure 10.6. Breast metastatic and mixed osteolytic and osteoblastic lesion at T9 in a patient presenting with severe back pain. (From J.M. Mathis, H. Deramond, and S.M. Belkoff [eds], Percutaneous Vertebroplasty. New York: Springer, 2002, with permission.)

Back pain described by the patient and detected on the clinical examination should be compared with the findings on plain radiographs, magnetic resonance imaging (MRI), computed tomography (CT), and nuclear medicine scans. These diagnostic studies should be assessed for osteolysis, the degree of collapse, extension of tumor into the epidural space and foramina, compression of the neural tissue, and diffusion of metastatic lesions on the spine and bones. Computed tomography is best for detecting destruction of the posterior vertebral wall and determining whether the lesion is osteolytic and/or osteoblastic. Computed tomography gives the percentage of vertebral body destruction: 50% or more of the vertebral body needs to be destroyed before there is a substantial risk of collapse (Figure 10.3).

Once the patient has been found to meet the criteria indicating a need for PV, the procedure should be completely discussed with the patient and his or her family. This discussion should include the potential benefits of PV, its palliative nature, and the risks associated with the procedure. Finally, the patients should undergo a preanesthetic evaluation: electrocardiogram (ECG) and laboratory screen (complete blood cell count/platelets, electrolytes, prothrombin time/partial thromboplastin time, and blood urea nitrogen/creatinine).

Technique

The technique for PV of malignant lesions is the same as that used for other indications (see Chapter 7). When the primary cancer is not known or if there is a doubt about the cause of the vertebral lesion, a biopsy should precede the injection of cement. The cannula placed for cement injection will accommodate a 15- to 18-gauge biopsy device. These two procedures can be performed in one session because the presence of malignancy does not preclude PV.

To obtain good structural reinforcement of a partially destroyed vertebral body, both the osteolytic and normal parts of the vertebra should be filled with cement (Figures 10.1 and 10.2). Therefore, a bilateral transpedicular approach is usually required to achieve maximal filling of malignant lesions.

The distribution of cement must be monitored in real time with a high-quality fluoroscope. It is most important to examine the lateral view because this projection reveals leaks that occur posteriorly toward the epidural or foraminal space or anteriorly toward veins. Cement injection should be stopped immediately when the cement approaches the projection of the posterior vertebral wall or fills a vein anterior to the projection of the anterior vertebral cortex. It is not important that the fill be homogeneous in distribution. A partial fill of the vertebral body can provide good pain relief. Pain relief has not been shown to be related to the quantity of cement injected (12,13).

However, if too little cement is injected, there remains the possibility of additional vertebral compression with weight bearing. Belkoff et al. (15) have shown in vitro that 4 to 6 mL of cement is needed to restore initial stiffness to osteoporotic vertebra (without osteolytic destruction). Their study provides an approximation of the minimal volume that may be desired for structural reinforcement at the lumbar level. Another reason to fill the metastatic lesion as much as possible is to try to get the best antitumoral effect of PV. This antitumoral effect could be related to the ischemia or thermal necrosis due to the exothermic polymerization of the cement. The bigger the core of cement, the better will be the antitumoral effect. This is important if the patient is contraindicated for complementary local radiation therapy.

Martin et al. (16) performed PV by using an access route via the lysed pedicle for the treatment of lytic lesions involving the pedicle. If the pedicle was not visible or was partially visible, the position of the pedicle was deduced from the position of the contralateral pedicle and the position of pedicles above and below the level to be treated. After treatment of the vertebral body, the needle is withdrawn stepwise through the pedicle, and the injection of cement can be obtained by introducing the stylet into the needle: 0.7 cc of cement is then delivered. In most of the procedures this amount of cement is sufficient to get a good filling of the osteolytic pedicle. The filling is considered satisfactory if the cement fills the metastasis and extends from the body through the affected pedicle.

The standard needle size varies from 10 to 13 gauge for the lumbar and thoracic spine. A 15-gauge needle is normally used in the cervical region. Smaller 18-gauge needles have been used, but the cement needs to be less viscous (17–19). Although we believe this technique is associated with a higher risk of cement leakage and resultant clinical cervical complications, a technique to reduce the risk of leaks is to insert several needles into different parts of the osteolytic lesion and inject small amounts of cement through each needle. At the cervical level, insertion of only one 15-gauge needle in the center of the osteolytic lesion using an anterolateral approach permits good filling of the vertebra.

Results

In 1989, Lapras et al. (17) were the first to report the use of PV for a L1 painful metastatic lesion. This early experience was encouraging because the patient experienced good pain relief and was able to resume walking. This report was followed by that of Kaemmerlen et al. (18,19), who found that 80% of 20 patients experienced substantial pain relief within 48 hours from PV for malignant lesions. In 1996, Weill et al. (12) reported that more than 75% of the patients in their series experienced pain relief and improved quality of life after PV. The results were sustained for 6 months or longer in 73% of the patients. Cortet et al. (20) reported a 97% positive response rate for patients with malignant lesions within 48 hours after PV. Pain relief was complete in 13.5% and substantially improved in 55%. The remaining 30% of patients rated their improvement as moderate. The improvement was unchanged in 75% of the patients 6 months later. Nevertheless, although substantial, the quality and quantity of pain relief after PV for malignant lesions appears to be less than that found for osteoporotic lesions treated by PV.

More recently, Fourney et al. (21) reviewed a consecutive group of cancer patients (21 with myeloma and 35 with other primary malignancies) undergoing vertebro- and kyphoplasty at their institution. Improvement or complete pain relief was noted in 84% of the patients. No patient's pain was worsened by the procedure. Analgesic consumption was reduced at 1 month, and there was a durable analgesic effect at each follow-up interval up to 1 year.

The mechanisms of pain relief in patients with malignant lesions are not completely known. Stabilization of microfractures and reduction of mechanical forces are certainly the main factors. Tumor ischemia induced by the injection of cement into a solid lesion may also play a role. Destruction of the nerve endings in response to chemical (cytotoxic effect of the monomer) and thermal (exothermic reaction of the cement) forces has been postulated, but these mechanisms likely play a relatively minor role (22). The necrotizing effect of the cement on the tumor mass may extend for a short distance beyond the limits of the margins of the PMMA (23) and may be a factor in the low rate of recurrence at the site of the PV even without complementary treatments.

Side Effects and Complications

A more complete description of the potential complications associated with PV is provided in Chapter 13. It is known that the incidence of cement leaks with PV for metastatic lesions is much higher than that associated with osteoporotic fractures. This fact is almost surely attributable to the cortical destruction frequent in metastatic lesions. The rate of complications is about 10% and the incidence of radiculopathy is about 5% after PV for metastatic lesions (11–13,24). Our personal experience with the most recent 200 patients indicates a complication rate less than 5%, and most of these complications are transient.

Problems that create pain may be transient and amenable to therapy with nonsteroidal anti-inflammatory medications or local steroid injections. Persistent radiculopathy may require surgical intervention to remove cement that might be compressing nerve roots (Figure 10.7). Any side effect (mild or major) should prompt re-examination to determine the cause and initiate the adequate treatment. Usually, a CT scan is the most direct study for identifying a cement leak.

Percutaneous Vertebroplasty and Other Therapies

Radiation therapy alone can give partial or complete pain relief in 75% to 90% of patients (25,26). However, it takes 2–10 days to see improvement in pain following half-body irradiation and 1–2 weeks following external beam radiotherapy (27), and there is little strengthening of the vertebra, which leaves the vertebra at long-term risk for additional collapse and pain. In situations when immediate pain relief is desired, such as intractable pain, or for patients with short life expectancy, vertebroplasty may provide an ideal solution. Percutaneous vertebroplasty does not diminish the positive effects of radiation (28). Percutaneous vertebroplasty can be used to obtain rapid pain relief and to

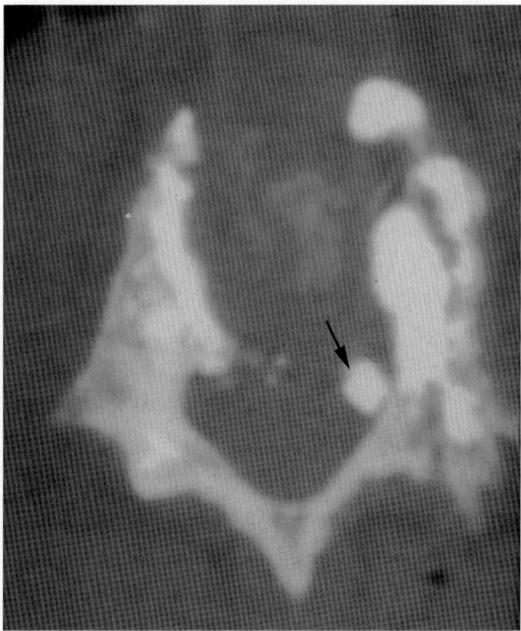

Figure 10.7. L4 breast cancer osteolytic metastatic lesion. Cement leaked into the radicular canal (black arrow), inducing severe radiculopathy that resolved after surgical removal of the extravasated cement. (From J.M. Mathis, H. Deramond, and S.M. Belkoff [eds], Percutaneous Vertebroplasty. New York: Springer, 2002, with permission.)

induce reinforcement of the involved vertebra. Radiation therapy should help reduce local tumor recurrence. Vertebroplasty and radiation therapy should be considered complementary procedures.

When there are clinical signs of nerve or cord compression in patients with spinal metastases presenting with neurologic symptoms, PV is contraindicated and surgery usually indicated. Surgery may require both anterior and posterior approaches to accomplish corporectomy and place instrumentation for spinal stabilization (29). Analysis of vertebral involvement may occasionally indicate that appropriate use of PV can reduce the amount of surgery needed. Percutaneous reinforcement of involved vertebra may eliminate the need for an anterior approach in some patients (11,12). With the anterior column support provided by PV, a posterior approach can be used for laminectomy to decompress the spinal cord and stabilize the spine with posterior instrumentation. For patients with a shortened expected life span, this less invasive procedure should provide palliative improvement and a shorter period of convalescence.

The main concern when planning PV and chemotherapy is the effect of the chemotherapy on platelets, coagulation factors, and immunization. When possible, PV should precede chemotherapy.

Other local percutaneous therapies for metastatic lesions may be used. Thermal ablation or direct injection of absolute ethanol may be used for small lesions (30). Intraarterial embolization may be used for large and hypervascularized tumors (31). Percutaneous vertebroplasty represents a direct percutaneous embolization of these hypervascular tumors (renal cell or thyroid metastases) and can be combined with transarterial embolization if the amount of cement injected does not fill the volume of the lesion. Percutaneous vertebroplasty must be used or combined with these treatments if structural reinforcement is to be achieved.

Image-guided radiofrequency ablation (RFA) can be a safe modality in the therapy for nonresectable spine tumors (32,33). Using combined multislice CT and fluoroscopic guidance, instrumentation can be precisely placed to cause a controlled ablation. Gronemeyer et al. (32) combined treatment of spinal metastasis with RFA heat ablation and PV with good results. In their experience, PV immediately after RFA during the same procedure is very painful for nonsedated patients and is best performed several days after radiofrequency ablation.

Percutaneous Vertebroplasty and Multiple Myeloma

Pathology and Patient Demographics

Multiple myeloma is a monoclonal proliferation of malignant plasma cells that usually affects the bone marrow (34). The peak incidence occurs during the sixth decade of life. The median survival time is 3 years. This disease is slightly more common in men than in women and affects 3 in 100,000 persons annually (34).

Excessive bone resorption due to an increase of proinflammatory cytokines is a characteristic feature of the disease (35–37). Diffuse osteoporosis and focal osteolytic lesions are thought to be potential causes of fractures in patients with multiple myeloma, and such fractures most frequently involve the spine (38–40). Indeed, vertebral compression fractures are present in 55% to 70% of patients with multiple myeloma and represent the initial clinical sign in 34% to 64% of such patients (41–44). Despite major improvements in chemotherapy, bone pain and widespread vertebral collapses are responsible for disability, respiratory restriction, and (sometimes) neurologic complications (45). All of these conditions decrease the quality of life for patients with multiple myeloma.

In approximately 5% of patients with plasma cell myeloma, solitary bone plasmacytoma represents the only disease feature. The diagnosis requires histologic evidence of a monoclonal plasma cell infiltrate in one bone lesion, absence of other bone lesions on skeletal radiographs, and lack of marrow plasmacytosis elsewhere (46). Two thirds of such patients develop multiple myeloma within 3 years after the discovery of a plasmacytoma; one third have no tumor progression for more than 10 years after discovery (46–51). Early progression most likely results from occult generalized disease that was not recognized at diagnosis. Magnetic resonance imaging, which is more sensitive than conventional radiography for the detection of myeloma lesions, may indicate additional foci that represent occult myeloma (46).

Technique

The procedure (guidance for needle positioning, needle route, etc.) for myelomatous vertebral lesions is not substantially different from that for other indications (5,12,52,53). The transpedicular approach, when possible, is preferred. However, it should be remembered that the distribution of cement and the risk of cement leaks depend on the radiologic appearance of the vertebral lesions.

Most of the vertebral collapses in patients with myeloma appear benign on radiographs and MR imaging with a distribution similar to that observed in osteoporotic fractures (36). When PV is performed for such collapses, the distribution of PMMA is frequently homogeneous in the vertebral body, and a single injection of cement may be sufficient (Figure 10.8). The risk of leaks of cement is small, especially if the cement injected is more viscous than that normally used for PV. Venous leaks are commonly observed if cement with a liquid consistency is injected into such lesions (13).

When a lytic lesion is demonstrated on conventional radiographs or CT scan, the degree of lesion filling is more varied and the risk of cement leakage is higher, possibly because of the different texture of this type of lesion. However, a better distribution of cement is usually obtained than in osteolytic metastases (Figure 10.9).

Solitary bone plasmacytoma frequently appears as an osteolytic but trabeculated lesion (54) with cortical osteolysis frequently present only in some places. The quality of the distribution of cement usually is intermediate between the two previously described vertebral lesions (Figure 10.10).

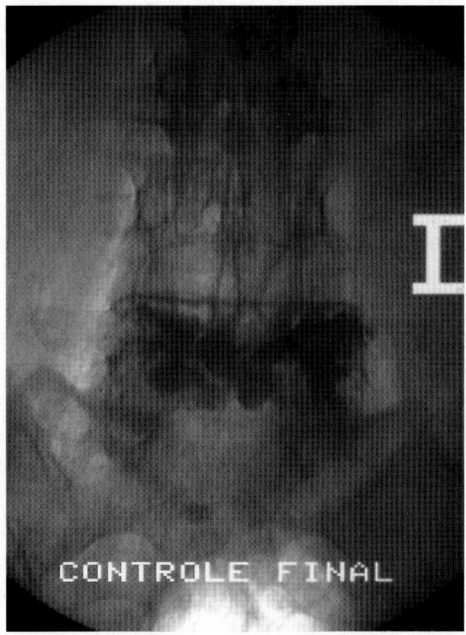

Figure 10.8. Homogeneous distribution of PMMA in the vertebral body of L5. (From J.M. Mathis, H. Deramond, and S.M. Belkoff [eds], Percutaneous Vertebroplasty. New York: Springer, 2002, with permission.)

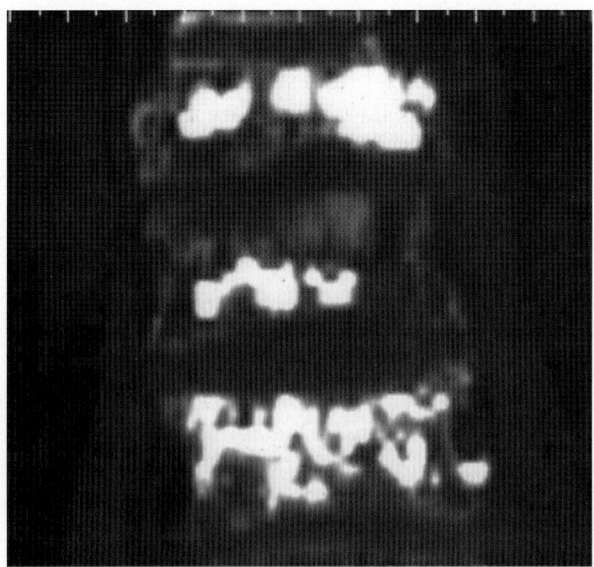

Figure 10.9. Three examples of inhomogeneous cement fill that may occur in myelomatous vertebral bodies. (From J.M. Mathis, H. Deramond, and S.M. Belkoff [eds], Percutaneous Vertebroplasty. New York: Springer, 2002, with permission.)

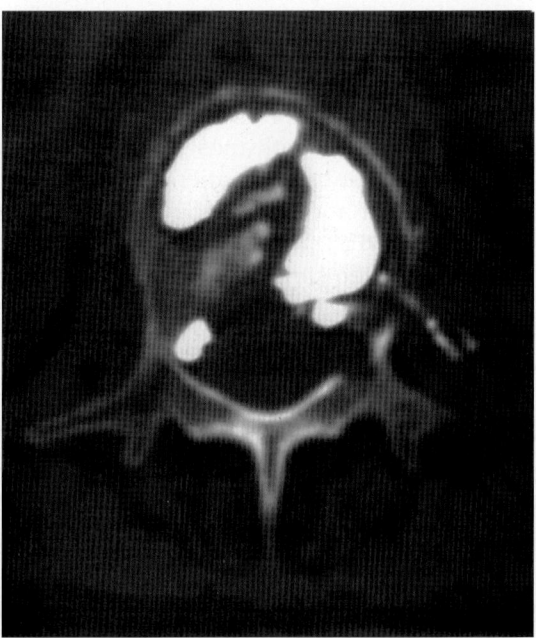

Figure 10.10. Solitary bone plasmocytoma. CT scan showing a small epidural leak. (From J.M. Mathis, H. Deramond, and S.M. Belkoff [eds], Percutaneous Vertebroplasty. New York: Springer, 2002, with permission.)

Results

As for metastases and osteoporotic vertebral collapses, pain relief after PV for myeloma occurs within hours or days (usually within 24 hours) after the procedure, sometimes after a transient worsening of pain. More than 70% of patients with multiple myeloma experience marked or complete pain relief (5,12,13,21,52,53).

Percutaneous Vertebroplasty and Other Procedures

Vertebrectomy is rarely performed for patients with myeloma because of the multifocal nature of the disease, but radiation therapy, in association with chemotherapy, plays a major role in the management of such patients. Even so, radiation and chemotherapy do not address several treatment issues completely. First, their rapid and highly effective therapeutic effect on epidural involvement and neurologic compression is well documented, and it is of great importance for patients at risk for spinal cord compression, which occurs in 10% to 15% of patients (55). Second, local radiation therapy is effective for solitary bone plasmacytoma because it may prevent tumor growth. However, patients with multiple marrow lesions respond less satisfactorily to local radiation therapy than do the patients with a single lesion, and either type of local tumor may recur. Third, radiation therapy has been associated with a reduced incidence of vertebral fractures and focal marrow lesions (56) and with bone healing, remodeling, and reossification resulting in local reinforcement (57). However, the bone reconstruction is minimal and delayed (2 to 4 months after the start of irradiation) and sometimes preceded by transitory osteoporosis, which increases the risk of vertebral collapse and consequently of neural compression. Finally, radiation therapy usually results in partial or complete pain relief, with most patients experiencing some relief within 10 to 14 days, but some patients (5% to 10%) may experience insufficient pain relief and may be unable to tolerate additional radiation therapy.

Therefore, PV has an interesting place in the management of focal complicated myeloma lesions: It may provide rapid pain relief and vertebral stabilization when the lesion threatens the stability of the spine. Because such vertebral lesions are of clinical importance to the quality of life of patients with myeloma, PV may prevent some of the morbidity and mortality associated with the disease (45). However, because in this clinical setting PV is a palliative procedure that does not prevent tumor growth, it should be used in conjunction, whenever possible, with radiation and chemotherapy for patients with myeloma.

Percutaneous Vertebroplasty and Benign Lesions

Pathology and Patient Demographics

Vertebral hemangiomas are common abnormalities. They have been found in 10% of spines at autopsy (58) or incidentally discovered on imaging studies. In rare cases, they can be aggressive lesions in terms of clinical and/or radiographic findings.

From a clinical point of view, aggressive VHs can be differentiated as painful VHs and VHs with neurologic symptoms. The most frequent symptom is severe, mechanical back pain that increases with movement, even minimal movement such as shifting position in a chair. The tumor's progression is associated with deterioration in the quality of life. Neurologic signs can be related to nerve root and/or spinal cord compression by the VH invading the neural foramina or the epidural space. These neurologic signs can be acute or progressive.

Asymptomatic VHs can be diagnosed on plain films, CT scan, and/or MRI studies. Plain radiographs show localized and regular vertical striation of the vertebral body affected by the VH (Figure 10.11A). The diagnostic CT scan shows a loss of the trabecular bone and thickening of the remaining vertical osseous network. The hypodense areas that appear surrounding the trabeculae on CT are fatty tissue that has replaced degenerated VH (Figure 10.11B). The fatty component could be evidence of the nonprogressive nature of that part of the lesion (59). Magnetic resonance imaging shows a typical hypersignal on T1-weighted images induced by the fatty stroma of the lesion (Figure 10.11C). All these modalities show a well-demarcated lesion in part or all of the vertebral body, without involvement of the cortical bone. Most of these lesions (which can occur singly or at multiple levels) are asymptomatic and discovered only incidentally.

Aggressive VHs are characterized by the involvement of the whole vertebral body, location (frequently) in the thoracic area, an irregular

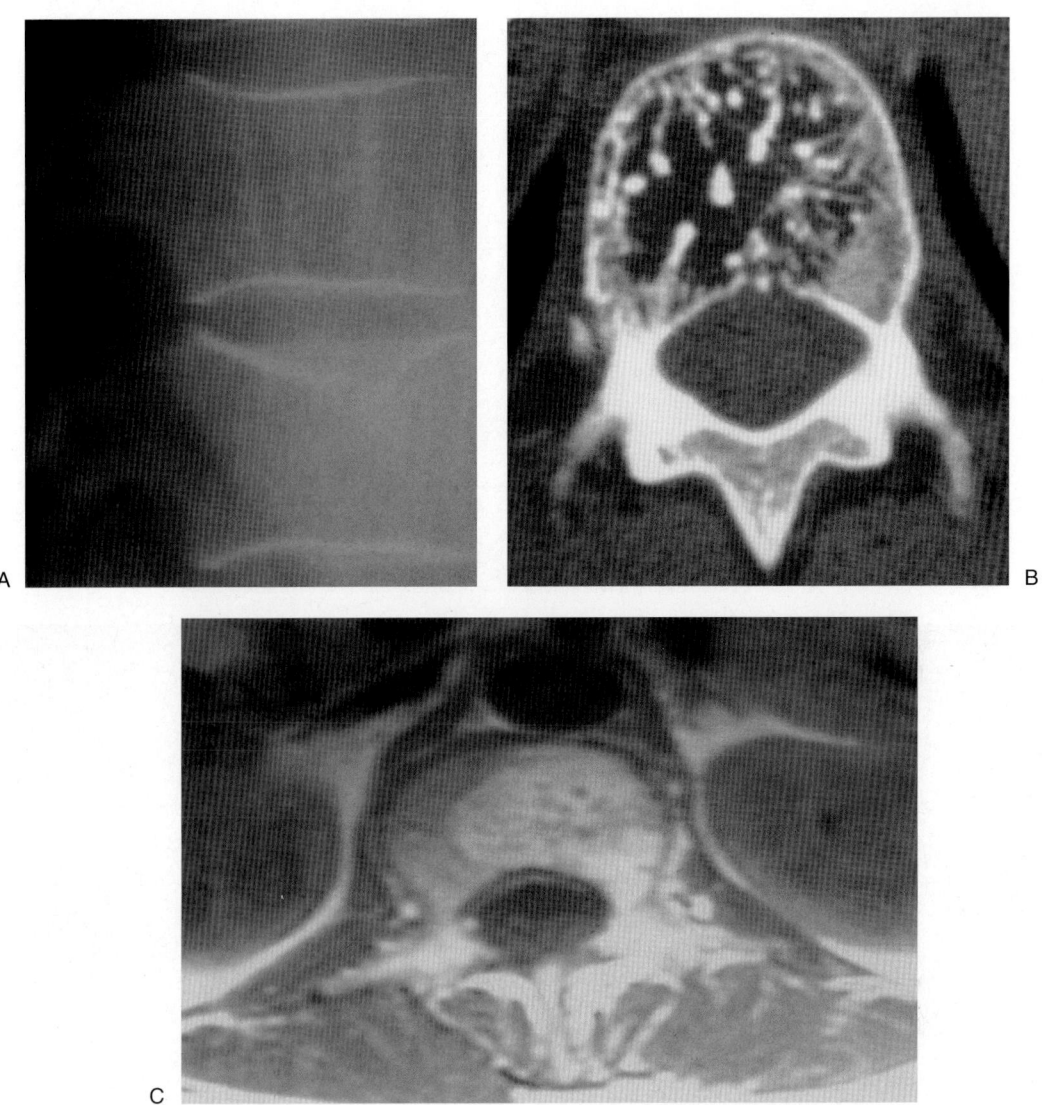

Figure 10.11. Nonaggressive VH. **(A)** Lateral radiograph showing localized and regular vertical striation of the vertebral body. **(B)** Axial CT scan showing loss of the trabecular bone and thickening of the remaining vertical osseous network, containing predominantly fatty stoma. **(C)** Axial T1-weighted MR image showing high signal intensity stroma related to fatty degeneration of a VH. (From J.M. Mathis, H. Deramond, and S.M. Belkoff [eds], Percutaneous Vertebroplasty. New York: Springer, 2002, with permission.)

honeycomb appearance of trabeculation, an expended and poorly defined cortical bone, and swelling of the soft tissues (60). On CT scans (Figure 10.12A) and MR images (Figure 10.12B), there is little or none of the fatty component usually seen with nonaggressive VHs. Computed tomography and MR imaging provide the best delineation of the extension of the VH to the paravertebral tissues. The epidural extension is best seen after intravenous injection of contrast (Figure 10.12C). This epidural involvement can induce spinal cord and/or nerve root

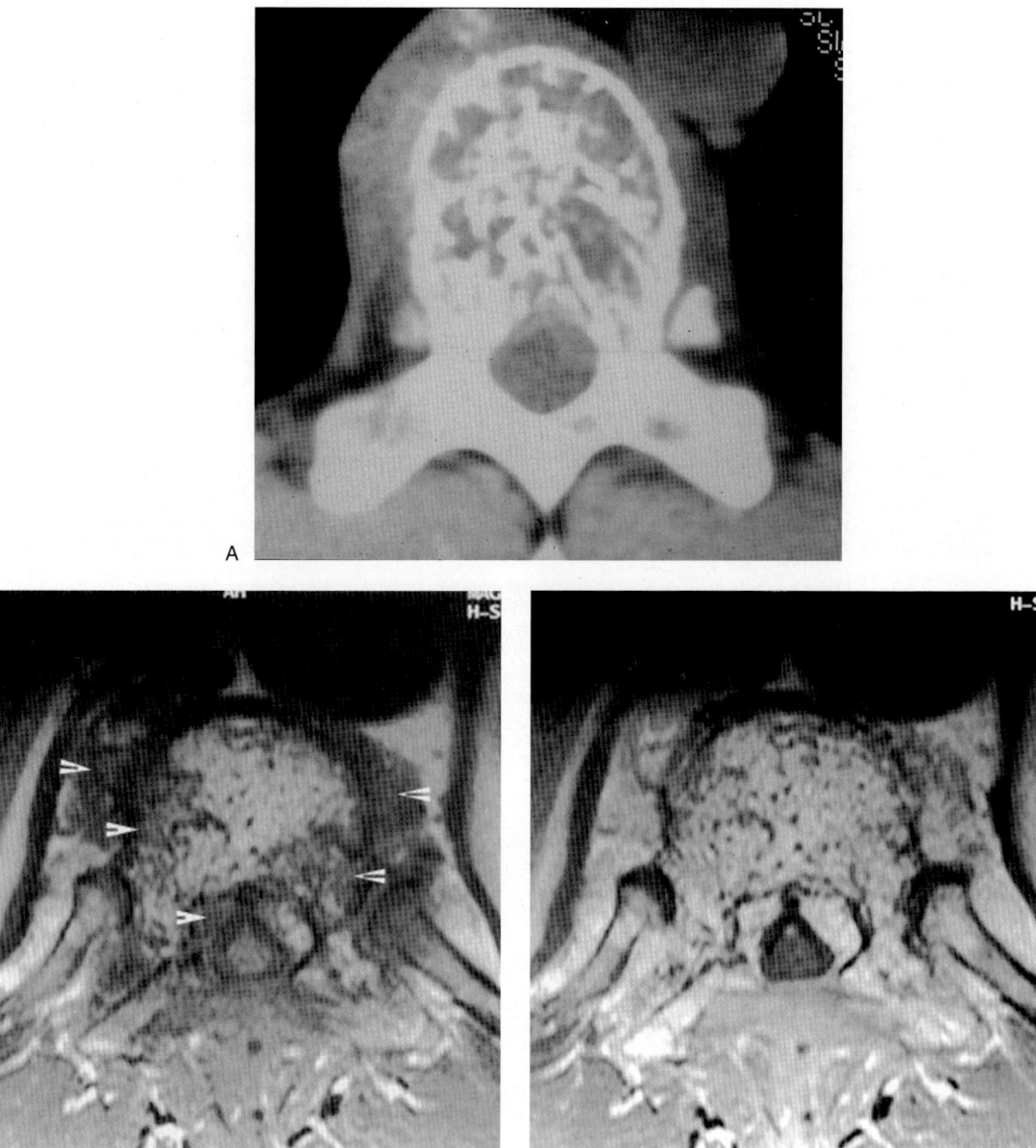

Figure 10.12. Aggressive VH. **(A)** Axial CT scan showing involvement of the whole vertebra with epidural and paravertebral extension. **(B)** Axial T1-weighted MR image showing epidural and paravertebral extension. The progressive parts of the lesion appear as an isosignal on noncontrast images (white arrowheads). **(C)** contrast-enhanced axial T1-weighted MR image showing hyperdense signal of the highly vascularized lesion. (From J.M. Mathis, H. Deramond, and S.M. Belkoff [eds], Percutaneous Vertebroplasty. New York: Springer, 2002, with permission.)

compression. Vertebral hemangiomas frequently extend to the posterior neural arch, involving the whole vertebra (Figure 10.12A).

Other signs of an aggressive VH include an increase in the size of the VH on two successive radiographic examinations; expansion of the cortical bone, or a periosteal osseous formation that induces a spinal canal stenosis; and a weakened vertebral body and possible vertebral collapse occurring spontaneously or secondary to low-energy trauma (Figure 10.13).

In most cases, VHs with radiographic signs of aggressiveness are symptomatic. Aggressive VHs can occur (singly or at multiple levels) in combination with the nonaggressive form.

Classification and Indications

Vertebral hemangiomas can be classified into one of four groups depending on their clinical and radiographic presentation (53): (1) asymptomatic VH without radiographic signs of aggressiveness (incidental discovery); (2) symptomatic (i.e., severe back pain) VH without radiographic signs of aggressiveness; (3) asymptomatic VH with radiographic signs of aggressiveness (incidental discovery); and (4) symptomatic VH with radiographic signs of aggressiveness. Group 4 can be divided into two subgroups: (a) VH with epidural extension and (b) VH without epidural extension, but inducing severe back pain.

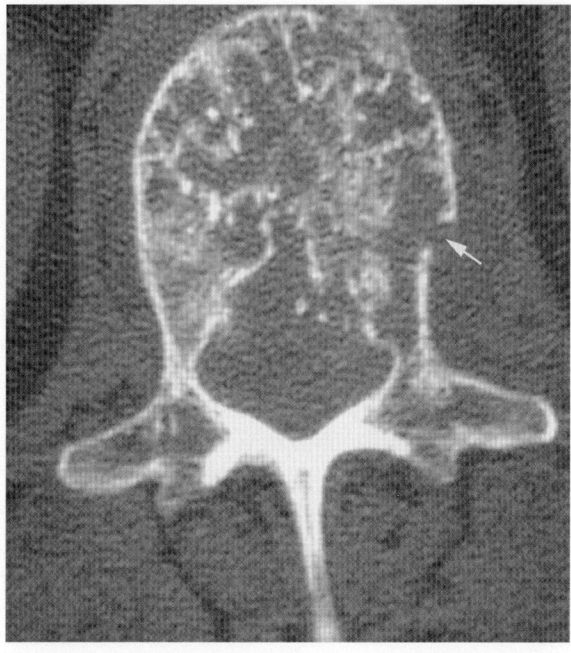

Figure 10.13. Aggressive VH. This axial CT scan of a patient presenting with severe back pain after falling on her back showed a VCF (white arrow). (From J.M. Mathis, H. Deramond, and S.M. Belkoff [eds], Percutaneous Vertebroplasty. New York: Springer, 2002, with permission.)

There are no indications for PV treatment for patients in group 1. For patients in group 2, PV is indicated because of severe back pain related to a VH, even in the absence of radiographic signs of aggressiveness. The indication is easier to confirm in the thoracic region when there is only an isolated VH to explain the back pain. It is often difficult to appreciate the role of such a VH in the cervical region and even more so at the lumbar region where associated degenerative disorders can induce the same pain.

Patients in group 3 require close monitoring with annual clinical and MR imaging examinations for progression of the VH. Percutaneous vertebroplasty is indicated only for patients for whom regular, long-term follow-up is not possible or for whom the VH becomes symptomatic or presents an evolution on successive radiographic studies.

Percutaneous vertebroplasty is indicated for all patients in group 4: The technique will vary depending on the progressive nature and severity of the neurologic signs. Patients with an acute myelopathy or cauda equina syndrome should be treated by a combination of PV and surgery (see "Technique," below). Patients presenting with progressive neurologic signs should be treated with PV and percutaneous injection of absolute ethanol (see "Technique," below). For a symptomatic patient with an aggressive VH but without epidural extension, PV alone is the treatment of choice.

Patient Evaluation

In general, patients present for evaluation for one of three reasons: (1) incidental imaging diagnosis of an asymptomatic VH, (2) severe back pain related to a VH, or (3) neurologic signs related to a VH. Evaluation of the patient should include all available clinical information. The clinical examination should elucidate focal pain or neurologic signs that correlate with the lesion in order for the lesion to be considered for PV. Pain should be documented with measurement instruments such as a visual analog scale or quality-of-life questionnaires (e.g., SF36) (61).

The pain described by the patient and detected on the clinical examination should be compared with the findings on plain radiographs, MR imaging, and CT. At the lumbar and cervical levels, particularly in patients with radiographically nonaggressive VH, the clinician should attempt to confirm the relationship between the pain and the VH, that is, exclude degenerative lesions as the possible origin of the pain, for PV to be indicated. The MR images and CT scans should be assessed to differentiate between aggressive and nonaggressive VH, to determine any extension of the VH into the epidural space and neural foramina, and to evaluate for compression of neural tissue.

Once the criteria for PV are met, the procedure should be completely discussed with the patient and his or her family. The discussion should include the potential benefits of PV and the risks associated with the procedure. Finally, the patient should undergo a preanesthetic evaluation, ECG, and laboratory screen (complete blood count/platelets, electrolytes, prothrombin time, partial thromboplastin time, blood urea nitrogen/creatinine).

Technique

According to the clinical presentation and radiographic signs, PV can be performed with acrylic cement alone or a combined treatment of acrylic cement followed by injection of glue or absolute ethanol (3,53,62,63).

Percutaneous Vertebroplasty
When a VH presents without epidural involvement in patients complaining of pain, the treatment goals are to fill the defect (Figure 10.14), obtain a structural reinforcement of the vertebral body, and provide pain relief. The needle must be inserted into the anterior part of the VH by a transpedicular approach. If the VH involves only a part of the vertebral body, it is possible to fill the whole malformation with only one injection and a single puncture (Figure 10.15). If the whole vertebral body is involved, a bilateral transpedicular approach is usually required to fill the lesion.

Percutaneous Vertebroplasty with Complementary Injection of Ethanol
When a VH invades the anterior epidural space with no or only minor neurologic symptoms, a complementary injection of absolute ethanol

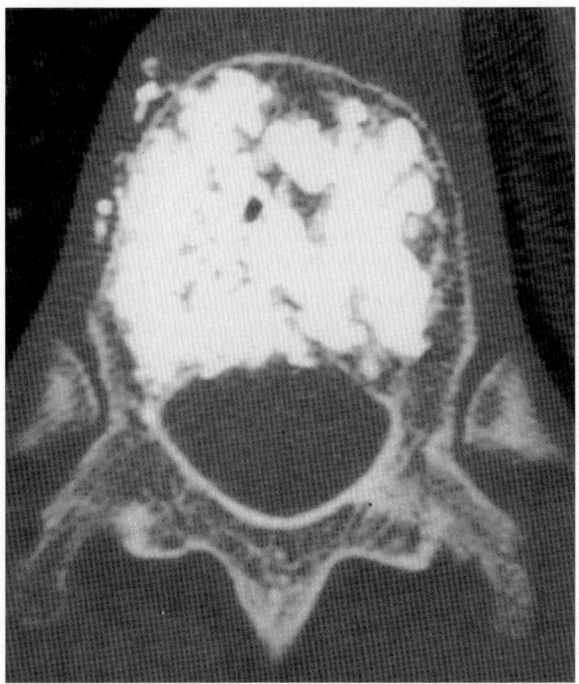

Figure 10.14. Axial CT scan after an injection of acrylic cement into a VH. (From J.M. Mathis, H. Deramond, and S.M. Belkoff [eds], Percutaneous Vertebroplasty. New York: Springer, 2002, with permission.)

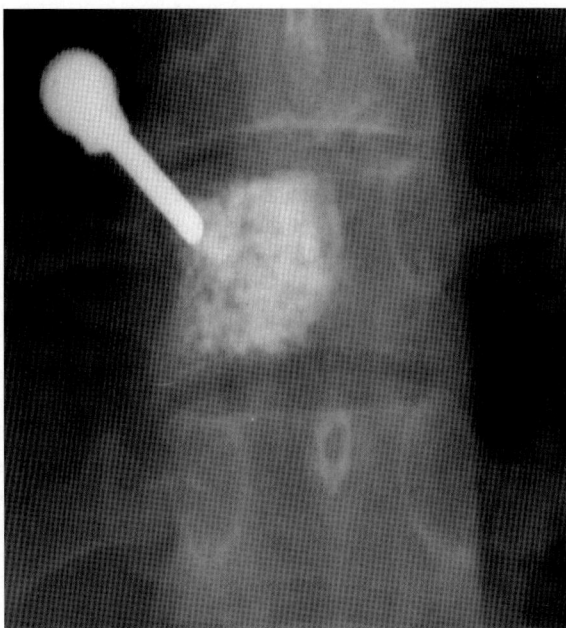

Figure 10.15. This AP radiograph showed a VH involving three quarters of the vertebral body, which was filled with acrylic cement using a unilateral transpedicular approach. (From J.M. Mathis, H. Deramond, and S.M. Belkoff [eds], Percutaneous Vertebroplasty. New York: Springer, 2002, with permission.)

may be used to sclerose the lesion completely. This procedure is accomplished in four steps. First, the affected vertebral body is injected with acrylic cement via a unilateral or bilateral transpedicular approach. Second, a site is found around or in the vertebral body that has not been injected with cement, and an 18-gauge needle is inserted into it (Figure 10.16). Third, the potential distribution of the sclerosing agent is checked by slow injection of 1 to 4 mL of contrast media; the quantity needed to inject the epidural component is noted and defines the amount to be used for the subsequent injection of ethanol. Fourth, the absolute ethanol, usually no more than 4 mL, is slowly injected. If the VH involves the posterior neural arch, it is possible in the same procedure to puncture that component using one or several needles and to obtain a complete sclerosis of the malformation, injecting no more than 1 mL of ethanol by each needle.

Heiss et al. (64) were the first to report the use of absolute ethanol (up to 50 mL) for the sclerosis of aggressive VH. However, they did not use an accompanying injection of acrylic cement. Two years later, they reported that two of seven patients had additional VCFs, presumably related to focal vertebral osteonecrosis secondary to the injection of a large amount of ethanol (40 and 50 mL, respectively) (65). Use of PV before the injection of ethanol prevents such a complication by providing structural reinforcement of the vertebral body and by decreasing the amount of alcohol needed for sclerosing the VH (no more than 4 mL in our experience).

Percutaneous Vertebroplasty with Complementary Injection of Glue
In the presence of VH associated with an epidural component and acute clinical signs of compression of the spinal cord or cauda equina, the goal of PV is to reinforce the vertebral body and to make laminectomy and surgical excision of the epidural hemangioma easier by completely devascularizing the VH. This goal is accomplished by combining a PV procedure accompanied by an injection of N-butyl cyanoacrylate glue (opacified) on day 1 and surgery on day 2 (53,63).

The PV with glue procedure has five steps. First, the vertebral body invaded by the VH (Figure 10.17A) is injected with acrylic cement via a unilateral or bilateral transpedicular approach. Second, an 18-gauge needle is inserted into the remaining VH that has not been injected with acrylic cement (Figure 10.17B). Third, the predictable distribution of the glue is checked by the slow injection of up to 4 mL of contrast media. Fourth, after having carefully washed the needle with a nonionic solution (glucose serum) to avoid the early polymerization of the glue in the needle, 3 to 5 mL of the glue mixture is slowly injected under fluoroscopic control to fill the compressive epidural component of the lesion (Figure 10.17C). Fifth (if necessary), the percutaneous embolization of the remaining component of the VH is completed by injecting glue via one or several needles inserted into the posterior neural arch (Figure 10.17D,E). Laminectomy and surgical excision of the epidural component of the VH (simplified by the PV) is usually planned for the following day (Figure 10.17F). (Editor's note: Thus far this aggressive therapy has only been reported in France).

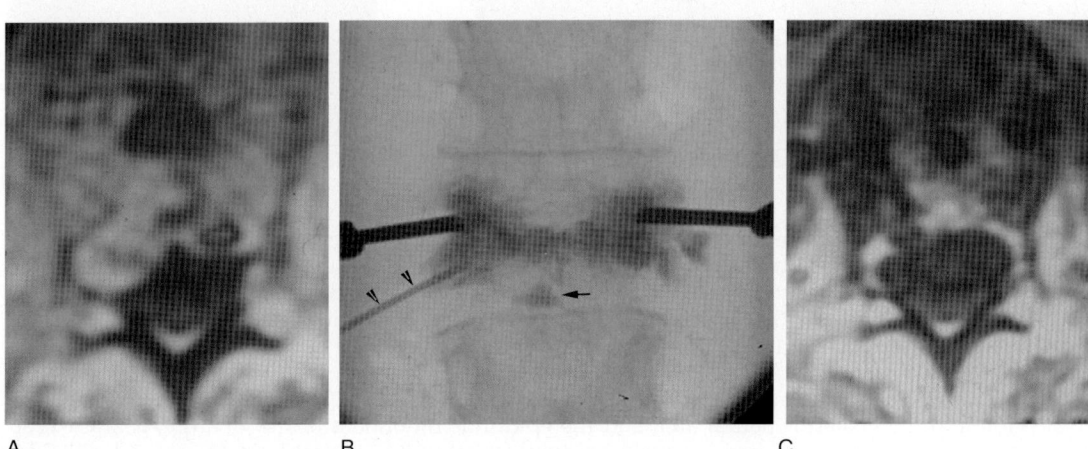

Figure 10.16. This patient had an aggressive VH with an epidural component. **(A)** Preoperative T1-weighted MR image. **(B)** Anteroposterior view showing injection of the vertebral body part of the VH with acrylic cement. An 18-gauge needle was inserted into a part of the vertebral body that was not injected with cement (black arrowheads), and alcohol was injected into the remaining part of the VH. Note the leakage of cement into the adjacent discs (black arrow). **(C)** Resolution of the epidural VH 3 months after PV. (From J.M. Mathis, H. Deramond, and S.M. Belkoff [eds], Percutaneous Vertebroplasty. New York: Springer, 2002, with permission.)

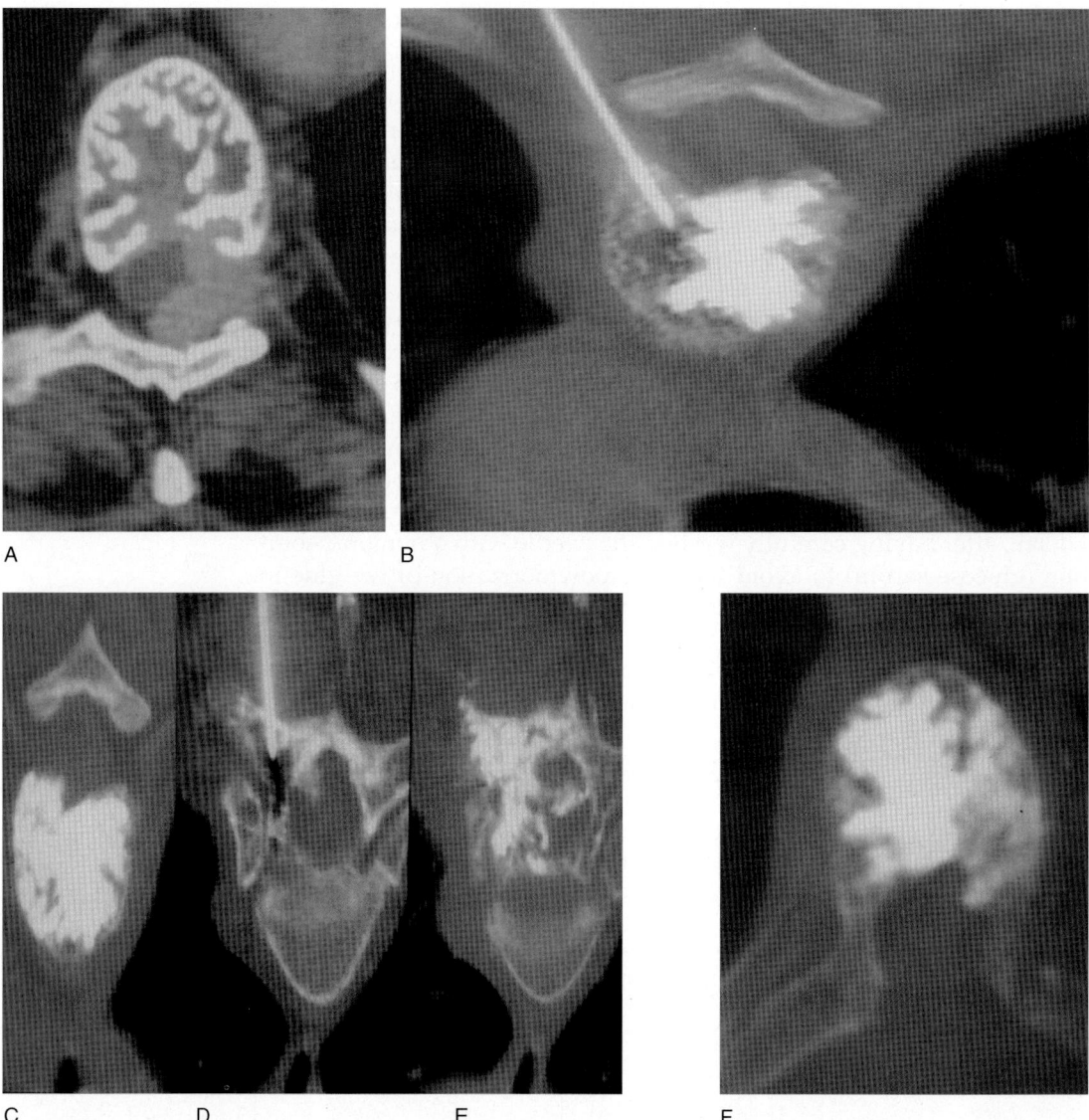

Figure 10.17. This patient presented with an acute spinal cord compression related to an aggressive thoracic VH. **(A)** Axial CT scan before PV. **(B)** Axial CT scan of the injection of acrylic cement into three quarters of the vertebral body part affected by the VH. Under CT guidance, an 18-gauge needle was inserted into the portion of the vertebral body lesion not injected with cement. **(C)** Axial CT scan showing the distribution of glue in the remaining part of the vertebral body but without injection of the epidural component. **(D)** Axial CT scan showing the insertion under CT guidance of an 18-gauge needle into the posterior neural arch invaded by the VH. **(E)** Axial CT scan showing the distribution of the glue into the posterior neural arch and the epidural component of the VH. **(F)** Axial CT scan after surgical laminectomy and excision of the epidural VH. (From J.M. Mathis, H. Deramond, and S.M. Belkoff [eds], Percutaneous Vertebroplasty. New York: Springer, 2002, with permission.)

Alcohol or glue? In our experience, we think it might be possible to avoid surgery by using the PV with ethanol procedure, and using a sclerosing agent could allow a progressive and complete improvement of the neurologic signs and avoid the need for surgery.

Percutaneous Vertebroplasty with Computed Tomography
Gangi et al. (66) described the technique for PV using CT: The needle is placed precisely and safely under CT guidance, and the cement injection is performed under real-time fluoroscopic control. Most of the time, a good biplane fluoroscopy unit allows a fast and safe procedure for PV. However, when a complementary injection of absolute ethanol or glue is needed for the treatment of VHs, checking the distribution of the acrylic cement into the vertebral body and setting the 18-gauge needle into a part of the vertebral body not injected with cement or into the posterior neural arch requires the use of CT (Figure 10.17).

Results

In the first published cases, PV was used to treat VHs (3,62). Of those first 11 patients, 10 had complete relief of pain after the PV procedure. The literature documents substantial pain reduction in more than 80% of patients whose VHs were treated by PV (53,64,67,68).

Deramond et al. (53) have treated 61 patients with symptomatic VH. With a long-term follow-up period (up to 15 years), structural reinforcement was obtained in all patients, there was no change in the shape of the vertebral body, and relief of severe back pain was obtained by more than 90%. Only once did evolution of the epidural part of the VH occur. In that case, PV was conducted at the C2 level, and acrylic cement alone (with no sclerosing agent) was injected into the vertebral body. Early results were good, but after 3 years the epidural component suddenly increased, and the growth continued despite radiation therapy. The patient died 4 years later from neurologic complications (56).

A review of the results in terms of the classification groups described above shows the following: group 2 (38 patients; treated with PV), complete pain relief in more than 90% (35 patients), with no recurrence of the lesion; group 4a-i (12 patients; all treated with PV, five also treated with ethanol injection), all had cessation of progressive neurologic signs, no evolution (3 to 7 years of follow up) or recurrence of the epidural component (except for the first patient already described), and the epidural component disappeared in two of the five treated with ethanol; group 4a-ii (four patients; treated with PV, glue, and laminectomy), no evolution (3 to 7 years of follow up) or recurrence of epidural component, and disappearance of acute neurologic signs; group 4b (seven patients; treated with PV), complete relief of back pain in all patients and no change in the lesion.

Side Effects and Complications

In the first group of 54 patients with VH treated by PV, there were only two complications: both were intercostal neuralgias that healed after local injection with steroids and anesthetic (53). These complications were related to leakage of cement into foraminal veins and occurred among the first patients treated. One patient had been injected with cement having a low radio-opacity; the method was subsequently improved by adding tantalum powder (62). In the second patient, intercostal neuralgia was related to a leakage of cement along the track of a needle inserted via an intercostal posterolateral approach (Craig technique) (69), which irritated the adjacent nerve root. The transpedicular approach avoids this complication.

Percutaneous Vertebroplasty and Other Therapies

Radiation Therapy
Radiation therapy alone with fractionated doses under 4,000 cGy has been used to treat VH. (70,71). With these low doses, the risk of complication is low, but the rate of recurrence is approximately 50% (72). These considerations, combined with the efficacy of PV, have led us to believe that radiation therapy is no longer indicated for the treatment of VHs.

Laminectomy and Surgical Excision
Laminectomy and surgical excision of the epidural component of the lesion was the classic treatment for VH with neurologic signs (73,74). However, this surgery is often difficult because of the vascular nature of the lesion. In our experience, PV before surgery makes the excision easier and less risky. In addition, we think that for most patients with acute neurologic signs, PV combined with ethanol injection may obviate surgery.

Transarterial Embolization
Transarterial embolization (75) provides excellent short-term results for aggressive VHs. However, evolution and recurrence of the VH is frequent. It is the classic treatment before surgery, with the goal of decreasing preoperative bleeding, but it has variable efficacy. Moreover, transarterial embolization can be impossible or dangerous, with the risk of spinal cord infarction when a common artery supplies the VH and the spinal cord. In the early days of PV treatment, embolization was performed before PV (62,63), but it quickly became evident that that procedure was unnecessary because PV provides a far more efficient in situ filling of the vascular malformation.

References

1. Parlier-Cuau C, Champsaur P, Nizard R, et al. Percutaneous removal of osteoid osteoma. Radiol Clin North Am 1998; 36(3):559–566.
2. Gladden ML, Jr, Gillingham BL, Hennrikus W, et al. Aneurysmal bone cyst of the first cervical vertebrae in a child treated with percutaneous intralesional injection of calcitonin and methylprednisolone. A case report. Spine 2000; 25(4):527–530.
3. Galibert P, Deramond H, Rosat P, et al. [Preliminary note on the treatment of vertebral angioma by percutaneous acrylic vertebroplasty.] Neurochirurgie 1987; 33(2):166–168.

4. Cardon T, Hachulla E, Flipo RM, et al. Percutaneous vertebroplasty with acrylic cement in the treatment of a Langerhans cell vertebral histiocytosis. Clin Rheumatol 1994; 13(3):518–521.
5. Cotten A, Boutry N, Cortet B, et al. Percutaneous vertebroplasty: state of the art. RadioGraphics 1998; 18(2):311–323.
6. Abrams HL, Spiro R, Goldstein N. Metastases in carcinoma. Analysis of 1000 autopsied cases. Cancer 1950; 3:74–85.
7. Malawer MM, Delandy TF. Treatment of metastatic cancer to bone. In Cancer: Principles and Practice of Oncology, 8th Ed. VT DeVita, S Hellman, SA Rosenberg (eds). Philadelphia: JB Lippincott Co, 1989:2298–2317.
8. Bontoux D, Azais I. Cancer secondaire des os. Clinique et epidemiologie. In Cancer Secondaire des Os. D Bontoux, M Alcalay (eds). Paris: Expansion Scientifique Francaise, 1997:19–27.
9. Tubiana-Hulin M. Incidence, prevalence and distribution of bone metastases. Bone 1991; 12(Suppl 1):S9–S10.
10. Tatsui H, Onomura T, Morishita S, et al. Survival rates of patients with metastatic spinal cancer after scintigraphic detection of abnormal radioactive accumulation. Spine 1996; 21(18):2143–2148.
11. Deramond H, Depriester C, Toussaint P. [Vertebroplasty and percutaneous interventional radiology in bone metastases: techniques, indications, contra-indications.] Bull Cancer Radiother 1996; 83(4):277–282.
12. Weill A, Chiras J, Simon JM, et al. Spinal metastases: indications for and results of percutaneous injection of acrylic surgical cement. Radiology 1996; 199(1):241–247.
13. Cotten A, Dewatre F, Cortet B, et al. Percutaneous vertebroplasty for osteolytic metastases and myeloma: effects of the percentage of lesion filling and the leakage of methyl methacrylate at clinical follow-up. Radiology 1996; 200(2):525–530.
14. Shimony JS, Gilula LA, Zeller AJ, Brown DB. Percutaneous vertebroplasty for malignant compression fractures with epidural involvement. Radiology 2004; 232(3):846–853.
15. Belkoff SM, Mathis JM, Jasper LE, et al. The biomechanics of vertebroplasty: the effect of cement volume on mechanical behavior. Spine 2001; 26(14): 1537–1541.
16. Martin JB, Wetzel SG, Seium Y, et al. Percutaneous vertebroplasty in metastatic disease: transpedicular access and treatment of lysed pedicles. Initial experience. Radiology 2003; 229:593–597.
17. Lapras C, Mottolese C, Deruty R, et al. [Percutaneous injection of methylmethacrylate in osteoporosis and severe vertebral osteolysis (Galibert's technic).] Ann Chir 1989; 43(5):371–376.
18. Kaemmerlen P, Thiesse P, Bouvard H, et al. [Percutaneous vertebroplasty in the treatment of metastases. Technic and results.] J Radiol 1989; 70(10):557–562.
19. Kaemmerlen P, Thiesse P, Jonas P, et al. Percutaneous injection of orthopedic cement in metastatic vertebral lesions [letter]. N Engl J Med 1989; 321(2):121.
20. Cortet B, Cotten A, Boutry N, et al. Percutaneous vertebroplasty in patients with osteolytic metastases or multiple myeloma [see comments]. Rev Rhum Engl Ed 1997; 64(3):177–183.
21. Fourney DR, Schomer DF, Nader R, et al. Percutaneous vertebroplasty and kyphoplasty for painful vertebral body fractures in cancer patients. J Neurosurg Spine 2003; 98(1):21–30.
22. Deramond H, Wright NT, Belkoff SM. Temperature elevation caused by bone cement polymerization during vertebroplasty. Bone 1999; 25(Suppl 2):17S–21S.

23. San Millan RD, Burkhardt K, Jean B, et al. Pathology findings with acrylic implants. Bone 1999; 25(Suppl 2):85S–90S.
24. Chiras J, Depriester C, Weill A, et al. [Percutaneous vertebral surgery. Technics and indications.] J Neuroradiol 1997; 24(1):45–59.
25. Shepherd S. Radiotherapy and the management of metastatic bone pain. Clin Radiol 1988; 39(5):547–550.
26. Salazar OM, Rubin P, Hendrickson FR, et al. Single-dose half-body irradiation for the palliation of multiple bone metastases from solid tumors: a preliminary report. Int J Radiat Oncol Biol Phys 1981; 7:773–781.
27. Chow E, Holden L, Danjoux C, et al. Successful salvage using percutaneous vertebroplasty in cancer patients with painful spinal metastases or osteoporotic compression fractures. Radiother Oncol 2004; 70(3):265–267.
28. Murray JA, Bruels MC, Lindberg RD. Irradiation of polymethylmethacrylate. In vitro gamma radiation effect. J Bone Joint Surg 1974; 56A(2):311–312.
29. Riley LH, Frassica DA, Kostuik JP, et al. Metastatic disease to the spine: diagnosis and treatment. Instr Course Lect 2000; 49:471–477.
30. Gangi A, Guth S, Dietemann JL, et al. Interventional musculoskeletal procedures. RadioGraphics 2001; 21(2):520.
31. Meder JF, Reizine D, Chiras J, et al. Apport de l'artériographie dans le diagnostic et la traitement des tumeurs du rachis. Rachis 1992; 4(4):215–228.
32. Gronemeyer DH, Schirp S, Gevargez A. Image-guided radiofrequency ablation of spinal tumors: preliminary experience with an expandable array electrode. Cancer J 2002; 8(1):33–39.
33. Schaefer O, Lohrmann C, Markmiller M, et al. Technical innovation. Combined treatment of a spinal metastasis with radiofrequency heat ablation and vertebroplasty. Am J Roentgenol 2003; 180(4):1075–1077.
34. Longo DL. Plasma cell disorders. In Harrison's Principles of Internal medicine, 12th Ed. JD Wilson, E Braunwald, KJ Isselbacher, et al (eds). New York: McGraw-Hill, 1991:1412–1416.
35. Bataille R, Chappard D, Klein B. Mechanisms of bone lesions in multiple myeloma. Hematol Oncol Clin North Am 1992; 6(2):285–295.
36. Lecouvet FE, Van de Berg BC, Maldague BE, et al. Vertebral compression fractures in multiple myeloma. Part I. Distribution and appearance at MR imaging [see comments]. Radiology 1997; 204(1):195–199.
37. Salmon SE, Cassady JR. Plasma cell neoplasms. In Cancer: Principles and Practice of Oncology, 4th Ed. VT DeVita, S Hellman, SA Rosenberg (eds). Philadelphia: JB Lippincott Co, 1993:1984–2025.
38. de Gramont A, Benitez O, Brissaud P, et al. Quantification of bone lytic lesions and prognosis in myelomatosis. Scand J Haematol 1985; 34(1):78–82.
39. Kanis JA, McCloskey EV. Disorders of calcium metabolism and their management. In Myeloma: Biology and Management. JS Malpas, DE Bergsagel, RA Kyle (eds). New York: Oxford University Press, 1995: 375–396.
40. Kapadia SB. Multiple myeloma: a clinicopathologic study of 62 consecutively autopsied cases. Medicine (Baltimore) 1980; 59(5):380–392.
41. Kyle RA. Multiple myeloma: review of 869 cases. Mayo Clin Proc 1975; 50(1):29–40.
42. Carson CP, Ackerman LV, Maltby JD. Plasma cell myeloma: a clinical, pathologic, and roentgenologic review of 90 cases. Am J Clin Pathol 1955; 25:849–888.
43. Riccardi A, Gobbi PG, Ucci G, et al. Changing clinical presentation of multiple myeloma. Eur J Cancer 1991; 27(11):1401–1405.
44. Spiess JL, Adelstein DJ, Hines JD. Multiple myeloma presenting with spinal cord compression. Oncology 1988; 45(2):88–92.

45. Lecouvet FE, Malghem J, Michaux L, et al. Vertebral compression fractures in multiple myeloma. Part II. Assessment of fracture risk with MR imaging of spinal bone marrow [see comments]. Radiology 1997; 204(1):201–205.
46. Moulopoulos LA, Dimopoulos MA, Weber D, et al. Magnetic resonance imaging in the staging of solitary plasmacytoma of bone. J Clin Oncol 1993; 11(7):1311–1315.
47. Knowling MA, Harwood AR, Bergsagel DE. Comparison of extramedullary plasmacytomas with solitary and multiple plasma cell tumors of bone. J Clin Oncol 1983; 1(4):255–262.
48. Chak LY, Cox RS, Bostwick DG, et al. Solitary plasmacytoma of bone: treatment, progression, and survival. J Clin Oncol 1987; 5(11):1811–1815.
49. Frassica DA, Frassica FJ, Schray MF, et al. Solitary plasmacytoma of bone: Mayo Clinic experience. Int J Radiat Oncol Biol Phys 1989; 16(1):43–48.
50. Dimopoulos MA, Goldstein J, Fuller L, et al. Curability of solitary bone plasmacytoma. J Clin Oncol 1992; 10(4):587–590.
51. Holland J, Trenkner DA, Wasserman TH, et al. Plasmacytoma. Treatment results and conversion to myeloma. Cancer 1992; 69(6):1513–1517.
52. Murphy KJ, Deramond H. Percutaneous vertebroplasty in benign and malignant disease. Neuroimaging Clin North Am 2000; 10(3):535–545.
53. Deramond H, Depriester C, Galibert P, et al. Percutaneous vertebroplasty with polymethylmethacrylate. Technique, indications, and results. Radiol Clin North Am 1998; 36(3):533–546.
54. Huvos HG. Multiple myeloma including solitary osseous myeloma. In Bone Tumors: Diagnosis, Treatment, and Prognosis. Philadelphia: WB Saunders Co, 1992:653–676.
55. Plowman PN. Radiotherapy of myeloma. In Myeloma: Biology and Management. JS Malpas, DE Bergsagel, RA Kyle (eds). New York: Oxford University Press, 1995:314–321.
56. Lecouvet F, Richard F, Vande Berg B, et al. Long-term effects of localized spinal radiation therapy on vertebral fractures and focal lesions appearance in patients with multiple myeloma. Br J Haematol 1997; 96(4):743–745.
57. Hoskin PJ. Radiotherapy in the management of bone pain. Clin Orthop 1995; 312:105–119.
58. Schmorl G, Junghans H. The Human Spine in Health and Disease, 2nd Ed. EF Besemann (ed, tr). New York: Grune & Stratton, 1971.
59. Laredo JD, Assouline E, Gelbert F, et al. Vertebral hemangiomas: fat content as a sign of aggressiveness. Radiology 1990; 177(2):467–472.
60. Laredo JD, Reizine D, Bard M, et al. Vertebral hemangiomas: radiologic evaluation. Radiology 1986; 161(1):183–189.
61. Ware JE, Jr., Snow KK, Kosinski M, et al. SF-36 Health Survey. Manual and Interpretation Guide. Boston: The Health Institute, 1993.
62. Deramond H, Darrason R, Galibert P. [Percutaneous vertebroplasty with acrylic cement in the treatment of aggressive spinal angiomas.] Rachis 1989; 1(2):143–153.
63. Cotten A, Deramond H, Cortet B, et al. Preoperative percutaneous injection of methyl methacrylate and N-butyl cyanoacrylate in vertebral hemangiomas. Am J Neuroradiol 1996; 17(1):137–142.
64. Heiss JD, Doppman JL, Oldfield EH. Brief report: relief of spinal cord compression from vertebral hemangioma by intralesional injection of absolute ethanol [see comments]. N Engl J Med 1994; 331(8):508–511.
65. Heiss JD, Doppman JL, Oldfield EH. Treatment of vertebral hemangioma by intralesional injection of absolute ethanol [letter; comment]. N Engl J Med 1996; 334(20):1340.

66. Gangi A, Kastler BA, Dietemann JL. Percutaneous vertebroplasty guided by a combination of CT and fluoroscopy. Am J Neuroradiol 1994; 15(1): 83–86.
67. Ide C, Gangi A, Rimmelin A, et al. Vertebral haemangiomas with spinal cord compression: the place of preoperative percutaneous vertebroplasty with methyl methacrylate. Neuroradiology 1996; 38(6):585–589.
68. Martin JB, Jean B, Sugiu K, et al. Vertebroplasty: clinical experience and follow-up results. Bone 1999; 25(Suppl 2):11S–15S.
69. Craig FS. Vertebral-body biopsy. J Bone Joint Surg 1956; 38A(1):93–102.
70. Yang ZY, Zhang LJ, Chen ZX, et al. Hemangioma of the vertebral column. A report on twenty-three patients with special reference to functional recovery after radiation therapy. Acta Radiol Oncol 1985; 24(2):129–132.
71. Pavlovitch JM, Nguyen JP, Djindjian M, et al. Radiotherapy of compressive vertebral hemangiomas. Neurochirurgie 1989; 35:296–298.
72. Nguyen JP, Djindjian M, Pavlovitch JM, et al. Vertebral hemangiomas with neurologic symptoms. Treatment. Results of the "Societe Francaise de Neuro-Chirurgie" series. Neurochirurgie 1989; 35:299–303.
73. Nguyen JP, Djindjian M, Gaston A, et al. Vertebral hemangiomas presenting with neurologic symptoms. Surg Neurol 1987; 27(4):391–397.
74. Nguyen JP, Djindjian M, Badiane S. Vertebral hemangiomas with neurologic symptoms. Clinical presentation. Results of the "Societe Francaise de Neurochirurgie" series. Neurochirurgie 1989; 35:270–274.
75. Picard L, Bracard S, Roland J, et al. [Embolization of vertebral hemangioma. Technic-indications-results.] Embolisation des hemangiomes vertebraux. Technique-indications-resultats. Neurochirurgie 1989; 35(5):289–293.

11
Extreme Vertebroplasty: Techniques for Treating Difficult Lesions

John D. Barr and John M. Mathis

For most patients, the standard techniques for performing percutaneous vertebroplasty (PV) work very well. However, for patients with malignant disease causing severe cortical destruction, the usual techniques may be associated with a high incidence of cement extravasation and complications. Osteoporotic patients presenting with very severe vertebral body compression are also a treatment challenge. Certain modifications of the usual techniques may provide a better treatment for both of these types of patients.

Computed Tomography and Fluoroscopy

Percutaneous vertebroplasty is useful for selected patients with pain due to vertebral column malignancies, particularly patients who are poor surgical candidates and those with limited anticipated survival. Percutaneous vertebroplasty may be performed to provide analgesia, spinal stabilization, or both. With the traditional fluoroscopically guided technique, PV for neoplastic lesions results in more complications than PV for osteoporotic vertebral compression fractures (VCFs) (1). Most complications associated with PV for neoplastic lesions are secondary to extravasation of cement through cortical bone destroyed by the tumor or extrusion of tumor during cement injection. The probability of symptomatic cement extravasation increases markedly when an osteolytic lesion breaches the cortical barrier to the spinal canal or neural foramen (2,3). The risk that even small cement extravasations will be symptomatic is increased in the presence of spinal canal compromise (preexisting tumor invading the spinal canal) or when the treatment involves an upper thoracic or cervical vertebra (due to inherent anatomic factors, including small vertebrae and the presence of the spinal cord). To reduce the risk of extravasation, it is imperative that a properly opacified cement and high-quality imaging equipment are used. Even so, fluoroscopy alone may not provide sufficient resolution to visualize small, potentially symptomatic cement extravasations. In such complex and high-risk cases, that is, when the posterior vertebral wall is disrupted (Figure 11.1) or when upper thoracic and cervical vertebral bodies are to be treated, a procedure using combined computed tomography (CT) and fluoroscopic guidance may be useful (4).

Gangi and colleagues (5) were the first to describe the use of a combination of CT and fluoroscopic guidance for PV of both VCFs and osteolytic neoplasms. This technique typically uses a CT scanner in combination with a portable c-arm angiography system (4). The primary advantage of using CT with fluoroscopy is that the CT scanner provides images that allow the operating physician to assess the three-dimensional distribution of the injected cement in exquisite detail (Figure 11.2). By noting the proximity of the cement to the posterior vertebral margin (and epidural space), the operating physician can determine the need for, and safety of, injecting additional cement. The occurrence of posterior wall destruction increases the problem of cement extravasation during treatment. Additionally, tumor may be extruded through the bone defect and cause compression of the thecal sac and cord. The tumor is tissue dense and may be missed with either fluoroscopy or CT. Therefore, we recommend that the thecal sac be defined with myelographic contrast. In the lumbar spine, this may allow adequate visualization with fluoroscopy, as the myelographic contrast can be collected in the lumbar lordosis and any compression of the thecal may be seen (Figure 11.3). In other parts of the spine, the myelographic contrast may not be localized in sufficient quantity for fluoroscopic monitoring. In these cases, CT is again used to look for extravasation of either cement or tumor (Figure 11.4). To minimize the effect of extravasation during the injection, cement volumes injected

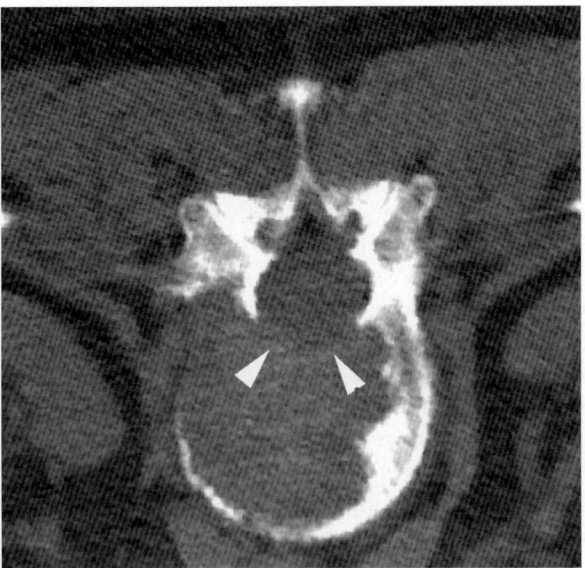

Figure 11.1. Computed tomography images of an L1 vertebra with trabecular and cortical destruction secondary to multiple myeloma. The preoperative scan shows complete destruction of the posterior cortical wall (white arrowheads).

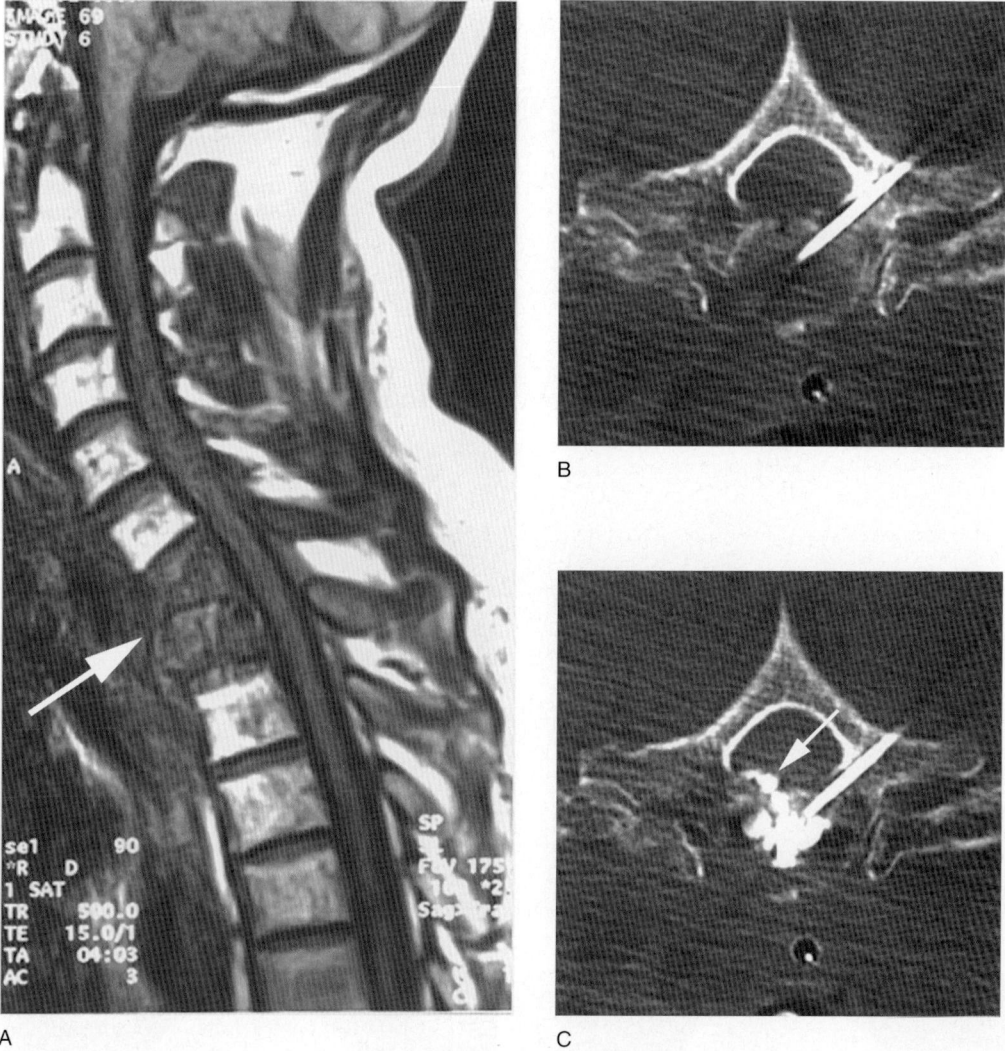

Figure 11.2. This patient's C7 and T1 were infiltrated by a metastatic, mediastinal sarcoma. **(A)** Sagittal T1-weighted magnetic resonance image showing tumor infiltration (white arrow) at C7 and T1. The collapse of these vertebrae was associated with intractable pain. Visualization of this area fluoroscopically was nearly impossible because of shoulders. **(B)** Computed tomography image showing needle placed via a posterior transpedicular approach. **(C)** Computed tomography image during PV revealed a very small epidural leak of cement (white arrow). The injection was terminated, and the patient had good pain relief without a clinical complication.

between CT scans are limited to 0.1–0.2 mL. Even if a leak occurs, these small volumes will protect against a clinically significant event.

When treating the small upper thoracic vertebrae (see Figure 11.2)—areas that are commonly obscured by the shoulders on fluoroscopic images—the operating physician can obtain CT images showing the precise location of the needles for cement delivery. Similarly, the imaging capability of CT may be needed for the cervical spine because

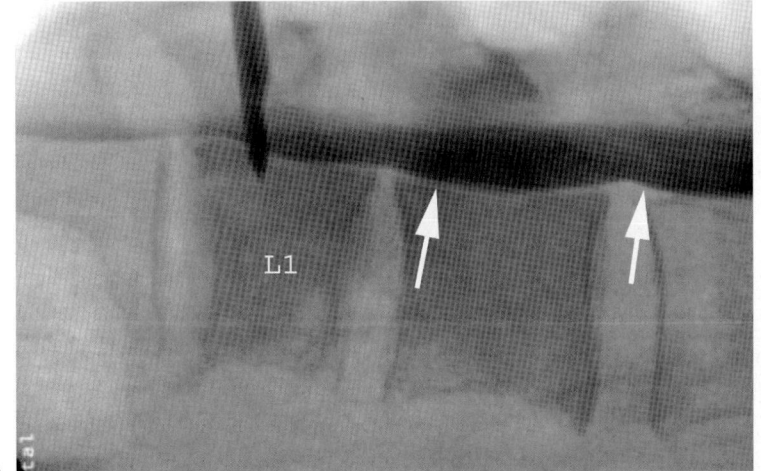

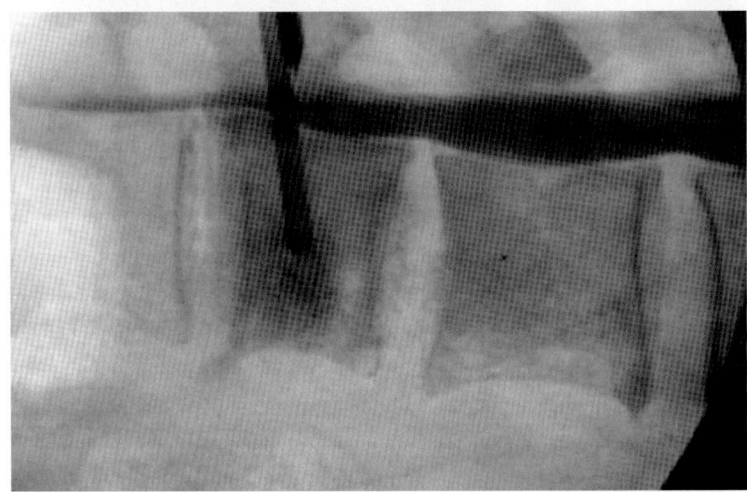

Figure 11.3. This patient had myeloma with compression of the L1 vertebra resulting in severe pain. **(A)** Lateral radiograph after the thecal sac was marked by injected myelographic contrast (white arrows). **(B)** During cement injection the contrast column marking the thecal sac can be observed for indentation or compression, which would indicate extrusion of tumor. None was seen during this procedure.

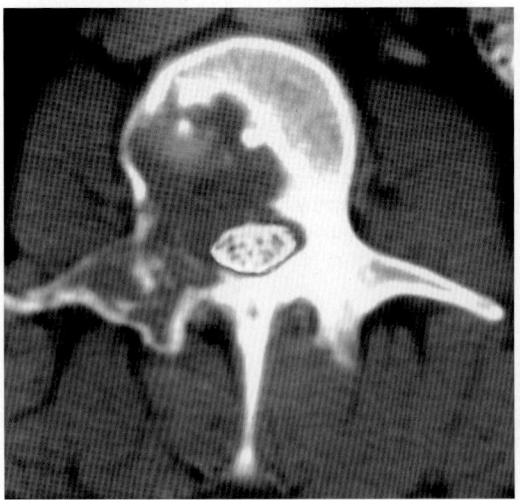 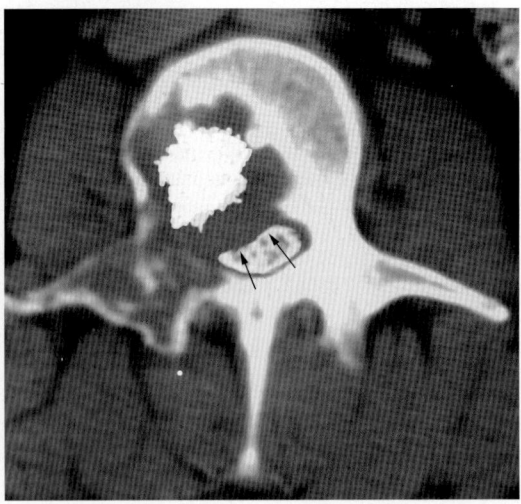

Figure 11.4. This patient has malignant destruction of a lumbar vertebra with absence of part of the posterior vertebral wall. **(A)** Computed tomography scan showing the partially destroyed vertebra and myelographic contrast present marking the thecal sac. **(B)** Computed tomography scan after bone cement has been injected. There is no cement leak, but tumor has been extruded into the epidural space by the cement, creating early deformity of the thecal sac (black arrows). Being able to see the thecal sac allows the operator to monitor the cement injection and stop injecting if either cement or tumor is displaced into areas that are not desired. (A, from J.M. Mathis, Am J Neuroradiol 24:1697–1706, 2003, with permission.)

of the small size of the vertebra and because of the critical structures that must be avoided (i.e., cervical cord and carotid and vertebral vessels).

With combined CT and fluoroscopic imaging, either fluoroscopy or CT is used for the initial needle placement. When precise anatomic visualization is needed for needle placement (e.g., near the carotid artery), the patient is positioned in the CT scanner and the needle is placed using CT guidance. Safe placement of the larger gauge cement delivery needle may be aided in this situation by first introducing a small 20- to 22-gauge guide needle. If a long needle (20 cm) is selected (and the hub removed) (Figure 11.5A), this smaller needle then becomes a guide for subsequent introduction of the larger cement delivery device using coaxial exchange (Figure 11.5C). After the larger needle is introduced to the bone surface over the guide needle, the guide is removed and the trocar or stylet reintroduced. The cement delivery needle is then introduced into the bone. The patient may be removed from the scanner so that cement injection can begin under fluoroscopic monitoring. Alternatively, cement can be injected using the CT for guidance. The injection of very small quantities (0.1 to 0.2 mL) of cement may take place with intermittent visualization with CT. This technique can detect leaks while still small and allows non-real-time monitoring with safety. Scans need to include more than just a central vertebral location to ensure that leaks outside the scan plane are not missed.

There are several disadvantages to the combined CT–fluoroscopy technique. Patients almost always need general anesthesia because most types of CT imaging are very sensitive to patient motion. Although transferring the patient in and out of the CT gantry can be done quickly with some practice, it is an added step and consumes time. It may be more efficient to leave the patient in the scan plane if CT alone is being used. Furthermore, when the patient is outside of the scanner, the fluoroscope is limited to producing images in the lateral plane because of interference caused by the CT table on which the patient is positioned. The use of CT is also markedly more expensive than fluoroscopy alone. For these reasons, the use of CT is limited to the extraordinary (not routine) cases.

Notwithstanding the above-mentioned disadvantages, combined CT and fluoroscopy may help reduce the incidence of complications in difficult cases. For example, Barr et al. (4) reported on eight patients who underwent treatment for malignant lesions in 13 vertebrae. Four vertebrae (in three patients) without cortical destruction were treated with the usual fluoroscopically guided technique. The modified technique of combined CT and fluoroscopic guidance was used to treat nine involved vertebrae in five patients. In four of these patients, eight vertebrae had posterior cortical disruption (see Figures 11.1 and 11.2). No symptomatic complications were observed in any of the patients so treated. Although these results are encouraging, the number of patients who have been managed with combined CT and fluoroscopy is too small to establish the efficacy of the procedure and make meaningful comparisons with the use of fluoroscopy alone.

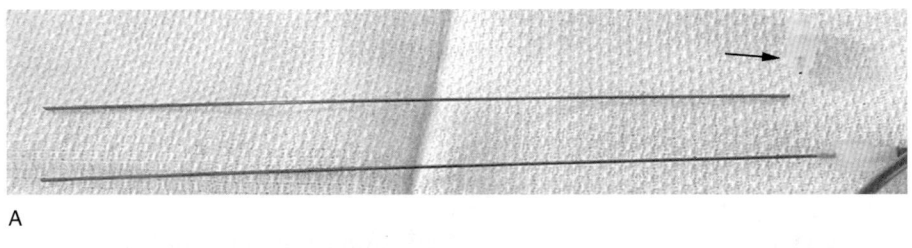

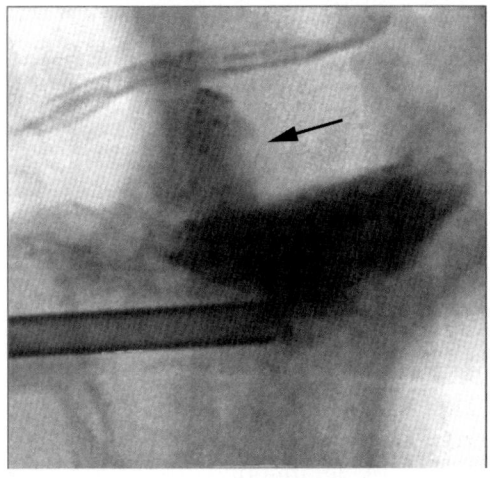

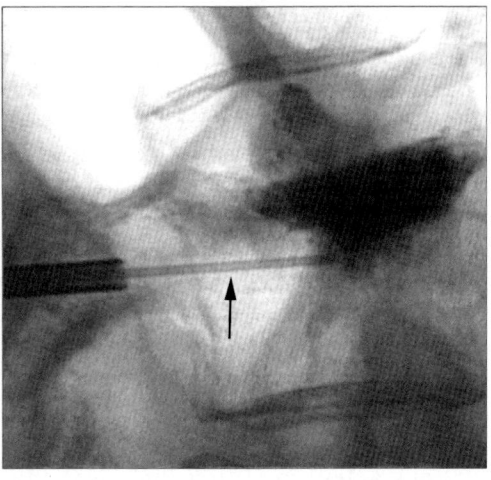

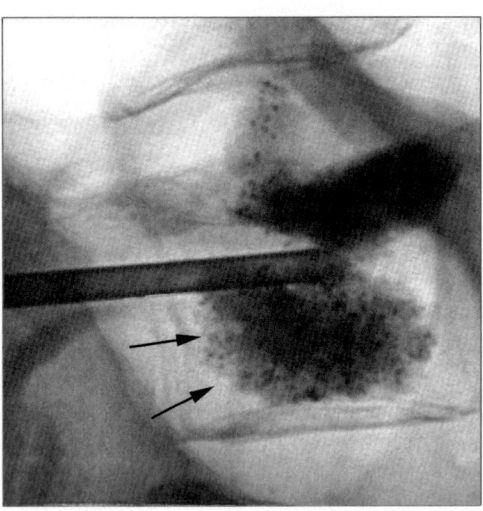

Figure 11.5. **(A)** A photograph of 10-inch, 20-gauge needles that can be used as guiding devices for cannula exchange. The hub must be removed (black arrow) to allow the cannula to slide over the wire. **(B)** A fluoroscopic image showing cement leak into the disc space (black arrow). The cement was allowed to harden and the cannula exchanged over a wire so that subsequent cement injection could take place. **(C)** The new cannula is being inserted over the wire (black arrow) used for the cannula exchange. **(D)** Additional cement injected (black arrows) now spreads into the bone and allows good filling of the vertebra without additional leak into the disc.

An alternative to combined CT and fluoroscopy is the use of CT-fluoroscopy, which allows real-time monitoring of the needle placement and cement injection (6). Limitations of this technique include the difficulty of positioning the needle and performing the cement injection with the patient in the CT scanner. If needle positioning and cement injection are prolonged, radiation doses to the physician and the patient may be undesirably high.

Coaxial Needle Placement and Exchange

Coaxial needle placement was described above. This technique may be used when extremely precise cannula placement is needed. Coaxial needle exchange consists of using a small-diameter needle to serve as a guide wire for the subsequent placement of a large-diameter cannula for cement injection (7). The small-diameter needle, typically a 20-gauge, 20-cm Chiba, is placed under fluoroscopic or CT guidance. Guide needle position can be confirmed before attempting to place the larger bore cement delivery needle. The Chiba needle can also be used to administer the local anesthetic for the subsequent PV procedure. Just before cannula placement, the hub of the needle is removed, and a small skin incision is made around the needle. The cannula of a 13-gauge needle is then advanced over the 20-gauge needle to the bone cortex. The 20-gauge needle, which served as a guide wire, is exchanged for the trocar of the 13-gauge needle. The 13-gauge needle (cannula and trocar) is then advanced into the vertebral body in the usual fashion (Figure 11.5).

Coaxial needle exchange is also helpful when cement injection is interrupted because of a cement leak. Because injected cement usually follows the path of least resistance, it is not uncommon for cement to flow though a vertebral endplate fracture into the disc space or through osteolytic defects in patients with neoplastic disease. Such extravasations, provided they are small, can serve a useful purpose. If injection is halted and the cement is allowed to polymerize, it may seal the cortical defects and prevent further extravasation of cement. Unfortunately, as the cement polymerizes, it will also occlude the cannula being used for the injection. This problem can be overcome by exchanging the cement-filled cannula for a new cannula, allowing more cement to be injected subsequently. To achieve an easy exchange, a 20-gauge Chiba needle is placed through the cement-filled cannula into the vertebral body. The cannula is then removed. A new cannula is placed coaxially, using the Chiba needle as a guide wire. The Chiba needle is then removed. The small-diameter Chiba needle has insufficient surface area for cement adherence, and it can be easily removed even when touching hardened cement. After the initially injected cement has polymerized, the bone defect will have been sealed. A new batch of cement is usually necessary for the injection performed through the new cannula that has been placed by this exchange method. The needle exchange allows safe filling of the vertebra even when cement leaks are encountered.

Fracture Instability and Height Restoration

Technically successful PV results in lasting pain relief for most patients. However, pain is not the only clinically significant problem caused by VCFs. Based on data from a prospective 8-year study of 9,575 women, Kado and colleagues (8) reported a 23% to 34% increase in mortality for postmenopausal women with vertebral fractures (even if asymptomatic) relative to age-matched controls without fractures. Pulmonary disease, probably related to kyphosis, was the leading cause of death. Thus, restoration of vertebral height and the reduction or elimination of kyphosis are believed to be desirable therapeutic goals. Vertebral height restoration and reduction of kyphosis may be attained in some cases using patient positioning or external traction. Barr and Barr (9) noted that in some patients, there was fluoroscopically recognizable fracture instability that allowed vertebral body height restoration with hyperextension or traction (Figure 11.6). Thus, vertebral height loss and the resulting kyphosis may be a partially reversible effect of VCFs. (Indeed, height gain with PV seems to be generally similar to that reported with kyphoplasty.) Due to the generally frail structure of the spine in patients with osteoporosis, traction should be applied slowly and with the patient's cooperation to avoid injuries. Once vertebral body height has been regained and the patient is in hyperextension or in traction, the vertebral body can be injected with cement (Figure 11.6). Experience with VCF reduction using traction is limited, but acute fractures appear to be more reducible because they have not had time to undergo early healing. Even so, one 8-month-old fracture presenting as a nonunion was successfully reduced with this technique (9).

Treatment of Extreme Vertebral Collapse

In cases of extreme vertebral body collapse, that is, more than 70% loss of vertebral body height, PV becomes increasing difficult and kyphoplasty essentially impossible (10). The decision not to treat with PV was originally recommended because of the difficulty of needle placement in these severely collapsed vertebral bodies. However, recent experience suggests that accurate needle introduction into extremely collapsed vertebra is possible when using smaller (13-gauge or smaller) needles (11). Furthermore, it was noted that many of the extremely collapsed vertebral bodies are often more collapsed centrally (Figure 11.7; see Figure 2.17C) than laterally. The lateral sparing allows the operating physician to place needles into the remaining lateral trabecular space and to obtain acceptable and clinically useful vertebral reinforcement. Patients adequately treated in this manner may experience good pain relief (11). Even so, treating extremely collapsed vertebral bodies is more challenging than treating vertebral bodies with less height loss, and it likely carries a greater risk of technical or clinical failure. Patients with such conditions should be made aware of these risks, and the operating physician should attempt PV for such extreme

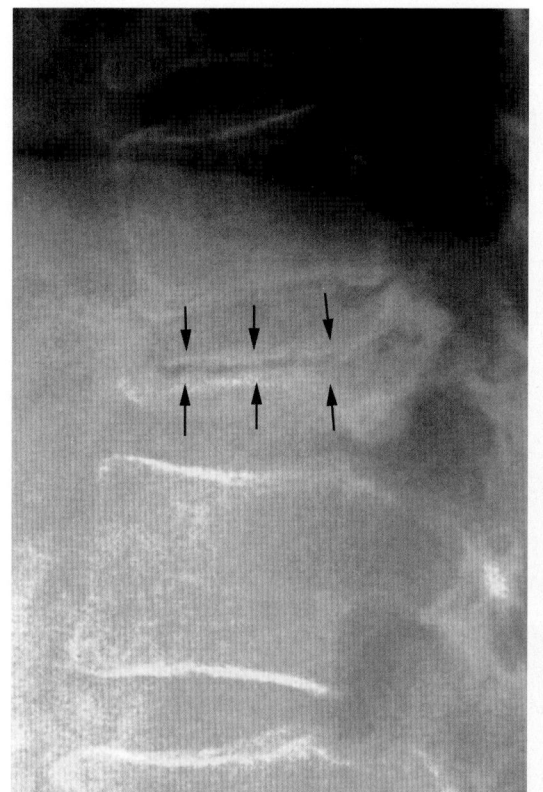
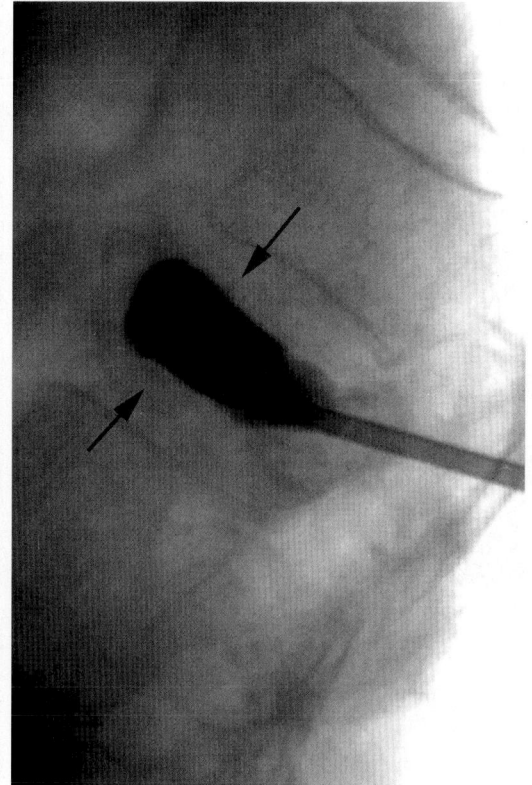
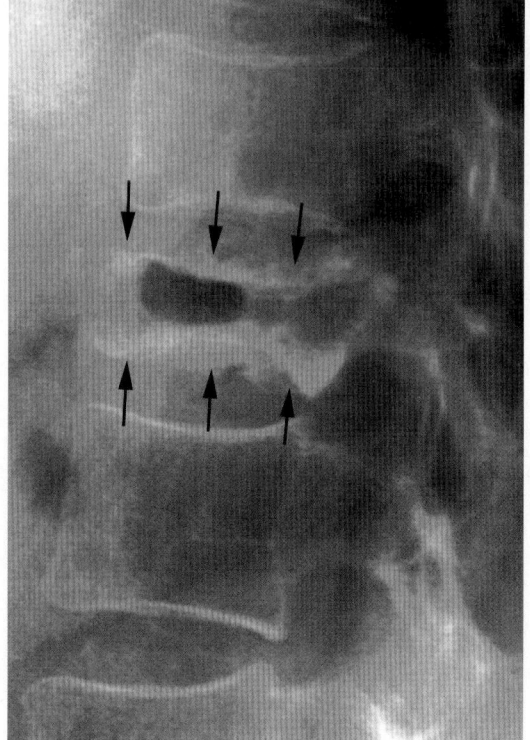

Figure 11.6. This patient had an extreme compression of T12 and continued severe pain 3 months after the fracture. **(A)** Lateral view showing the cortical margins of the compressed vertebra (black arrows). The faint dark line centrally was created by a central vacuum phenomenon. **(B)** Traction was applied to the shoulder and legs, and lateral fluoroscopy revealed partial height restoration of the T12 collapse. The black arrows highlight the cortical endplates. **(C)** Lateral fluoroscopic image during PV (after traction) shows cement filling the central cavity within the vertebra (black arrows). The height restoration achieved with traction was maintained. The patient's pain resolved after PV, and her clinical status was stable at 9 months follow-up.

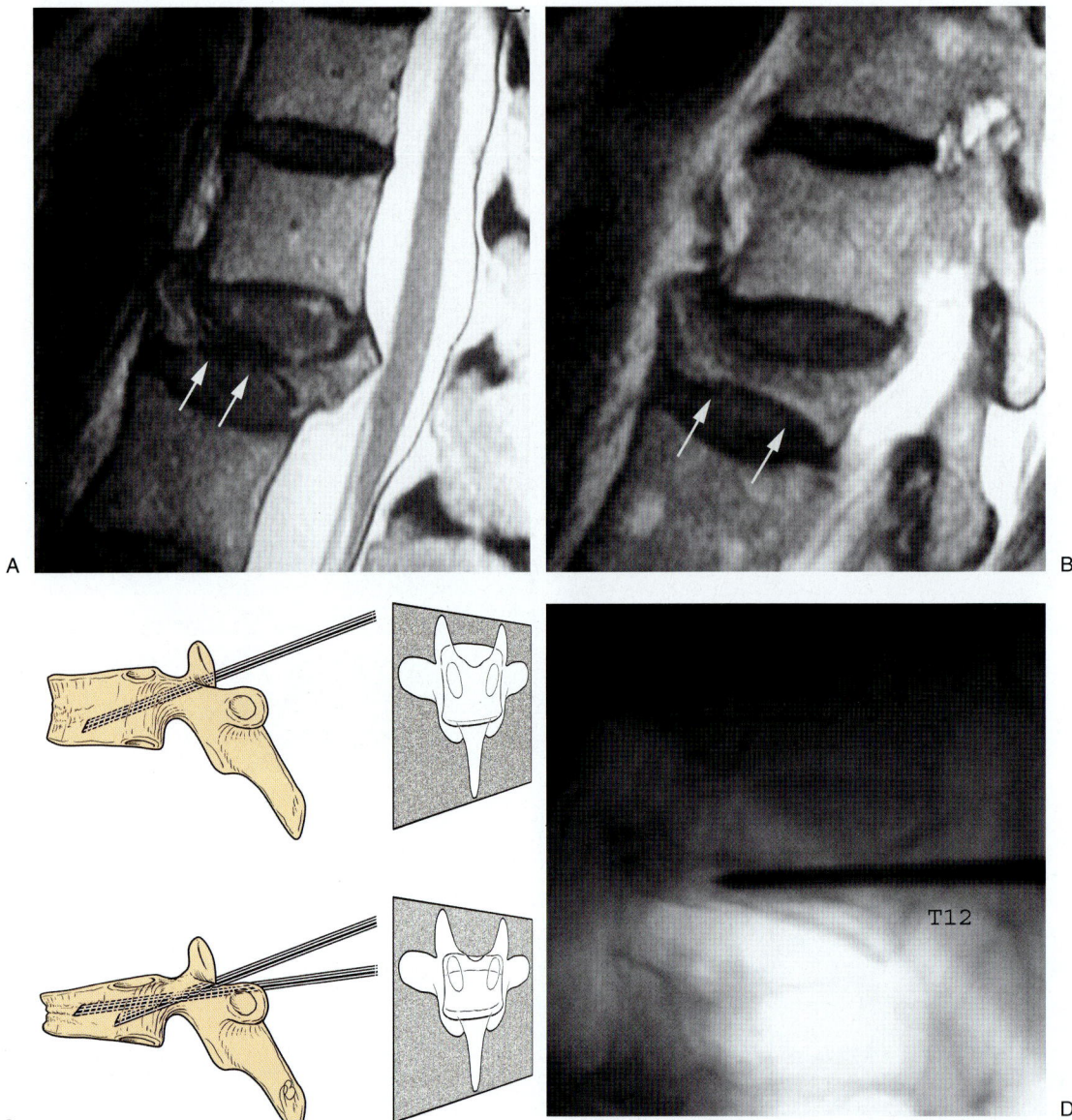

Figure 11.7. This patient had extreme compression of the T12 vertebra and severe pain at this level. **(A)** A T1-weighted sagittal magnetic resonance image (midline) showing severe central vertebral compression (white arrows). **(B)** A more lateral magnetic resonance image from the same series showing residual marrow space (white arrows) that would allow needle placement for PV. **(C)** Artist drawing shows how a less steep needle angle (one parallel to the vertebral endplates) is needed as compression increases. **(D,E)** Lateral **(D)** and anteroposterior **(E)** views of T12 after bilateral transpedicular needle placement (13-gauge needle). **(F,G)** Lateral images during and after PV show that a modest amount of cement was injected. This patient had good pain relief after this procedure.

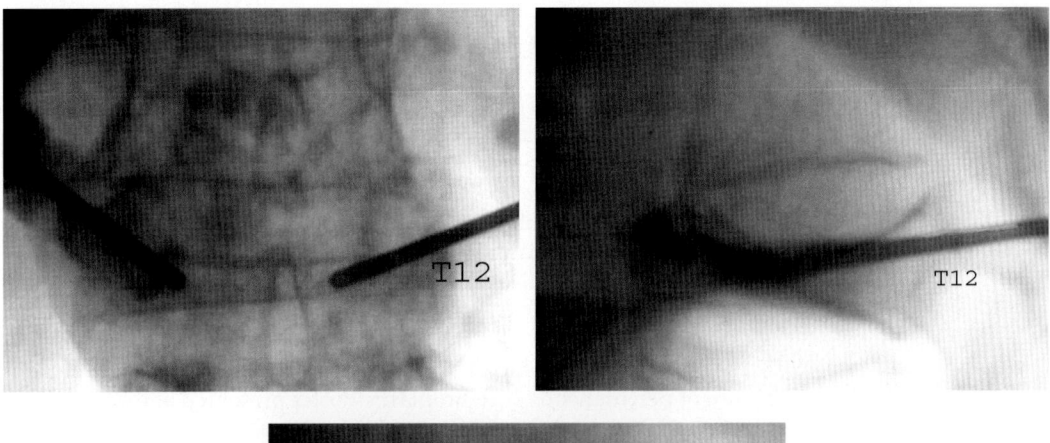

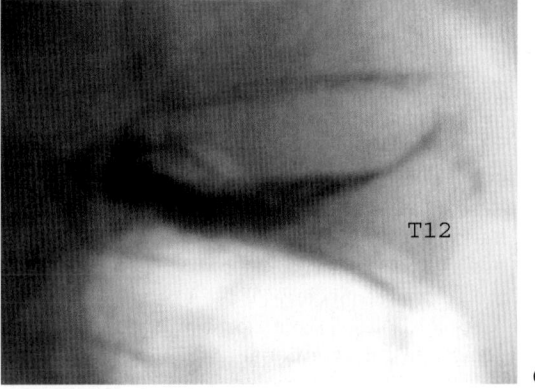

Figure 11.7. *Continued*

cases of collapse only after gaining substantial experience with more routine cases.

The severe collapse substantially alters the vertebral body anatomy. A bilateral transpedicular approach remains the preferred route for needle introduction. The fluoroscope must be positioned to visualize the pedicle over the collapsed vertebral body. Taking a trajectory through the lower aspect of the pedicle with an angle that allows one to access the anterior part of the vertebral body is crucial to successful needle placement (Figure 11.7C). This usually places the needle parallel to the residual endplates of the vertebra. The amount of cement that can be introduced into an extremely collapsed vertebra will be much smaller than is usually used for less collapsed vertebrae in the same spinal location (Figure 11.7F).

References

1. Chiras J, Depriester C, Weill A, et al. Percutaneous vertebral surgery. Technics and indications. J Neuroradiol 1997; 24(1):45–59.

2. Weill A, Chiras J, Simon JM, et al. Spinal metastases: indications for and results of percutaneous injection of acrylic surgical cement. Radiology 1996; 199(1):241–247.
3. Cotten A, Dewatre F, Cortet B, et al. Percutaneous vertebroplasty for osteolytic metastases and myeloma: effects of the percentage of lesion filling and the leakage of methyl methacrylate at clinical follow-up. Radiology 1996; 200(2):525–530.
4. Barr JD, Barr MS, Lemley TJ, et al. Percutaneous vertebroplasty for pain relief and spinal stabilization. Spine 2000; 25(8):923–928.
5. Gangi A, Kastler BA, Dietemann JL. Percutaneous vertebroplasty guided by a combination of CT and fluoroscopy. Am J Neuroradiol 1994; 15(1):83–86.
6. Barr JD, Barr MS, Lemley TJ. CT as the sole imaging modality for performance of percutaneous vertebroplasty. Poster presented at the 36th Annual Meeting of the American Society of Neuroradiology, Philadelphia, May 17–21, 1998.
7. Barr JD, Barr MS. Coaxial needle system for percutaneous vertebroplasty. Poster presented at the 38th Annual Meeting of the American Society of Neuroradiology, Atlanta, April 3–8, 2000.
8. Kado DM, Browner WS, Palermo L, et al. Vertebral fractures and mortality in older women: a prospective study. Study of Osteoporotic Fractures Research Group. Arch Intern Med 1999; 159(11):1215–1220.
9. Barr JD, Barr MS. Fluoroscopically visible vertebral fracture instability observed during vertebroplasty. Presented at the Joint Annual Meetings of the American Society of Neuroradiology, American Society of Head and Neck Radiology, American Society of Pediatric Neuroradiology, American Society of Interventional and Therapeutic Neuroradiology, and American Society of Spine Radiology, San Diego, May 23–28, 1999.
10. Mathis JM, Petri M, Naff N. Percutaneous vertebroplasty treatment of steroid-induced osteoporotic compression fractures. Arthritis Rheum 1998; 41(1):171–175.
11. Barr JD, Mervart M. Percutaneous vertebroplasty of vertebra plana. Poster presented at the 38th Annual Meeting of the American Society of Neuroradiology, Atlanta, April 3–8, 2000.

12
Sacroplasty

Keith Kortman, John M. Mathis, and A. Orlando Ortiz

Incidence

Spontaneous, pathologic fractures of the sacrum are now well known but were only recently described by Lourie (1) in 1982. Such injuries are often termed *insufficiency fractures*, indicating that bone strength is insufficient to withstand normal mechanical and physiologic forces (2). Sacral fractures may occur spontaneously in patients with osteoporosis, disorders of calcium metabolism, osseous metastatic disease, and prior radiation therapy. There is a strong (10:1) female predominance. The incidence of sacral insufficiency fractures is substantially less than that of osteoporotic fractures involving the lumbar and thoracic spine. Nevertheless, sacral fractures are estimated to make up 1%–2% of pathologic fractures involving the spine and pelvis. Thus, they are a frequent cause of debilitating pain, especially in elderly women.

Morbidity and Mortality

There are relatively few reported series of patients with sacral insufficiency fractures, the largest of which comprised 60 patients who required hospitalization for pain control (3). In that series, the average hospital stay of patients was 45 days. A long-term decrease in self-sufficiency was reported in 50% of patients. Twenty-five percent of patients were institutionalized, and there was a 14% 1-year mortality rate. Better outcomes have been reported in a number of smaller series (4–6).

Diagnosis

Sacral fractures are often misdiagnosed or go undiagnosed. This may be due to nonspecific symptomatology (7). Patients complain of severe low back and/or buttock pain, often acute in onset. A fall or direct trauma may be hard to elicit as part of the history. The pain is typically exacerbated by weight bearing. Referred pain to the hip or groin is common, especially in patients with concurrent fractures of the ischial and pubic rami. There can be coexistent vertebral compression fractures (Figure 12.1). Physical examination revealed nonspecific sacral tenderness and restricted mobility, indistinguishable from sacroiliac arthropathy and any number of other spinal and pelvic pathologic conditions.

Conventional spine radiographs are not sensitive enough to detect these fractures. Computed tomography is more sensitive (Figure 12.2) (8); however, acute, nondisplaced fractures without reactive sclerosis may still be relatively inconspicuous (9,10). Sacral fractures are typically well shown by bone scintigraphy (Figure 12.1) (10). An H-shaped pattern of increased uptake is typical and pathognomonic (11); however, radionuclide uptake along symmetric fracture lines may be mistaken for normal variation. Fracture patterns other than the typical

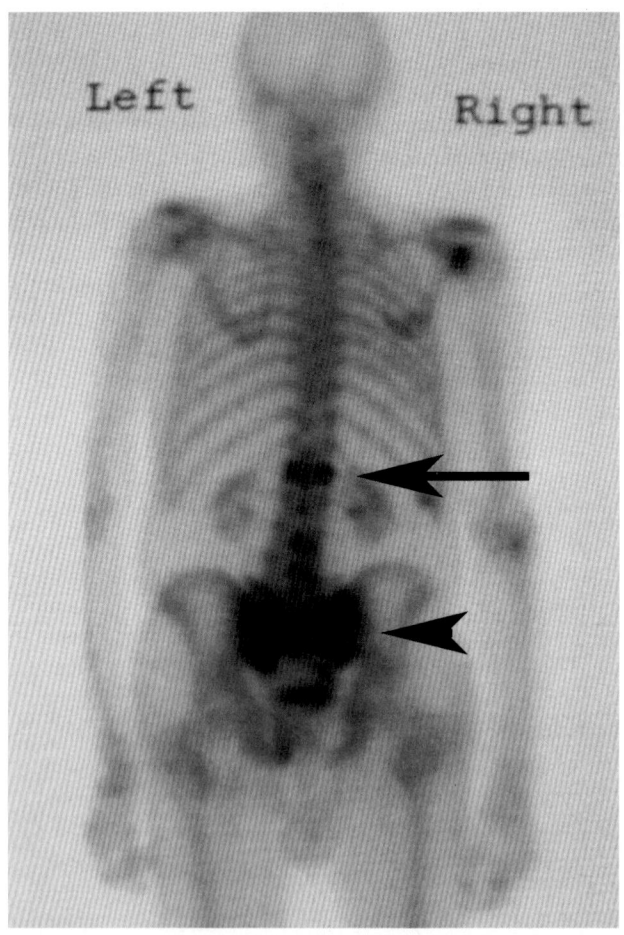

Figure 12.1. Bone scan showing the typical H-shaped sacral insufficiency fracture (black arrowhead) with abnormal activity in both sacral ala and the central body of the sacrum. A vertebral compression fracture coexists at L1 (black arrow).

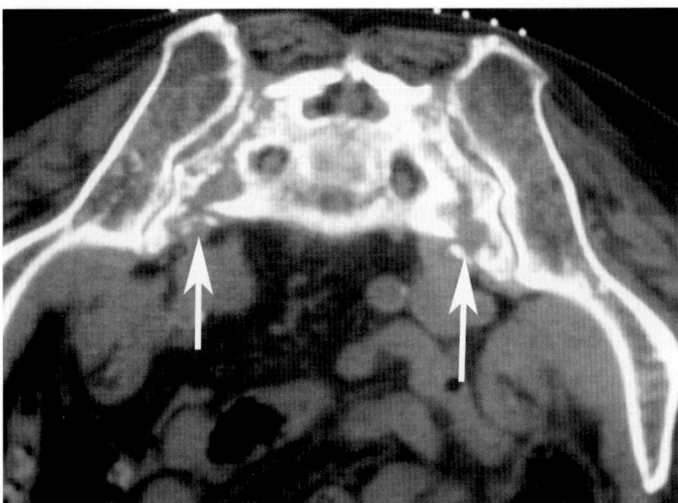

Figure 12.2. An axial CT scan of the sacrum shows bilateral fractures through the sacral ala (white arrows). The fracture lines are easily seen on CT.

H-shaped fracture also occur and may be more difficult to recognize with radionuclide scans.

Magnetic resonance imaging is both sensitive and specific in the demonstration of sacral fractures (12). Fractures are best shown in either sagittal or angled coronal planes. Marrow edema is conspicuously demonstrated on routine T1-weighted sequences (Figure 12.3A), with slightly greater sensitivity afforded by fat-suppressed T2-weighted or short T1 inversion recovery (STIR) sequences (Figure 12.3B). Sacral fractures are often detected as the result of a "corner call" at the bottom of a lumbar spine examination. When suspicion of a sacral fracture is sufficiently high, dedicated images centered on the sacrum with a small field-of-view are indicated.

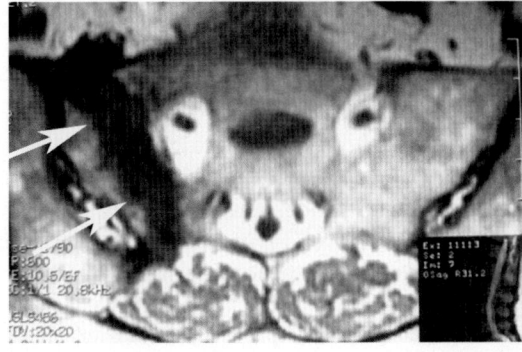 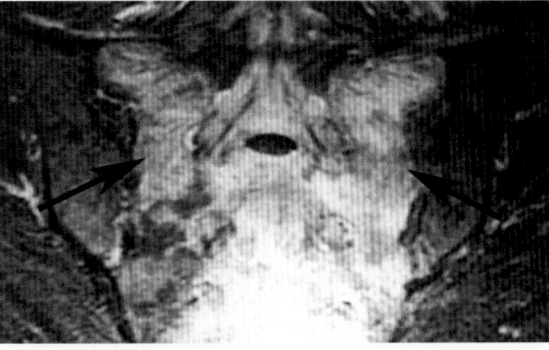

Figure 12.3. (A) Axial T1-weighted MRI demonstrates the low signal fracture through the right sacral wing (white arrows). The patient presented with a fracture on only one side. (B) Coronal inversion recovery magnetic resonance image shows high signal in both sacral ala (black arrows) and the central body. In this case, a typical H-shaped fracture is present.

A spectrum of fracture types can occur in the sacrum, with the H-shaped fracture being the paradigm. The H fracture involves both sacral ala and has a horizontal component that connects the two vertical or alar fractures (Figure 12.4A; see also Figure 2.21). The horizontal component can be absent, and the fracture can present with unilateral or bilateral alar components only (Figure 12.4B,D; see also Figure 2.21). When a unilateral component presents, it may progress over time to a bilateral or H-shaped fracture (Figure 12.4A; see also Figure 2.21). Finally, the horizontal component can present with a single unilateral alar fracture (Figure 12.4C; see also Figure 2.21). This multiplicity of fracture configurations can make identification difficult as well.

Conventional Treatment

Historically, patients with sacral insufficiency fractures have been treated with a regimen of bed rest, local warmth, and narcotic analgesics (13). More recently, mobilization and physical therapy have been utilized after a short period of initial bed rest (14). When appropriate, pharmacologic therapy of underlying osteoporosis should be promptly initiated. Response to therapy is usually slow, with prolonged pain and reduced mobility that can last for months (Figure 12.5B).

Sacroplasty

Percutaneous vertebroplasty (PV) has been proven effective in alleviating the pain associated with lumbar and thoracic vertebral body compression fractures (15–18). The proposed mechanism of pain relief is fracture stabilization that eliminates motion in the fractured bone. Although this should theoretically apply to sacral fractures as well, even experienced practitioners have been hesitant to apply vertebroplasty techniques at this level. This is in large part due to constraints imposed by the relatively complex sacral anatomy. The inherent difficulty in fluoroscopic visualization of important sacral landmarks, including the spinal canal and neural foramina, makes the detection of cement leaks into these spaces difficult.

Percutaneous sacroplasty (PS) was first described in France in the mid-1990s for osteoporosis and in 2000 as a treatment for patients with symptomatic metastatic disease (19,20). Subsequently, a single case (21) and a small series (22) of patients who underwent sacral vertebroplasty were reported. In three of the four patients included in these reports, PS was performed with fluoroscopic guidance. The remaining patient was treated with computed tomography (CT) guidance. All of the patients reported significantly decreased pain following the procedure. There were no reported complications.

Percutaneous sacroplasty is ideally suited for CT guidance, with or without fluoroscopy. Localizing images display sacral anatomy and fracture lines. This allows safe and effective placement of two, three, or more needles. After optimal needle tip position is confirmed by additional images, cement can be injected in small aliquots with interval CT

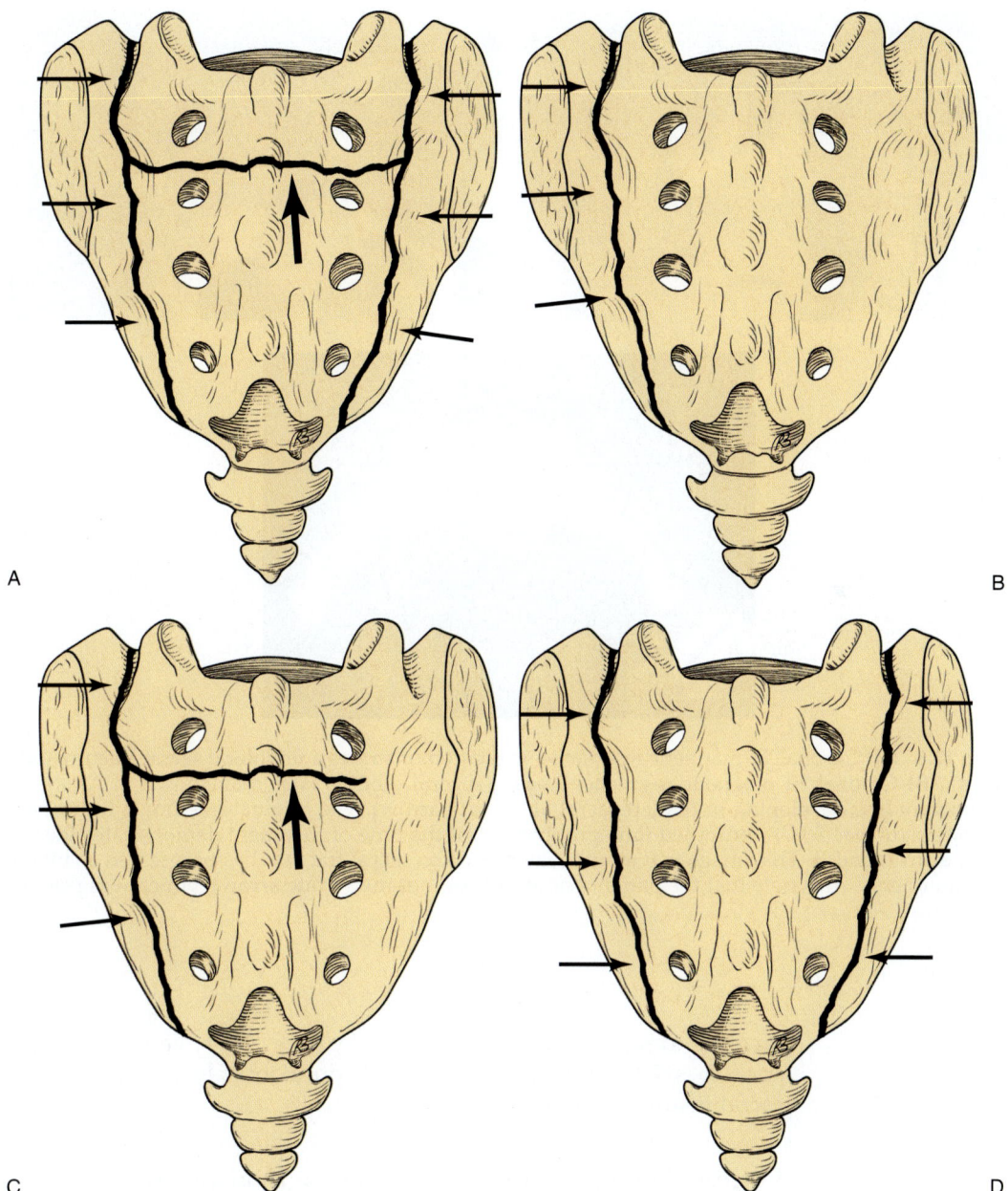

Figure 12.4. **(A)** Artist's sketch of sacrum showing the typical H-shaped fracture with bilateral vertical and connecting horizontal components (black arrows). **(B)** Unilateral sacral fracture (black arrows). **(C)** Combined unilateral vertical and horizontal fractures. **(D)** Bilateral vertical sacral fractures without the horizontal component.

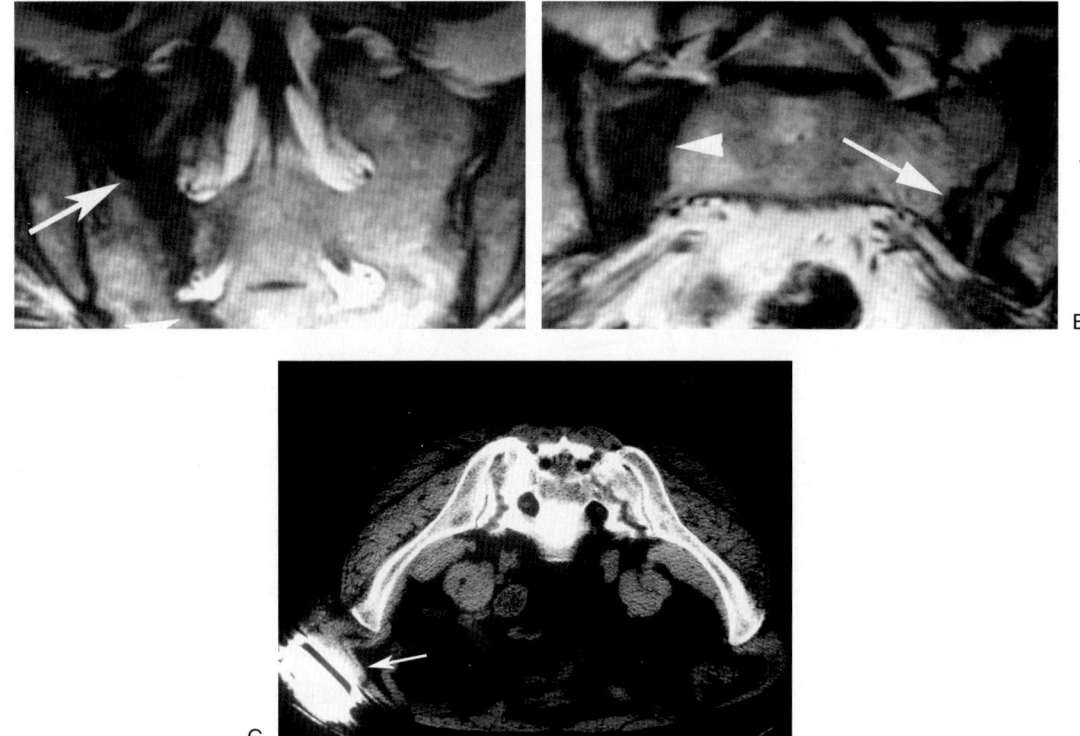

Figure 12.5. **(A)** Coronal T1 magnetic resonance image demonstrates a unilateral sacral fracture (white arrows). **(B)** Coronal T1 magnetic resonance image (several months later than shown in A) shows a new fracture line developing in the left sacral ala (white arrow). The original fracture is indicated by the white arrowhead. **(C)** Computed tomography scan at the time of treatment demonstrates the same patient as in A and B. This image is 6 months later, and the sacral fracture has progressed to bilateral alar components. Also note that the patient has an infusion pump (white arrow), which was put in for pain control.

imaging to monitor for extraosseous leakage. We have used CT guidance to safely and effectively treat approximately 30 patients with sacral insufficiency fractures.

Patient Selection and Preoperative Evaluation

As with PV elsewhere in the spine, appropriate patient selection is critical to ensure favorable outcomes. Percutaneous sacroplasty should be offered only to patients with severe pain poorly responsive to conventional medical therapy. Fractures should be documented by scintigraphy, CT, and/or magnetic resonance imaging (MRI). We prefer MRI for its combination of sensitivity, specificity, and anatomic detail. Healing fractures may remain "hot" on bone scan and appear sclerotic on CT. If marrow edema is limited or absent on MRI, we are hesitant to perform a PS. An alternative approach might be a sacroiliac joint injection or nerve block as indicated by the location and distribution of pain.

In addition to appropriate imaging, preoperative evaluation includes a focused history and physical examination, as well as routine laboratory studies. Patients with an active, untreated infection or coagulopathy should be deferred or excluded.

Informed written consent is obtained from eligible patients. In light of limited reported experience with PS, approval may be sought from the appropriate credentialing committee and/or investigational review board.

Technique

Computed Tomography Guidance Only

Patients are positioned prone on the CT table with care taken to avoid additional injury to these fragile patients during transfer. Protective padding may be applied to the shoulders, elbows, hips, knees, and ankles. Procedural sedation can be achieved with small divided doses of intravenous (IV) fentanyl and midazolam, titrated to the patient's needs. The patient's vital signs and oxygen saturation levels should be monitored throughout the procedure.

Intravenous antibiotics are recommended and should be given at the onset of the procedure. One gram of cephazolin supplies adequate coverage for most skin pathogens and can be given to all patients except those with a specific allergy to cephalosporins and/or a severe allergy to penicillin. Adding antibiotics to the cement is not required or recommended.

The patient's preprocedure imaging studies should be reviewed and accessible within the CT suite. Localizing noncontrast CT images are obtained at 3- or 5-mm intervals. Puncture sites are then chosen and, if desired, can be marked on the skin with an indelible marker. The low back and buttocks are then scrubbed with an antiseptic solution, and a surgical drape is applied. The physician and any personnel with direct access to the surgical site or equipment should observe conventional handwashing techniques and wear a surgical gown, cap, mask, and sterile gloves.

The choice of puncture sites depends on the fracture pattern and location of fracture lines (Figure 12.6; see also Figure 2.11). For H-shaped fractures, one may choose to attempt fixation along the horizontal component of the fracture, but injection of cement into this component of the fracture seems optional for pain relief. This component of the fracture is usually located at the S2 level. The horizontal component of the fracture can be accessed via a needle puncture posterolaterally through the SI joint (Figure 12.7A). An alternative approach places the puncture site over one of the ala with medial angulation of the needle between the spinal canal and the ipsilateral sacral foramen (Figure 12.7B). This needle is advanced into the sacral body to be treated.

Puncture sites to treat the lateral fracture components are chosen over each sacral ala at a somewhat medial location to allow mild lateral angulation of the needle along the fracture line, which is usually parallel to the sacroiliac joint (Figure 12.7C).

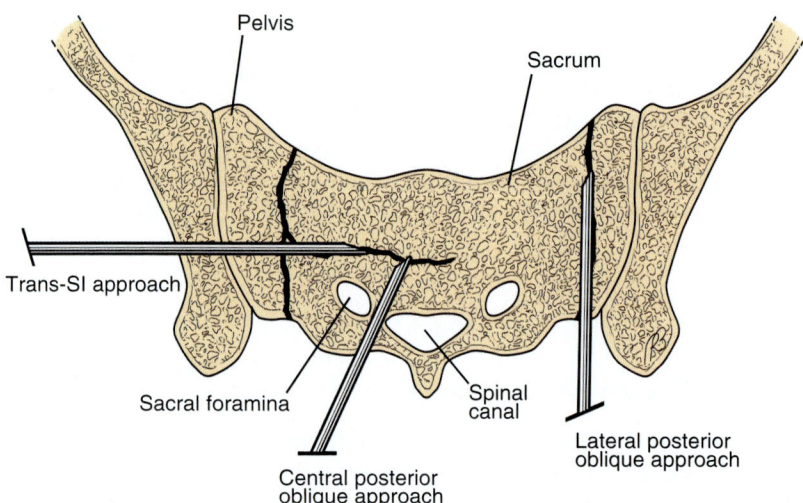

Figure 12.6. Sketch of axial section through the sacrum and pelvis. This shows the various needle trajectories that can be used to access the various components of the sacral insufficiency fractures. The central component can be reached by a trans-sacroiliac joint approach or a posterolateral approach between the foramina and the spinal canal. The alar fracture can be easily treated by a posterolateral approach, which usually parallels the sacroiliac joint and is lateral to the foramina.

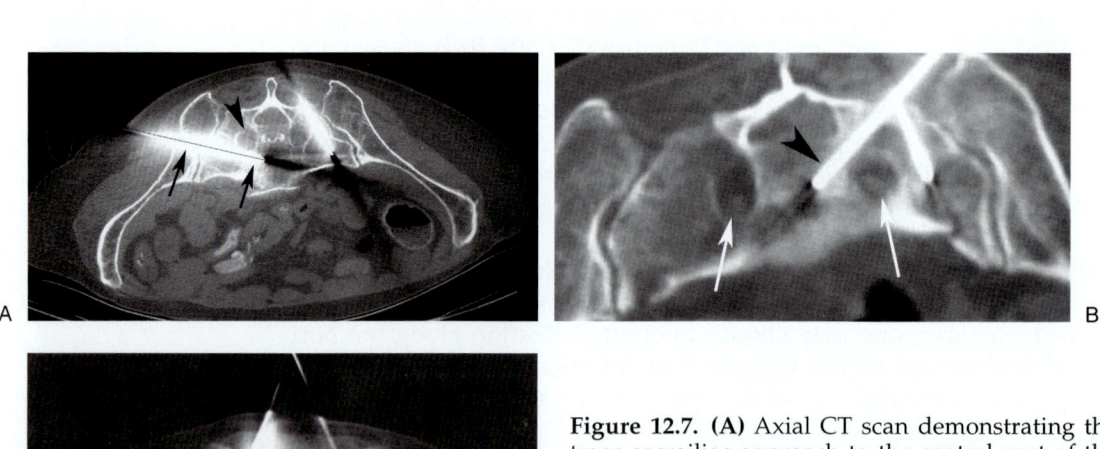

Figure 12.7. (A) Axial CT scan demonstrating the trans-sacroiliac approach to the central part of the sacrum (black arrows). Care must be taken to avoid the foramina (black arrowhead). (B) Axial CT scan shows the other approach to the central sacrum. This posterolateral approach places the needle (black arrowhead) between the foramina (white arrows) on the entry side and the spinal canal. (C) Axial CT of needles (white arrows) placed into the lateral fracture components bilaterally. This trajectory is parallel to the sacroiliac joint and avoids the foramina (black arrowhead).

At each puncture site, the skin, underlying soft tissues, and periosteum are first infiltrated with local anesthetic. A small dermatotomy is made at the intended puncture site with an 11-gauge scalpel blade. The cement delivery needle is advanced to the posterior sacral cortex. We prefer smaller (e.g., 13) gauge needles for all sacral procedures. The needle tip can be fixed in place by advancing it 2 to 3 mm into the cortex. Needle position is then checked by additional CT imaging. The cortical entry site and angulation are adjusted as needed. Initially the needle is advanced in small (5- to 10-mm) increments. Each advance is monitored by additional CT imaging. The needles can be advanced with manual pressure or by small taps with a sterile mallet. When a safe needle course is ensured, the needle can be advanced in 10-mm increments. The alar needles can be advanced to within 10 mm of the anterior sacral cortex.

Vertical sacral fractures (through the lateral ala) may be unilateral or bilateral. Puncture sites are chosen over each affected ala to allow fracture fixation along the vertical axis. Each puncture site is chosen to allow mild lateral angulation of the needle along the fracture line parallel to the sacroiliac joint, taking care to avoid the neural foramina (Figure 12.6; see also Figure 2.11).

After satisfactory needle position is confirmed by additional CT imaging, the cement is mixed. Because of the additional time required for CT monitoring, cement with a relatively long set-up time is preferred. As with conventional vertebroplasty, barium may be added to increase cement opacification, but less is needed due to the increased sensitivity of CT to differential bone/cement density. New bone cements (i.e., Spineplex; Howmedica, Kalamazoo, MI) that are Food and Drug Administration-approved for PV and kyphoplasty will be adequately opacified. Because cement is injected in small aliquots, 1-cc syringes are used rather than a bulky delivery system. Working time can be increased by storing filled syringes in a container of sterile iced saline.

The cement is injected sequentially through each needle in 0.5-cc aliquots, initially allowing for the volume of the cannula. After each aliquot, the distribution of cement is monitored by additional CT imaging (Figure 12.8A). If cement extravasates into the spinal canal or a neural foramen, no additional cement is injected through that needle (Figure 12.8B). During the injection, alar needles may be withdrawn along the fracture line in 1-cm increments to increase the cross-sectional area of cement fixation.

As with vertebroplasty elsewhere in the spine, the volume of cement injection does not directly correlate with pain relief. Typical total cement volumes range from 3 to 5 mL per side. The alar component of the fracture will accommodate a higher volume of cement than the central sacral body (Figure 12.8C). The distribution and amount of cement varies from patient to patient and is seldom symmetric (Figure 12.8D).

As cement hardens within the needle, further injection with a syringe may become difficult or impossible. If desired, the cement volume within the needle can be directed into the sacrum by advancing the

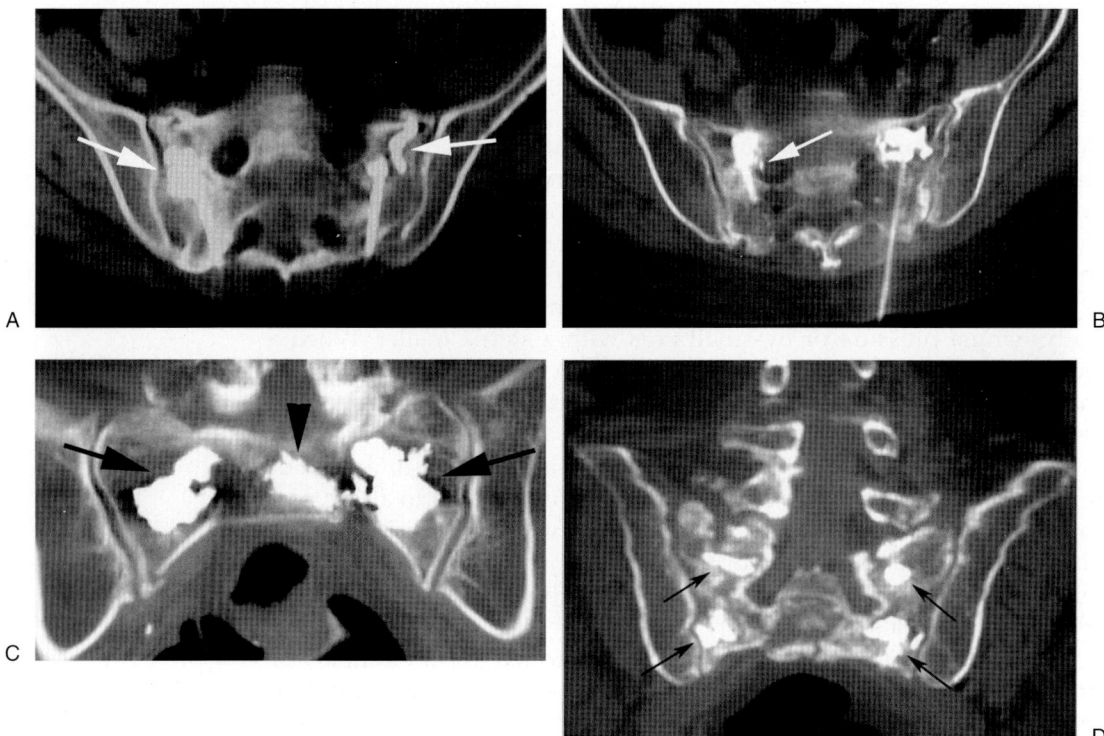

Figure 12.8. (A) Computed tomography scan showing early cement injections bilaterally (white arrows). Note the anatomic definition and easy visualization of the neural foramina. **(B)** Computed tomography scan of another patient reveals minimal extravasation of cement into the neural foramina (white arrow) long before the quantity is likely to create symptomatic nerve encroachment. **(C)** Coronal CT demonstrates cement in the central sacral body (black arrowhead) and lateral sacral wings (black arrows). A larger amount of cement was used laterally to secure the fractures in the sacral ala. **(D)** Coronal CT demonstrates four injections of cement (black arrows) that resulted in good pain relief for this patient following PS.

trocar through the cannula. Care must always be taken to avoid extraosseous or foraminal cement extravasation.

Procedure time is considerably decreased if CT fluoroscopy is utilized. In addition, "real-time" visualization afforded by CT fluoroscopy decreases the likelihood of cement extravasation and neurologic complication (23).

A small sample of cement may be used to assess cement hardening on the working table. When the cement is hardened ex vivo, the needles are removed and sterile dressings are placed over the puncture sites. The patient is carefully rolled supine onto a gurney. The patient can typically be ambulated and discharged after a short period of bed rest and monitoring (usually 1–2 hours).

Fluoroscopic Guidance

Fluoroscopic guidance (with or without CT) has been used for PS (21,22). Fluoroscopy alone may be faster than either CT alone or fluoroscopy in combination with CT, but it suffers from a lack of anatomic resolution. There typically is difficulty seeing the neural foramina with assurance. Cement can be visualized, but one does not always know whether cement is leaking into the foramina early enough to stop the injection and avoid complications (Figure 12.9). To identify the foramina better, some operators have introduced small-gauge spinal needles into the foramina before cement is injected. This aids the operator to identify the foramina even when the margins are not well seen with fluoroscopy during the procedure.

The use of fluoroscopy has not caused many complications to date. However, we believe that its use alone is problematic, and we have found CT to offer a greater margin of safety for identifying where cement is going during injection.

Additional Considerations

Patients with sacral insufficiency fractures may have additional injuries or conditions that contribute to their pain. Patients with unilateral alar fractures have a high incidence of ipsilateral pubic and ischial ramus fractures (5,24,25). Although there is no specific treatment for these injuries, the fractures should be documented and the patient informed regarding the likelihood of ongoing pain that may take weeks to resolve.

Concurrent osteoporotic fractures of the thoracic and lumbar spine are not uncommon (5) and should be treated with conventional vertebroplasty techniques. Sacroiliac pain is also common, especially opposite a unilateral alar fracture. If the patient is tender over the contralateral sacroiliac joint, an intraarticular corticosteroid injection can be easily performed with CT guidance at the time of the PS. As previously discussed, patients with healing fractures of the sacrum may

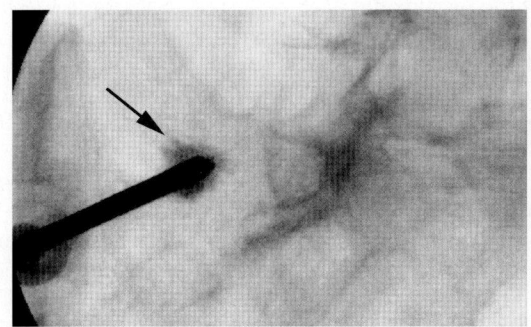 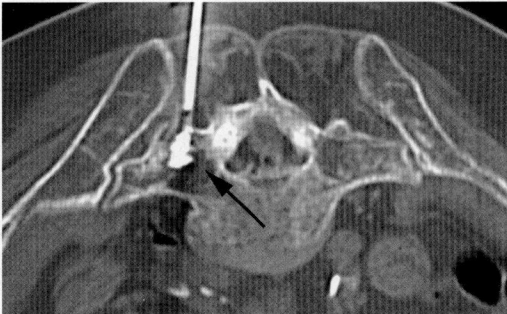

Figure 12.9. **(A)** Fluoroscopic image of an injection needle in the sacral wing and early cement injection (black arrow). Note the general lack of anatomic landmarks with this imaging method. Neural foramina are hard to see at best, making early detection of a cement leak almost impossible. **(B)** The same case viewed with CT demonstrates the anatomy in much better detail and allows accurate localization of cement (black arrow) as it is injected.

also develop sacroiliac joint pain. Distinguishing the exact source of pain is difficult in these patients. Typically, sacroiliac joint pain is less severe than that associated with a recent fracture and less exacerbated by weight bearing. Sacroiliac joint pain is characterized by morning stiffness and a fatigue-like stiffness brought on by prolonged standing or sitting. Certainly, in patients with persistent sacral level pain following vertebroplasty, sacroiliac arthropathy should be strongly considered.

Occasionally, sacral insufficiency fractures will result in S1 radiculopathy, although nerve root impingement by a fracture fragment is extremely uncommon in this patient population. For patients with the appropriate dermatomal distribution of pain, a selective S1 nerve root block may be considered. Computed tomography guidance is ideally suited for that procedure, and it can be performed in conjunction with PS.

References

1. Lourie H. Spontaneous osteoporotic fracture of the sacrum. An unrecognized syndrome of the elderly. JAMA 1982; 248:715–717.
2. Pentecost RL, Murray RA, Brindley HH. Fatigue, insufficiency, and pathologic fractures. JAMA 1964; 187:1001–1004.
3. Taillandier J, Langue F, Alemanni M, et al. Mortality and functional outcomes of pelvic insufficiency fracture in older patients. Joint Bone Spine 2003; 70(4):287–289.
4. Rawlings CE, Wilkins RH, Martinez S, et al. Osteoporotic sacral fractures: a clinical study. Neurosurgery 1988; 22:72–76.
5. Weber M, Hasler P, Gerber H. Insufficiency fractures of the sacrum: twenty cases and review of the literature. Spine 1993; 18(16):2507–2512.
6. Gotis-Graham I, McGuigan L, Diamond T, et al. Sacral insufficiency fractures in the elderly. J Bone Joint Surg 1994; 76-B(6):882–886.
7. Renner JB. Pelvic insufficiency fractures. Arthritis Rheum 1990; 33:426–430.
8. Gacetta DJ, Yandow DR. Computed tomography of spontaneous osteoporotic sacral fractures. J Comput Assist Tomogr 1984; 8:1190–1191.
9. Grangier C, Garcia J, Howarth NR, et al. Role of MRI in the diagnosis of insufficiency fractures of the sacrum and acetabular roof. Skel Radiol 1997; 26(9):517–524.
10. Schneider R, Yacavone J, Ghelman B. Unsuspected sacral fractures: detection by radionuclide bone scanning. AJR 1985; 144(2):337–341.
11. Ries T. Detection of osteoporotic sacral fractures with radionuclides. Radiology 1983; 146(3):783–785.
12. Brahme SK, Cervilla V, Vint V, et al. Magnetic resonance appearance of sacral insufficiency fractures. Skel Radiol 1990; 19:489–493.
13. Grasland A, Pouchot J, Mathieu A, et al. Sacral insufficiency fractures: an easily overlooked cause of back pain in elderly women. Arch Intern Med 1996; 156:668–674.
14. Babayev M, Lachmann E, Nagler W. The controversy surrounding sacral insufficiency fractures: to ambulate or not to ambulate? Am J Phys Med Rehabil 2000; 79:404–409.
15. Jensen ME, Evans AJ, Mathis JM, et al. Percutaneous polymethylmethacrylate vertebroplasty in the treatment of osteoporotic vertebral body compression fractures: technical aspects. AJNR 1997; 18:1897–1904.

16. Deramond H, Depriester C, Galibert P, et al. Percutaneous vertebroplasty with polymethylmethacrylate: technique, indications, and results. Radiol Clin North Am 1998; 36(3):533–546.
17. Cotton A, Boutry N, Cortet B, et al. Percutaneous vertebroplasty: state of the art. RadioGraphics 1998; 18:311–320.
18. Mathis J, Barr J, Belkoff S, et al. Percutaneous vertebroplasty: a developing standard of care for vertebral compression fractures. AJNR 2001; 22:373–381.
19. Dehdashti AR, Martin JB, Jean B, et al. PMMA cementoplasty in symptomatic lesions of the S1 vertebral body. Cardiovasc Intervent Radiol 2000; 23:235–237.
20. Marcy PY, Palussiere J, Descamps B, et al. Percutaneous cementoplasty for pelvic bone metastasis. Support Care Cancer 2000; 8:500–503.
21. Garant M. Sacroplasty: a new treatment for sacral insufficiency fracture. J Vasc Intervent Radiol 2002; 13:1265–1267.
22. Pommerscheim W, Huang-Hellinger F, Baker M, et al. Sacroplasty: a treatment for sacral insufficiency fractures. AJNR 2003; 24:1003–1007.
23. Pitton MB, Drees P, Schneider J, et al. Evaluation of percutaneous vertebroplasty in osteoporotic vertebral fractures using a combination of CT fluoroscopy and conventional lateral fluoroscopy. Rofo Fortschr Geb Rontgenstr N 2004; 176(7):1005–1012.
24. Davies AM, Evans NS, Struthers GR. Parasymphyseal and associated insufficiency fractures of the pelvis and sacrum. Br J Radiol 1988; 61(722):103–108.
25. Peh WC, Khong PL, Ho WY, et al. Sacral insufficiency fractures. Spectrum of radiological features. Clin Imaging 1995; 19(2):92–101.

13
Complications Associated with Vertebroplasty and Kyphoplasty

John M. Mathis and Hervé Deramond

Since percutaneous vertebroplasty (PV) was introduced in Europe in 1984, it has become an increasingly popular technique. It was introduced in the United States in the early 1990s, and since 1998 it has been the standard of care for painful compression fractures (1). Although less commonly used than PV, kyphoplasty (KP), or "balloon-assisted vertebroplasty," introduced in the late 1990s, has also become popular for treating the pain associated with vertebral compression fractures (VCFs). Both procedures are structurally similar and use percutaneously introduced bone cement to augment a fractured or destroyed vertebral body. This chapter evaluates the types of complications that have occurred with both procedures and indicates ways to avoid these complications.

Initially, training for both procedures was achieved through short (usually 1-day) cadaver courses given by experienced physicians worldwide. This ideally was followed by several proctored cases to get the "physician in training" off to a safe start. No formal training was offered in universities for residents until more recently. The first physicians doing the procedures progressed through their learning curves carefully as the procedure was cautiously applied. Few complications were initially experienced and reported. Severe or permanent complications were rare. However, since the procedures were first devised, complication reports have been collected and have identified definite risks of the procedures. Although complications cannot be eliminated completely, they can be minimized through good image guidance (high-quality fluoroscopic equipment or computed tomography), a thorough knowledge of the spinal anatomy involved in both PV and KP, and a complete understanding of the criteria for performing these procedures safely. This means appropriate patient selection, adherence to safe procedure technique, proper material selection, and good judgement that minimizes the patient risk while affording a high probability of successful outcome. It should be remembered that *preventing complications* is the key to a safe procedure.

Incidents and Complications

Incidents

An incident is an asymptomatic event that is unexpected or undesirable but that produces no measurable ill effect to the patient.

Cement Leakage

Cement leaks are not uncommon with either PV or KP. They are typically small and pose no risk to the patient. Leaks may occur through the vertebral wall due to a fracture fissure, destruction created by malignancy, or even a blow-out fracture through the vertebral wall created by the Kyphon balloon (Figure 13.1A). Leaks can also occur through connecting vascular structures because injecting into the intratrabecular space is effectively injecting into the intravascular, venous space. Small amounts of cement in the venous structures, paraspinous tissue, or the disc space are almost never associated with clinical symptoms. To minimize these leaks and keep them asymptomatic, they must be realized very early and while still small. This allows the operating physician to stop the cement injection. Cement should be viscous or thick before injection to ensure that it does not flow out of the vertebra except with the continued pressure of injection. Cement that is very liquid or cement that has a very long working time at room temperature (e.g., Cranioplastic, Vertebroplastic, or Secore) can remain liquid even after injection and present a risk for leak from the needle stick site and along the needle track (Figure 13.1B). Recognizing the leak and immediately stopping the injection will protect against a large and potentially symptomatic leak. Figure 13.1C shows a small leak through the posterior venous plexus into the epidural space on a computed tomographic (CT) scan obtained after the PV was completed. The fluoroscopic images obtained during the procedure (Figure 13.1D) show that cement appears to approach the posterior wall, but there is no initial evidence of leak. This highlights an important aspect of the vertebral anatomy: The vertebra is not a box with square borders, but rather has a concave posterior margin and a convex anterior margin. If cement extends to what appears to be the posterior margin on fluoroscopy, then it has likely already leaked beyond the true concave portion of the posterior wall. Cement therefore should be stopped when it reaches the posterior quarter of the vertebra.

The convex anterior margin is important also, as a laterally placed needle can breach the anterolateral wall before the tip of the needle appears to reach the anteriormost portion of the vertebra in the lateral projection (Figure 13.1E). The needle should be positioned beyond the midline at the junction of the middle and anterior thirds of the vertebra (in the lateral projection), but not all the way to the apparent anterior margin. At least mild angulation away from the lateral margin is optimal to avoid the lateral wall.

Asymptomatic Pulmonary Emboli

Essentially all PV and KP procedures will displace blood products and marrow fat during either balloon inflation or cement injection (2). Both

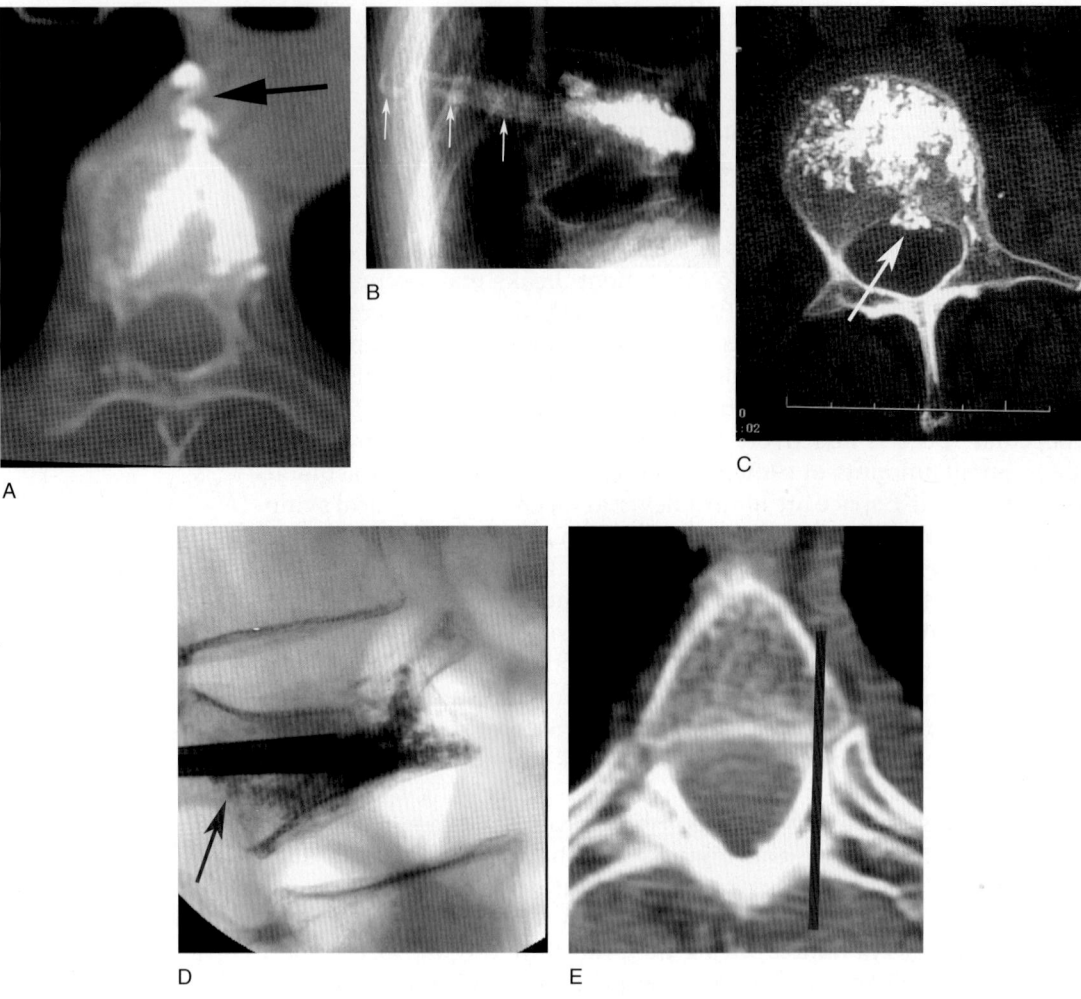

Figure 13.1. **(A)** Axial CT following KP. The lateral wall of the vertebra was ruptured by the balloon, and cement leaked through the hole into the mediastinum (black arrow) and created persistent pain that required several days of additional hospitalization and intravenous analgesics. **(B)** Lateral radiograph (postvertebroplasty) showing cement that has leaked along the needle tracts after the needles were removed (white arrows). This can be a source of local pain and can happen when the cement is very liquid, as is the case with long work time cements such as Cranioplastic, Vertebroplastic, and Secore. **(C)** Computed tomography scan (postprocedure) demonstrates a small, asymptomatic cement leak (white arrow). Note the concave posterior margin and the convex anterior margin of the vertebra. **(D)** The initial fluoroscopic images during the procedure demonstrate cement at what appears to be the posterior margin of the vertebra (black arrow). Injection should be stopped when the cement reaches the posterior quarter of the vertebra as seen on fluoroscopy to ensure that no leak through the posterior margin occurs. **(E)** This image shows a very triangular shape to the anterior vertebral margin, not uncommon in the upper thoracic spine. The black line indicates a potential lateral needle track that would breach the lateral wall considerably before the needle would reach the anterior margin of the vertebra, as seen in the lateral projection. (A–D, from Mathis [2], with permission.)

processes are hydraulic events and must expel a volume from the marrow equal to that of the cement injected. Under most circumstances this will create emboli of either fat or marrow elements, some of which are blood precursor that will not pass through the pulmonary capillary bed (3), to the lungs. Fortunately, the quantity of these emboli is small and almost always is of no clinical significance. This phenomenon cannot, however, be ignored. Patients with severe chronic obstructive pulmonary disease (COPD) with limited pulmonary reserve can experience cardiopulmonary failure with only a small volume of emboli that may be able to obstruct a significant portion of the remaining capillary bed. These patients are at higher than normal risk even when only a single level is treated and should be consented to accordingly. Every effort should be made to prepare for this rare event. At least one death has been reported to the authors and was found to be the result of fat emboli (no cement) after a one-level procedure in a patient with severe COPD.

Cement also can embolize via the connecting vascular system to the lungs (Figure 13.2). This usually occurs when cement is used before it begins to sufficiently polymerize and when it is still too thin. It can flow with the blood (without being pushed during injection). These emboli will also usually reach the lungs (Figure 13.2B,C). Once again, the body's reserve usually makes these small emboli asymptomatic. However, as described above, even small quantities of embolic material can be devastating to some individuals, so this situation should always be avoided by using cement that is as thick as possible during injection.

Disc Space Leaks

A vertebral fracture can extend into the superior or inferior endplate and make a leak into the disc possible. These are not infrequent and

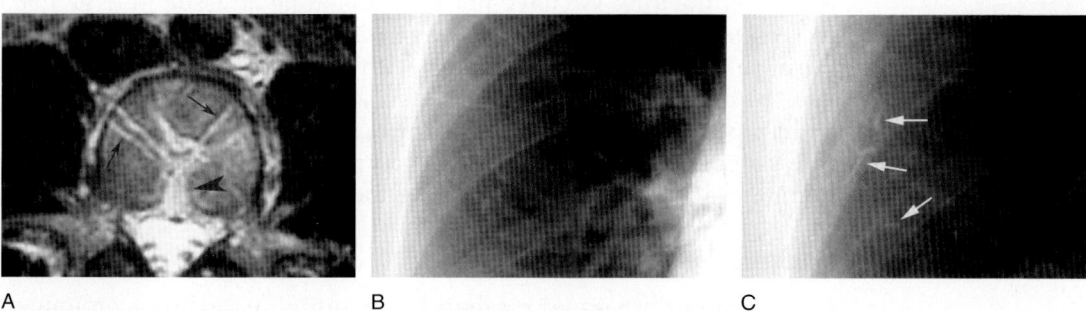

A B C

Figure 13.2. (A) Magnetic resonance image of a lumbar vertebra showing several vascular channels (black arrows) connecting to the paraspinous venous system. It is through these normal connections that emboli easily migrate to the lungs. Note also the large venous confluence in the posterior part of the vertebra (black arrowhead). This connects to the epidural venous system and indicates why the needle tip needs to be in the anterior part of the vertebra and away from this communication. **(B)** Radiograph of a segment of the right lung before PV. **(C)** Same area of the right lung post-PV shows small cement emboli (white arrows). These (and other) pulmonary emboli in this individual were totally asymptomatic and discovered incidentally on a radiograph obtained several weeks later for an unrelated problem.

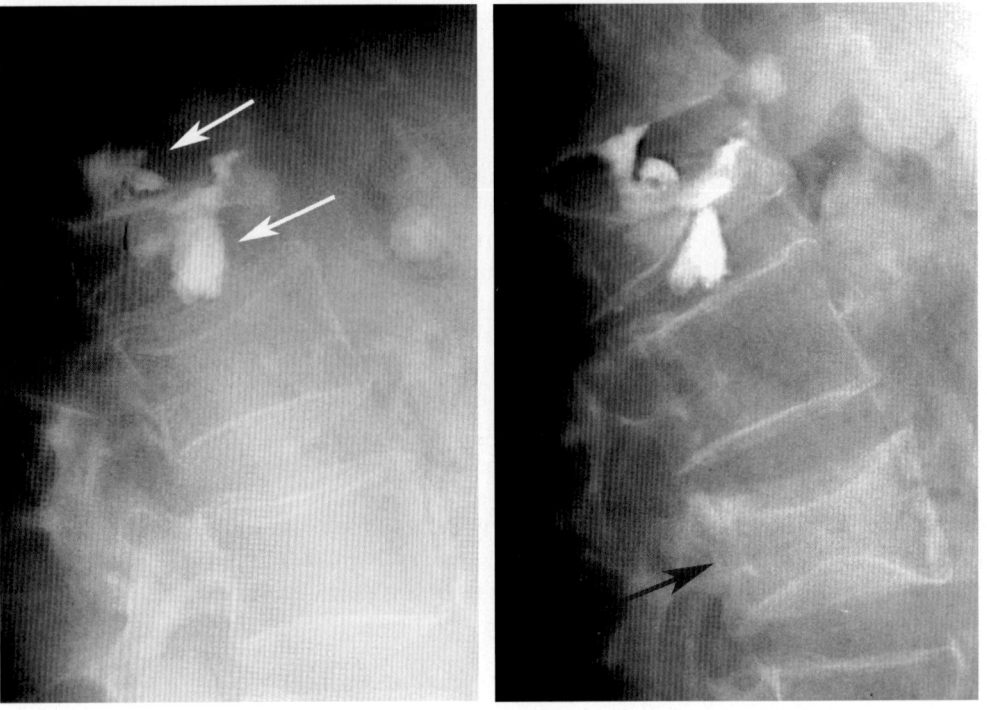

Figure 13.3. (A) Lateral radiograph post-PV shows large cement leaks into the superior and inferior disc space (white arrows). (B) Six months later the patient returned with a new compression fracture (black arrow) that is not at an adjacent level. Even though the cement leak into the disc was large, it did not predispose this patient to a fracture of an adjacent vertebral level.

seem to be of no clinical significance when small. There are no reports of complications associated with this event. However, there has been speculation that large disc leaks may predispose to an increase in adjacent level fracture. We have not seen this to be an issue in over 1,500 PV cases. Figure 13.3 shows a large disc leak that initially occurred during a PV. The patient did return with a new fracture some 6 months later, but the fracture was not in an adjacent level. To date, only anecdotal reports of adjacent level fractures are available, with no statistically significant proof that they occurred. It does seem prudent to minimize all cement leaks, including those that extend into the disc.

Complications

Complications are adverse events that require treatment or prolonged hospital stay. Fortunately, complications occur less frequently than do incidents. The complication rate is related to the specific indication for PV or KP treatment (osteoporosis, benign hemangioma, or malignant tumor). When PV is used to treat osteoporotic VCFs or vertebral hemangiomas (VH), the incidence of symptomatic complications is less than 1% (Table 13.1), whereas complication rates range from 5% to 10% when PV is performed to treat vertebral bodies that are infiltrated with malignant neoplasms (Table 13.2). Complications can be related to the

Table 13.1. Complications of Percutaneous Vertebroplasty in Osteoporotic Vertebral Fractures and Vertebral Hemangiomas.

Parameter	Grados et al. (16)*	Jensen et al. (5)*	Cortet et al. (17)*	Cyteval et al. (18)*	Chiras and Deramond (19)*	Deramond et al. (20)†
Number of patients	25	29	16	20	67	54
Number of PVs	34	47	20	23	76	55
Transitory worsening of the pain	1	0	0	0	1	0
Transitory fever	2	NS‡	0	0	NS‡	0
Transitory radiculopathy	2	0	0	0	1	2
Durable radiculopathy	0	0	0	1	1	0
Rib fracture	0	2	0	0	0	0
Infection	0	0	0	0	0	0
Spinal cord compression	0	0	0	0	0	0

* Osteoporotic vertebral fractures.
† Vertebral hemangioma.
‡ Not specified.

percutaneous approach or device chosen, the medical condition of the patient, and the injection of the bone cement polymethylmethacrylate (PMMA).

Spinal Infection

Spinal infection appears to be rare, as only one case has been reported (4). In that case, the patient treated with PV developed an infection (spondylitis) and presented with worsening back pain and fever a few weeks after the procedure. Treatment consisted of 3 months of medical management with intravenous antibiotics and immobilization, after which the infection completely resolved. Of course, the specific treatment plan for spinal infection depends on the imaging findings and on the presence or absence of neurologic symptoms. Intravenous antibiotics should be given to all patients before PV. Patients with signs of systemic infection should not be treated with PV until the infection is treated and resolved. Furthermore, for patients at high risk of infection because of poor medical status or who are immunocompromised,

Table 13.2. Complications of Percutaneous Vertebroplasty for Malignant Tumors in the Spine.

Parameter	Weill et al. (21)	Cotten et al. (22)	Chiras and Deramond (19)
Number of patients	37	37	113
Number of PVs	52	40	120
Transitory worsening of the pain	2	1	2
Transitory fever	NS*	0	NS*
Transitory radiculopathy	1	1	5
Durable radiculopathy	2	2	5
Infection	0	0	1
Spinal cord compression	0	0	1

* Not specified.

antibiotics introduced into the cement may be of benefit. This is not indicated in routine cases.

Transitory Increase in Pain
Transitory increase in pain is infrequent (<2%) (1) and may be related to manipulation during the procedure, injection of the cement at high pressure, or inflammatory reactions induced by the presence of the cement. In any case, such pain, in our experience, typically resolves in less than 24 hours with the use of nonsteroidal anti-inflammatory medications.

Transitory Fever
Transitory fever is rare and may be related to the same causes of transitory increase in pain mentioned above. In our experience, the fever resolves in less than 48 hours after a course of nonsteroidal anti-inflammatory medications.

Rib Fractures
There are two reports of rib fracture in the literature: one report with PV and one with KP (5,6). The fractures were likely a result of the thorax being compressed against the procedure table during needle insertion. For osteoporotic patients, it is not unreasonable to expect that such compression may cause rib fractures. Such fractures theoretically may be prevented by inserting the needles by tapping them with a small hammer. However, it must be noted that the efficacy of this insertion technique at reducing rib fractures has not been tested and that some patients experience more pain with the tapping than with the manual method of insertion.

Radiculopathy and Spinal Cord Compression
Radiculopathy is related to the leakage of cement into the foraminal veins or the foraminal space (Figure 13.4) (2). They usually resolve after local injection of steroids and anesthetic or after medical treatment with oral nonsteroidal anti-inflammatory medications. However, in rare instances, some radiculopathies can be recalcitrant to medical treatment and require surgical excision of the foraminal cement. Such radiculopathies are more often associated with malignant, osteolytic tumors (3% to 5%). The treatment of osteoporosis, or even myeloma and aggressive hemangioma, produces radiculopathy in less than 1% of patients as the vertebrae are usually intact.

Spinal Cord Compression
Literature reports of spinal cord compression with PV have been rare (2,7). It does seem that there may be more chance of this type of complication with metastatic disease because of the destruction of the vertebra that occurs, making cement leak more likely. Nussbaum et al. (7) found more cord-related, permanent complications reported to the Food and Drug Administration with KP than with PV. They reported 19 cases of cord compression and some degree of permanent neurologic compromise in 40,000–50,000 cases of KP. This number was much higher than the numbers reported for PV in the same series (1/150,000). The KP procedure has been marketed as safer than PV because cement

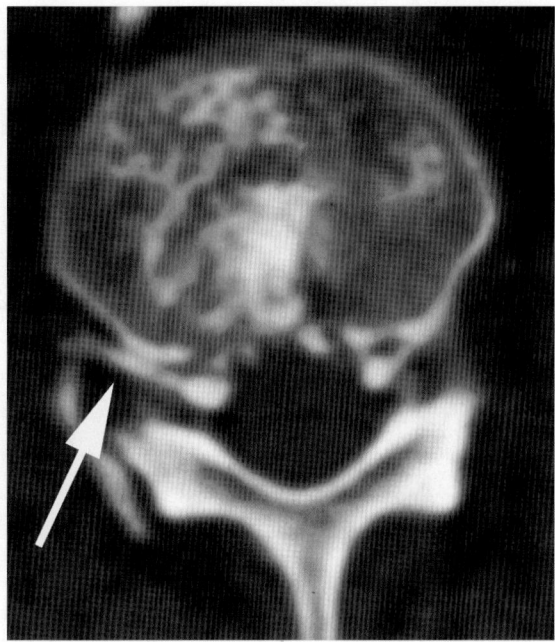

Figure 13.4. Computed tomography scan post-PV reveals a cement leak that extends into the epidural venous plexus and fills a vein in the lateral recess (white arrow). This type of leak can result in nerve root irritation.

is ultimately injected into a cavity made by the balloon. The cavity is said to help retard cement leaks and to allow injection at lower pressure than with PV. Laboratory analysis of the injection pressure found that intravertebral pressures are the same for PV and KP (8,9). Food and Drug Administration device-related complication data clearly dispute the KP marketing claim of improved safety compared with PV.

The major point is that both KP and PV can result in permanent neurologic injury due to spinal cord compression resulting from large cement leaks. Figure 13.5 shows cases of PV and KP that resulted in permanent paraplegia due to such cement leaks. These types of leaks must be recognized early and injection of cement terminated before cord compression occurs.

Cement leaks may occur more easily when there is vertebral wall destruction. When the posterior wall is absent, there is a direct route for cement to leak into the epidural space. As posterior wall destruction usually occurs due to destruction of the vertebra by tumor, there also exists the possibility of displacing tumor into spinal canal. Either cement or tumor can then cause cord compression. In Chapter 11, we describe a method to monitor the effects of tumor and cement on the thecal sac by putting myelographic contrast into the cerebrospinal fluid before cement injection. This allows us to see the effect of the injection on the thecal sac (Figure 13.6) and monitor for cement leak or tumor displacement causing cord or nerve root compression.

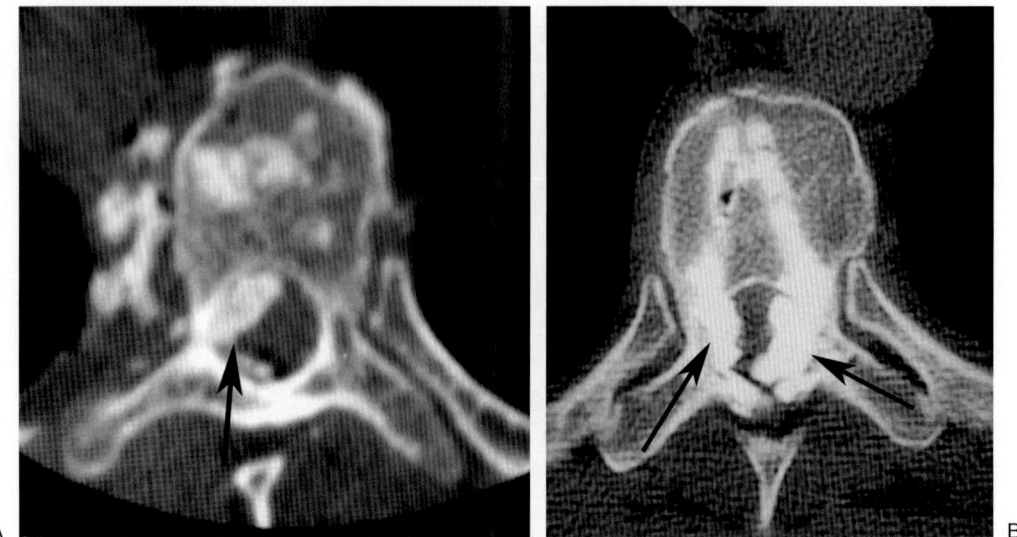

Figure 13.5. **(A)** Computed tomography scan post-PV reveals a large cement leak into the spinal canal (black arrow). This patient had permanent spinal cord injury following this leak. **(B)** Computed tomography scan post-KP also shows a large cement leak into the spinal canal (black arrows). Again, permanent spinal cord injury and paraplegia resulted from this complication.

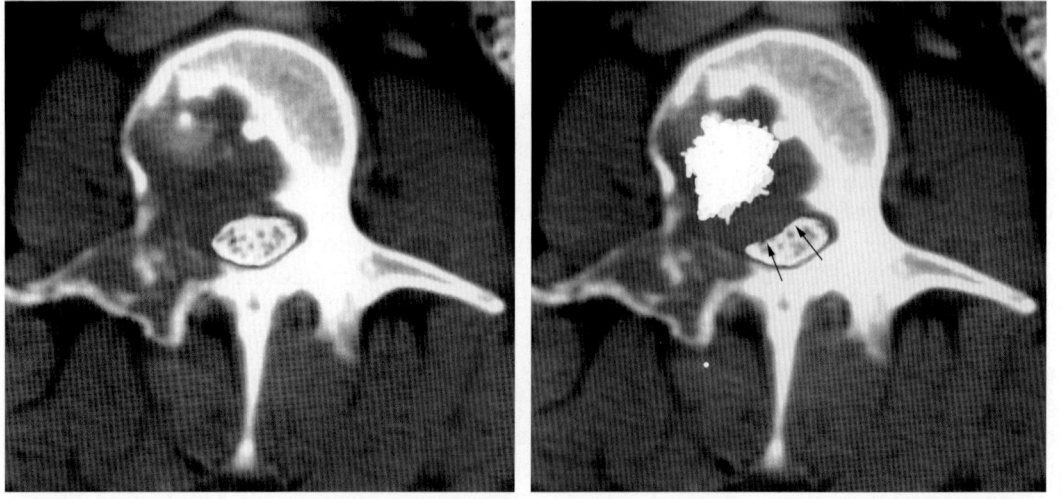

Figure 13.6. **(A)** Computed tomography scan before PV shows destruction of the posterior vertebral wall. The thecal sac is well seen after the introduction of myelographic contrast. **(B)** After PV, the CT reveals early compression of the thecal sac (black arrows) by tumor that has been displaced through a defect in the posterior vertebral wall caused by the cement. This finding allows the operator to stop the cement injection before significant compression occurs.

Figure 13.7. This patient presented with retroperitoneal hematoma 2 days after PV performed via a parapedicular route at two vertebral levels. Contrast was injected via an 18-gauge needle inserted into the pedicle. **(A)** Nonsubtracted transosseous venogram showing leak of contrast medium through the previous parapedicular hole (arrow). **(B)** Subtracted radiographic image. The leak was sealed by injecting glue via the needle. (From J.M. Mathis, H. Deramond, S.M. Belkoff [eds], Percutaneous Vertebroplasty. New York: Springer, 2002, with permision.)

Symptomatic Pulmonary Embolism

It was well known that pulmonary emboli occurred with each PV and KP procedure due to marrow products (blood precursors and marrow fat) that were displaced by balloon inflation (KP) or during cement injection (PV). These are almost always asymptomatic. Even when small amounts of cement migrate to the lungs, there is usually no clinical side effect (Figure 13.2A,B). Pulmonary infarct has been reported due to cement emboli (10). Additionally, this complication has become more common in the 4 years since the first edition of this book (11–15). It is now clear that patients should be categorized into high- and low-risk groups with regard to this problem. Patients with respiratory disease may be made worse (or develop full cardiorespiratory failure) if small quantities of emboli reach the residual pulmonary capillary bed. The effect may be so severe that death occurs. This complication should be discussed specifically with such patients at risk, and appropriate support should be available during the procedure. Low-risk patients are those who have no known pulmonary disease and no complex anatomy that would make leaks more likely.

Hemorrhage

Hemorrhage can occur in patients with coagulopathy. One of the authors (H.D.) treated a patient with such a complication (4). That patient presented with myeloma, hypercalcemia, and severe pain. Despite the presence of coagulation disorders, PV was indicated before chemotherapy to provide pain relief and allow the patient to remain ambulatory. Percutaneous vertebroplasty was performed with a single needle using a parapedicular approach. Two days later, the patient complained of abdominal pain, and a CT scan revealed a retroperitoneal hematoma related to leakage of blood secondary to the needle puncture. The puncture was sealed by injecting glue via a transpedicular percutaneous route (Figure 13.7). In general, whenever possible,

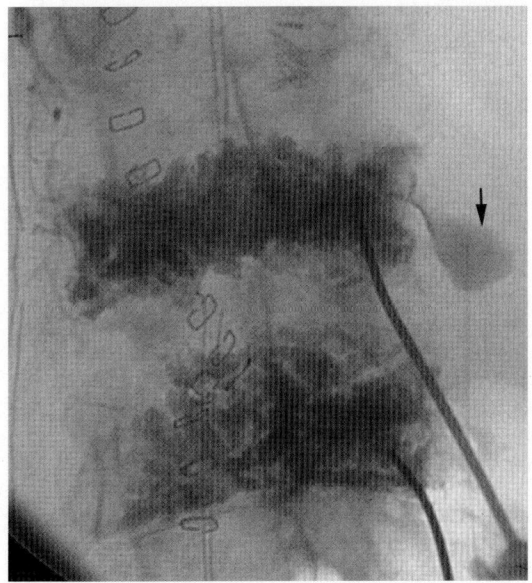

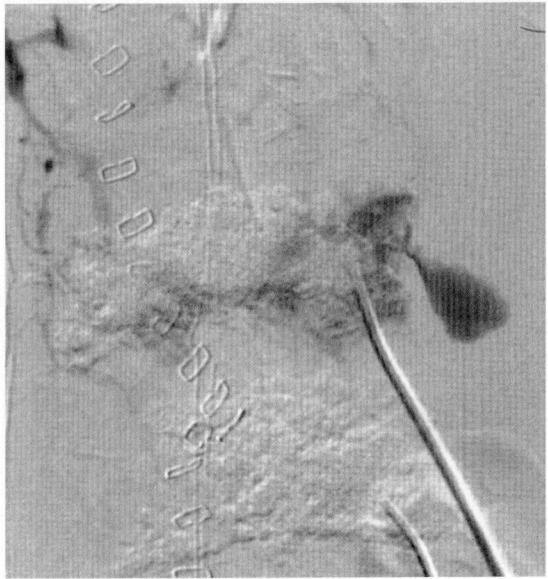

A

B

coagulation disorders should be corrected before PV. As discussed in previous chapters (on anatomy and technique), the parapedicular approach makes bleeding more likely than does the transpedicular approach. This occurs both because of large vessels that run along the paraspinous portions of the vertebrae (Figure 13.8) and because the stick site is along the lateral aspect of the vertebra and pressure cannot be applied for hemostasis (after needle removal) as can be accomplished when using the transpedicular approach.

Death

Fortunately, death is a rare complication of PV and KP. It has been reported with both procedures (8,15), with an equal incidence of approximately 1/50,000 cases each. The etiology of this complication

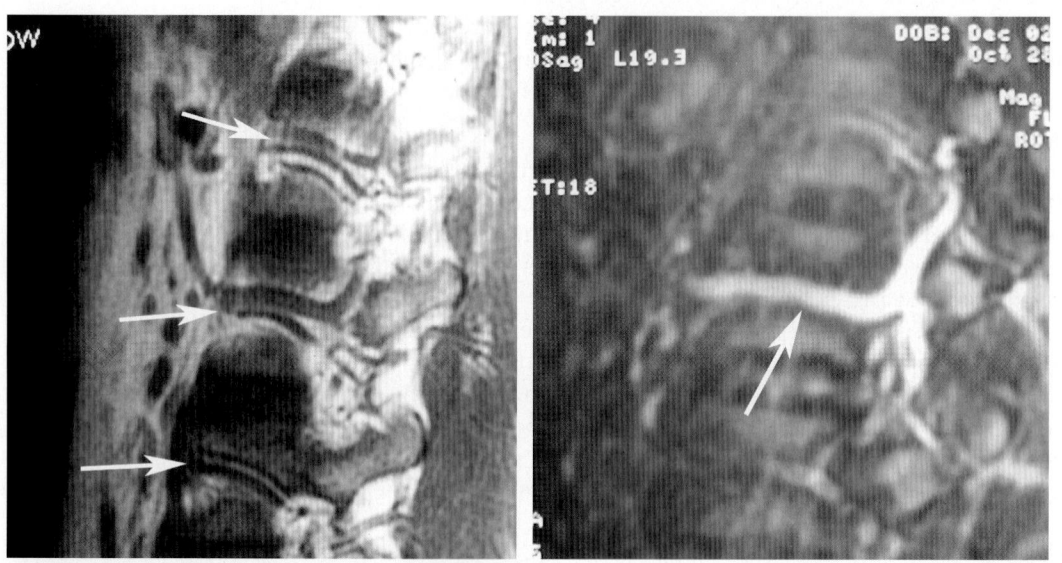

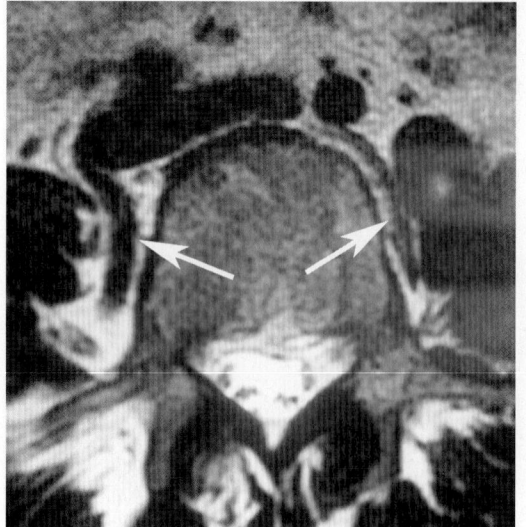

Figure 13.8. (A,B) Lateral MRI images (T1 and inversion recovery) demonstrate the large venous and arterial vascular structures (white arrows) that run along the lateral aspect of the vertebra. These vessels connect the anterior vascular systems (vena cava and aorta) with the epidural vessels. The vessels can be quite large, and injury can result in a large hematoma. **(C)** An axial MRI demonstrating the paravertebral vessels (white arrows) in this projection. It is easy to see how the parapedicular approach makes damage to these vessels possible.

is not completely clear, but it is believed that some cases are related to severe allergic reactions.

Cardiopulmonary compromise from pulmonary emboli in high-risk patients is also a contributing cause. As previously discussed, it can occur secondary to cement or fat emboli after PV or KP. Also, some patients are at increased risk of cardiopulmonary compromise. Severe COPD and known allergies to materials used during KP or PV should be considered when determining the appropriateness of therapy. Cardiopulmonary compromise, though rare, should be discussed as part of the consenting process, as it remains an idiosyncratic complication that cannot be completely eliminated.

References

1. Mathis JM, Barr JD, Belkoff SM, et al. Percutaneous vertebroplasty: a developing standard of care for vertebral compression fractures. Am J Neuroradiol 2001; 22:373–381.
2. Mathis JM. Percutaneous vertebroplasty: complication avoidance and technique optimization. Am J Neuroradiol 2003; 24:1697–1706.
3. Aebli N, Kreb J, Davis C, et al. Fat embolism and acute hypotension during vertebroplasty: an experimental study in sheep. Spine 2002; 27:460–466.
4. Deramond H, Dion J, Chiras J. Complications of percutaneous vertebroplasty. In Percutaneous Vertebroplasty. JM Mathis, H Deramond, SM Belkoff (eds). New York: Springer, 2001:165–174.
5. Jensen ME, Evans AJ, Mathis JM, et al. Percutaneous polymethylmethacrylate vertebroplasty in the treatment of osteoporotic vertebral body compression fractures: technical aspects. Am J Neuroradiol 1997; 18(10):1897–1904.
6. Liberman IH, Dudeney S, Reinhardt MK, et al. Initial outcome and efficacy of kyphoplasty in the treatment of painful osteoporotic vertebral compression fractures. Spine 2001; 26:1631–1638.
7. Nussbaum DA, Gailloud P, Murphy K. A review of complications associated with vertebroplasty and kyphoplasty as reported to the Food and Drug Administration medical device related web site. J Vasc Intervent Radiol 2004; 15:1185–1192.
8. Agris JM, Zoarski GH, Stallmeyer MJB, Ortiz O. Intravertebral pressure during vertebroplasty: a study comparing multiple delivery systems. Presented at the annual meeting of the American Society of Spine Radiology, Scottsdale, AZ, February 19–23, 2003.
9. Tomita S, Malloy S, Abe M, Belkoff SM. Ex vivo measurement of intramedullary pressure during vertebroplasty. Spine 2004; 29:723–725.
10. Padovani B, Kasriel O, Brunner P, et al. Pulmonary embolism caused by acrylic cement: a rare complication of percutaneous vertebroplasty. Am J Neuroradiol 1999; 20(3):375–377.
11. Yoo KY, Jeong SW, Yoon W, Lee J. Acute respiratory distress syndrome associated with pulmonary cement embolus following percutaneous vertebroplasty and polymethylmethacrylate. Spine 2004; 15:294–297.
12. Stricker K, Orler R, Yen K, et al. Severe hypercapnia due to pulmonary embolism of polymethylmethacrylate during vertebroplasty. Anesth Analg 2004; 98:1184–1186
13. Koessler MJ, Aebli N, Pitto RP. Fat and bone marrow embolism during percutaneous vertebroplasty. Anesth Analg 2003; 97:293.

14. Jang JS, Lee SH, Jung SK. Pulmonary embolism of polymethylmethacrylate after percutaneous vertebroplasty. A report of three cases. Spine 2002; 27:416–418.
15. Chen HL, Wong CS, Ho ST, et al. A lethal pulmonary embolism during percutaneous vertebroplasty. Anesth Analg 2002; 95:1060–1062.
16. Grados F, Depriester C, Cayrolle G, et al. Long-term observations of vertebral osteoporotic fractures treated by percutaneous vertebroplasty. Rheumatology 2000; 39:1410–1414.
17. Cortet B, Cotten A, Boutry N, et al. Percutaneous vertebroplasty in the treatment of osteoporotic vertebral compression fractures: an open prospective study. J Rheumatol 1999; 26(10):2222–2228.
18. Cyteval C, Sarrabere MP, Roux JO, et al. Acute osteoporotic vertebral collapse: open study on percutaneous injection of acrylic surgical cement in 20 patients. Am J Roentgenol 1999; 173(6):1685–1690.
19. Chiras J, Deramond H. Complications des vertebroplasties. In Echecs et Complications de la Chirurgie du Rachis: Chirurgie de Reprise. G Saillant, C Laville C (eds). Paris, France: Sauramps Medical, 1995:149–153.
20. Deramond H, Depriester C, Galibert P, et al. Percutaneous vertebroplasty with polymethylmethacrylate. Technique, indications, and results. Radiol Clin North Am 1998; 36(3):533–546.
21. Weill A, Chiras J, Simon JM, et al. Spinal metastases: indications for and results of percutaneous injection of acrylic surgical cement. Radiology 1996; 199(1):241–247.
22. Cotten A, Dewatre F, Cortet B, et al. Percutaneous vertebroplasty for osteolytic metastases and myeloma: effects of the percentage of lesion filling and the leakage of methyl methacrylate at clinical follow-up. Radiology 1996; 200(2):525–530.

14

Standards for the Performance of Percutaneous Vertebroplasty: American College of Radiology and Society of Interventional Radiology Guidelines

Part I STANDARD FOR THE PERFORMANCE OF PERCUTANEOUS VERTEBROPLASTY[*,†]

The American College of Radiology, with more than 30,000 members, is the principal organization of radiologists, radiation oncologists, and clinical medical physicists in the United States. The College is a non-profit professional society whose primary purposes are to advance the science of radiology, improve radiologic services to the patient, study the socioeconomic aspects of the practice of radiology, and encourage continuing education for radiologists, radiation oncologists, medical physicists, and persons practicing in allied professional fields.

The American College of Radiology will periodically define new standards for radiologic practice to help advance the science of radiology and to improve the quality of service to patients throughout the United States. Existing standards will be reviewed for revision or renewal, as appropriate, on their fifth anniversary or sooner, if indicated.

---

[*] This standard (Res. 14, which became effective on January 1, 2001) has been included in its unaltered entirety. However, it should be noted that there are some errors in reference citations that are undergoing correction.

[†] Reprinted with permission of the American College of Radiology. No other representation of this document is authorized without express written permission from the American College of Radiology.

Each standard, representing a policy statement by the College, has undergone a thorough consensus process in which it has been subjected to extensive review, requiring the approval of the Commission on Standards and Accreditation, as well as the American College of Radiology (ACR) Board of Chancellors, the ACR Council Steering Committee, and the ACR Council. The standards recognize that the safe and effective use of diagnostic and therapeutic radiology requires specific training, skills, and techniques, as described in each document. Reproduction or modification of the published standard by those entities not providing these services is not authorized.

The standards of the ACR are not rules, but are guidelines that attempt to define principles of practice to produce high-quality radiologic care. The physician and medical physicist may modify an existing standard as determined by the individual patient and available resources. Adherence to ACR standards will not ensure a successful outcome in every situation. The standards should not be deemed inclusive of all proper methods of care or exclusive of other methods of care reasonably directed to obtaining the same results. The standards are not intended to establish a legal standard of care or conduct, and deviation from a standard does not, in and of itself, indicate or imply that such medical practice is below an acceptable level of care. The ultimate judgment regarding the propriety of any specific procedure or course of conduct must be made by the physician and medical physicist in light of all circumstances presented by the individual situation.

Standard for the Performance of Percutaneous Vertebroplasty

Developed by a collaborative panel of the American College of Radiology, the American Society of Neuroradiology, the American Society of Interventional and Therapeutic Neuroradiology, and the American Society of Spine Radiology.

I. Introduction

This Standard for the Performance of Percutaneous Vertebroplasty was developed by a consensus of recognized pioneers of the technique in the United States. Physicians from the fields of interventional neuroradiology, musculoskeletal radiology, neurosurgery, and orthopedic surgery participated in the development process. A thorough review of the literature was performed. When published data were felt to be inadequate, data from the expert panel members' own quality assurance programs were used to supplement. Thresholds for quality assurance were difficult to set due to the relative paucity of data and lack of uniform reporting of clinical outcomes and complications.

Percutaneous vertebroplasty is being performed with rapidly increasing frequency in the United States. We anticipate that more data regarding outcomes and complications will be collected and published in the near future. Therefore, we recommend that this standard be reviewed and, if necessary, revised within the next 24 months in order to remain current with this rapidly progressing technique.

Developed by Galibert and colleagues in France in the late 1980s (1), percutaneous vertebroplasty entails injection of polymethylmethacrylate (PMMA) cement into the collapsed vertebra. Although this procedure does not reexpand the collapsed vertebra, reinforcing and stabilizing the fracture seems to alleviate pain.

Radiologic imaging has been a critical part of percutaneous vertebroplasty from its inception. Most procedures are performed utilizing fluoroscopic guidance for needle placement and to monitor cement injection. The use of computed tomography (CT) has also been described for these purposes.

Percutaneous vertebroplasty is an established, safe, and effective procedure for selected patients. Extensive experience documents the safety and efficacy of this procedure (1–20). As with any invasive procedure, the patient is most likely to benefit when the procedure is performed in an appropriate environment by qualified physicians.

II. Overview

Vertebral compression fractures are a common and often debilitating complication of osteoporosis (21–25). Although most fractures heal within a few weeks or months, a minority of patients continue to suffer pain that does not respond to conservative therapy (26,27). Vertebral compression fractures are a leading cause of nursing home admission. Open surgical fixation is rarely employed to treat these fractures. The poor quality of bone at the adjacent unfractured levels does not provide a good anchor for surgical hardware, and the advanced age of most affected patients increases the risk of major surgery.

Initial success with percutaneous vertebroplasty for treatment of aggressive hemangiomas (1,2) and osteolytic neoplasms (3,4) led to extension of the indications to include osteoporotic compression fractures refractory to medical therapy (5–19).

III. Indications and Contraindications

A. Indications

1. Painful osteoporotic vertebral compression fracture(s) refractory to medical therapy. Failure of medical therapy is defined as minimal or no pain relief with the administration of physician-prescribed analgesics or achievement of adequate pain relief only with narcotic dosages that induce excessive and intolerable sedation, confusion, or constipation. Associated major disability such as inability to walk, transfer, or perform activities of daily living is almost always present.

2. Painful vertebral fracture or severe osteolysis with impending fracture related to benign or malignant tumor, such as hemangioma, myeloma, or metastasis.

3. Painful vertebral fracture associated with osteonecrosis (Kummell's disease).
4. Unstable compression fracture with demonstration of movement at the wedge deformity.
5. Patients with multiple compression deformities resulting from osteoporotic collapse for whom further collapse would likely result in pulmonary compromise, gastrointestinal tract dysfunction, or altered center of gravity with associated increased risk of falling as a result of deformity of the spine.
6. Chronic traumatic fractures in normal bone with nonunion of fracture fragments or internal cystic changes.

B. Absolute Contraindications

1. Asymptomatic stable fracture.
2. Patient clearly improving on medical therapy.
3. Prophylaxis in osteopenic patients with no evidence of acute fracture.
4. Osteomyelitis of target vertebra.
5. Acute traumatic fracture of nonosteoporotic vertebra.
6. Uncorrectable coagulopathy or hemorrhagic diathesis.
7. Allergy to any component required for the procedure.

C. Relative Contraindications

1. Radicular pain or radiculopathy, significantly in excess of vertebral pain, caused by a compressive syndrome unrelated to vertebral body collapse. In such circumstances, preoperative vertebroplasty may be indicated if a spinal destabilization procedure is planned.
2. Retropulsion of fracture fragment causing significant spinal canal compromise.
3. Tumor extension into the epidural space with significant spinal canal compromise.
4. Severe vertebral body collapse.
5. Stable fracture without pain and known to be more than 2 years old.
6. Treatment of more than three levels performed at one time.

200 Appendix I

The threshold for these indications is 95%. When fewer than 95% of the procedures are for these indications, the institution should review the process of patient selection.

IV. Qualifications and Responsibilities of Personnel

A. Physician

1. In general, the requirements for the performance of percutaneous vertebroplasty (see Section IV.A.3) may be met by adhering to the recommendations listed below:

a. Certification in Radiology or Diagnostic Radiology by the American Board of Radiology, the American Osteopathic Board of Radiology, or the Royal College of Physicians and Surgeons of Canada.

and

b. Completion of an Accreditation Council for Graduate Medical Education (ACGME) accredited residency or fellowship program that included 6 months training in cross-sectional imaging, including CT and MR imaging, and 4 months training in image-guided interventional radiologic techniques including percutaneous vertebroplasty, biopsy and drainage procedures, and vascular embolization. This must include performance (under the supervision of a qualified physician) of at least 10 percutaneous vertebroplasties with acceptable success and complication rates documented by a log of cases performed as described in this document (see Section VII.C).

Physicians whose residency or fellowship training did not include the above-described experience with percutaneous vertebroplasty may be considered as satisfying the qualifications for this procedure if they meet all other requirements and have performed at least 10 percutaneous vertebroplasties with acceptable success and complication rates documented by a log of cases performed as described in this document (see Section VII.C).

2. In the absence of appropriate ACGME approved residency or fellowship training (as listed in Section IV.A.1.a above) or other postgraduate training that included comparable instruction and experience, physicians may meet the requirements listed in Section IV.A.1 by adhering to the following recommendations:

a. Documentation of "hands-on" training in the performance of percutaneous vertebroplasty.

and

b. Performance and completion of at least two successful and uncomplicated percutaneous vertebroplasty procedures as principal operator under the supervision of an on-site, qualified physician with acceptable success and complication rates and (see Section VII.C).

c. Substantiation in writing by the Director of the Department of Radiology, the Chief of the Medical Staff, or the Chair of the Credentials Committee of the institution in which the procedures were performed that the physician is familiar with all of the following:

1. Indications and contraindications for percutaneous vertebroplasty.
2. Preprocedural assessment and intraprocedural monitoring of the patient.
3. Appropriate use and operation of fluoroscopic and radiographic equipment, digital subtraction systems, and other electronic imaging systems.

4. Principles of radiation protection, hazards of radiation exposure to the patient and the radiologic personnel, and radiation monitoring requirements.
5. Anatomy, physiology, and pathophysiology of the spine, spinal cord, and nerve roots.
6. Pharmacology of contrast agents and of polymethylmethacrylate and recognition and treatment of adverse reactions to these substances.
7. Technical aspects of performing this procedure.
8. Postprocedural patient management, particularly the recognition and initial management of procedural complications.

3. Certain fundamental knowledge and skills are required for the appropriate application and safe performance of percutaneous vertebroplasty:

　a. In addition to a basic understanding of spinal anatomy, physiology, and pathophysiology, the physician must have sufficient knowledge of the clinical and imaging evaluation of patients with spinal disorders to determine those for whom percutaneous vertebroplasty is indicated.

and

　b. The physician must fully appreciate the benefits and risks of percutaneous vertebroplasty and the alternatives to the procedure.

and

　c. The physician is required to be competent in the use of fluoroscopy, computed tomography (CT), and magnetic resonance imaging (MRI); modalities employed to evaluate potential patients and to guide the percutaneous vertebroplasty procedure.

and

　d. Operator should be able to recognize, interpret, and act immediately on image findings.

and

　e. The physician must have the ability, skills, and knowledge to evaluate the patient's clinical status and to identify those patients who might be at increased risk, who may require additional pre- or postprocedural care, or who have relative contraindications to the procedure.

and

　f. The physician must be capable of providing the initial clinical management of complications of percutaneous vertebroplasty, including administration of basic life support, treatment of pneumothorax, and recognition of spinal cord compression.

and

　g. Training in radiation physics and safety is an important component of these requirements. Such training is important to maximize both patient and physician safety. It is highly recommended that the physician have adequate training in and be familiar with the principles of radiation exposure, the hazards of radiation exposure to both patients and radiologic personnel, and the radiation monitoring requirements for the imaging methods listed above.

4. Maintenance of competence. Maintenance of competence requires regular continuing clinical activity, including:
   a. Regular performance of imaging-guided percutaneous interventions, including sufficient numbers of percutaneous vertebroplasties to maintain success and complication rates as outlined below.
   b. Participation in a quality improvement program that monitors these rates.
   c. Participation in postgraduate courses that provide continuing education on diagnostic and technical advances in percutaneous vertebroplasty.
   d. The physician's continuing education should be in accordance with the ACR Standard for Continuing Medical Education (CME).

B. Medical Physicist

A Qualified Medical Physicist is an individual who is competent to practice independently in one or more of the subfields in medical physics. The American College of Radiology considers that certification and continuing education in the appropriate subfield(s) demonstrate that an individual is competent to practice one or more of the subfields in medical physics, and to be a Qualified Medical Physicist. The ACR recommends that the individual be certified in the appropriate subfield(s) by the American Board of Radiology (ABR).

The appropriate subfields in medical physics for this standard are Radiological Physics and Diagnostic Radiological Physics. The continuing education of a Qualified Medical Physicist should be in accordance with the ACR Standard for Continuing Medical Education (CME).

C. Radiological Technologist

The technologist, together with the physician and the nursing personnel, should have responsibility for patient comfort. The technologist should be able to prepare and position the patient for the vertebroplasty procedure, and together with the nurse, monitor the patient during the procedure. The technologist should obtain the imaging data in a manner prescribed by the supervising physician. The technologist should also perform regular quality control testing of the equipment under the supervision of the medical physicist. The technologist should have documented training and experience in the percutaneous vertebroplasty procedure or similar interventional procedures and be certified by the American Registry of Radiologic Technologists (ARRT) or have an unrestricted state license.

D. Nursing Services

Nursing services are an integral part of the team for pre- and postprocedural patient management and education and may assist the physician in monitoring the patient during the percutaneous vertebroplasty procedure.

V. Specifications of the Procedure

A. Technical Requirements

There are several technical requirements that are necessary to ensure safe and successful percutaneous vertebroplasties. These include adequate institutional facilities, imaging and monitoring equipment, and support personnel. The following are minimum facility requirements for any institution in which percutaneous vertebroplasty is to be performed:

1. A procedure suite large enough to allow easy transfer of the patient from bed to procedural table with sufficient space for appropriate positioning of patient monitoring equipment, anesthesia equipment, respirators, etc. There should be adequate space for the operating team to work unencumbered on either side of the patient and for the circulation of other staff within the room without contaminating the sterile conditions.

2. A high-resolution image intensifier and video system with adequate shielding capable of rapid imaging in orthogonal planes and capabilities for permanent image recording is essential. Imaging findings are acquired and stored either on conventional film or digitally on computerized storage media. Imaging and image recording must be consistent with the as low as reasonably achievable (ALARA) radiation safety guidelines. Operator should be able to recognize, interpret, and act immediately on image finding.

3. Immediate access to CT and MR imaging is necessary to allow evaluation of potential complications. This may be particularly desirable if percutaneous vertebroplasty is planned in patients with osteolytic vertebral metastasis and/or with significant preexisting spinal canal compromise. CT is desirable for evaluation of the spinal canal and intervertebral foramina if significant extravasation of cement is suspected, even if the patient remains asymptomatic.

4. The facility must provide adequate resources for observing patients during and after percutaneous vertebroplasty. Physiologic monitoring devices appropriate to the patient's needs—including blood pressure monitoring, pulse oximetry, and electrocardiography—and equipment for cardiopulmonary resuscitation must be available in the procedural suite.

B. Surgical and Emergency Support

Although serious complications of percutaneous vertebroplasty are infrequent, there should be prompt access to surgical, interventional, and medical management of complications.

C. Patient Care

1. *Preprocedural care*
   a. The clinical history and findings, including the indications for the procedure, must be reviewed and recorded in the patient's medical record by the physician performing the procedure. Specific inquiry should be made with respect to relevant medications, prior allergic reactions, and bleeding/clotting status.
   b. The vital signs and results of physical and neurological examinations must be obtained and recorded.
   c. The indication(s) for the procedure, including (if applicable) documentation of failed medical therapy, must be recorded.
   d. The indication(s) for treatment of the fracture should have documentation of imaging correlation and confirmation.
2. *Procedural care*
   a. Vital signs should be obtained at regular intervals during the course of the procedure, and a record of these measurements should be maintained.
   b. Patients undergoing percutaneous vertebroplasty must have intravenous access in place for the administration of fluids and medications as needed.
   c. If the patient is to receive conscious sedation, pulse oximetry must be used. Administration of sedation for percutaneous vertebroplasty should be in accordance with the ACR Standard for Adult Sedation/Analgesia. A registered nurse or other appropriately trained personnel should be present and have primary responsibility for monitoring the patient. A record of medication doses and times of administration should be maintained.
3. *Postprocedural care*
   a. A procedural note should be written in the patient's medical record summarizing the course of the procedure and what was accomplished, any immediate complications, and the patient's status at the conclusion of the procedure (see Section VII.A.2 below). This note may be brief if the formal report will be available within a few hours. This information should be communicated to the referring physician in a timely manner. A more detailed summary of the procedure should be written in the medical record if the formal typed report will not be on the medical record within the same day.
   b. All patients should be at bed rest and observed during the initial postprocedural period. The length of this period will depend on the patient's medical condition.
   c. During the immediate postprocedural period, skilled nurses or other appropriately trained personnel should monitor the patient's vital signs, urinary output, sensorium, and motor strength. Neurological status should be assessed frequently at regular intervals. Initial ambulation of the patient must be carefully supervised.

d. The operating physician or a qualified designee (another physician or a nurse) should evaluate the patient after the initial postprocedural period, and these findings should be summarized in a progress note on the patient's medical record. The physician or designee must be available for continuing care during hospitalization and after discharge.

VI. Equipment Quality Control

Each facility should have documented policies and procedures for monitoring and evaluating the effective management, safety, and proper performance of imaging and interventional equipment. The quality control program should be designed to maximize the quality of the diagnostic information. This may be accomplished as part of a routine preventive maintenance program.

VII. Quality Improvement and Documentation

A. Documentation

Results of percutaneous vertebroplasty procedures should be monitored on a continuous basis. Records should be kept of both immediate and long-term results and complications. The number of complications should be documented. Any biopsies performed in conjunction with percutaneous vertebroplasty should be followed up to detect and record any false negative and false positive results.

A permanent record of percutaneous vertebroplasty procedures should be maintained on a retrievable image storage format.

1. Image labeling should include permanent identification containing:
   a. Facility name and location.
   b. Examination date.
   c. Patient's first and last names.
   d. Patient's identification number and/or date of birth.
2. The physician's report of a percutaneous vertebroplasty procedure should include:
   a. Procedure undertaken and its purpose.
   b. Local anesthesia, if used, listing agent and amount.
   c. Conscious sedation, if used, listing medications and amounts.
   d. Listing of level(s) treated and amount of cement injected at each level.
   e. Immediate complications, if any, including treatment and outcome. Reporting should be in accordance with the ACR Standard on Communication: Diagnostic Radiology.
3. Follow-up documentation:
   a. Evaluation of long-term patient response (pain relief, mobility improvement). Standardized assessment tools such as the SF-36 and the Roland scale may be useful for both pre- and postoperative patient evaluation.

b. Delayed complications, if any, including treatment and outcome.
   c. Pathology (biopsy) results, if any.
   d. Record of communications with patient and referring physician.
   e. Patient disposition.

B. Informed Consent and Procedural Risk

Informed consent or emergency administrative consent must be obtained and must be in compliance with state law. Risks cited should include infection; bleeding; allergic reaction; fracture; pneumothorax (for appropriate levels); and extravasation of cement into the adjacent epidural or paravertebral veins resulting in worsening pain or paralysis, spinal cord or nerve injury, or pulmonary compromise. The potential need for immediate surgical intervention should be discussed. The possibility that the patient may not experience significant pain relief should also be discussed.

C. Complication Rates and Thresholds (1–20)

While practicing physicians should strive to achieve perfect outcomes (i.e., 100% success, 0% complications), in practice all physicians will fall short of this ideal to a variable extent. Thus, indicator thresholds may be used to assess the efficacy of ongoing quality improvement programs. For the purposes of this standard, a threshold is a specific level of an indicator (e.g., complication rate) that should prompt a review. When complication rates exceed a maximum threshold, a review should be performed to determine causes and to implement changes, if necessary.

Routine periodic review of all cases having less than perfect outcomes is strongly encouraged. Serious complications of percutaneous vertebroplasty are infrequent. A review is therefore recommended for all instances of death, infection, and symptomatic pulmonary embolus.

A review may be prompted when a complication rate surpasses the threshold values outlined below (suggested thresholds are listed in parentheses):

1. *Clinical complications*
   a. Death (0%).
   b. Permanent (duration >30 days) neurological deficit (other than radicular pain):
      1. osteoporosis (0%)
      2. neoplasm (5%)
   c. Transient (duration ≤30 days) neurological deficit (other than radicular pain) or radicular pain syndrome (either permanent or transient):
      1. osteoporosis (5%)
      2. neoplasm (10%)
   d. Symptomatic pulmonary cement embolus (0%).
   e. Symptomatic epidural venous cement embolus (5%).
   f. Infection (0%).
   g. Fracture of rib or vertebra (5%)

h. Significant hemorrhage or vascular injury (0%).
i. Allergic or idiosyncratic reaction (1%)
2. *Technical/procedural complications*
   a. Failure to obtain proper informed consent (0%).
   b. Cement embolus to pulmonary vasculature without clinical sequela and estimated volume >0.25 mL (5%).
   c. Cement embolus to epidural veins without clinical sequela and producing >10% spinal canal compromise or estimated volume >0.25 mL (10%).

D. **Clinical Outcomes**

1. Achievement of significant pain relief and improved mobility (osteoporosis) (80%).
2. Achievement of significant pain relief and improved mobility (neoplasm) (50%) (when treatment is performed primarily for spinal stabilization, not pain relief, this threshold would not apply).

VIII. Quality Control and Improvement, Safety, Infection Control, and Patient Education Concerns

Policies and procedures related to quality, patient education, infection control, and safety should be developed and implemented in accordance with the ACR policy on Quality Control and Improvement, Safety, Infection Control, and Patient Education Concerns appearing elsewhere in this publication.

Acknowledgments

This Standard was developed according to the process described elsewhere in this publication by the Standards and Accreditation Committee of the Commission on Neuroradiology and MR in collaboration with the American Society of Neuroradiology, the American Society of Interventional and Therapeutic Neuroradiology, and the American Society of Spine Radiology.

Principal Drafters

John D. Barr, MD, Co-Chair
John M. Mathis, MD, MSc, Co-Chair
Michelle S. Barr, MD
Andrew J. Denardo, MD
Jacques E. Dion, MD
Lee R. Guterman, MD, PhD
M. Lee Jensen, MD
Isador H. Lieberman, MD
Wayne J. Olan, MD
Wade Wong, DO

Standards and Accreditation Committee

Stephen A. Kieffer, MD, Chair
John D. Barr, MD
Richard S. Boyer, MD
John J. Connors, MD
Robert Dawson, III, MD
Robert Hurst, MD
Richard E. Latchaw, MD
Andrew W. Litt, MD
Gordon K. Sze, MD
H. Denny Taylor, MD
Patrick A. Turski, MD
Robert C. Wallace, MD
Jeffrey C. Weinreb, MD
William G. Bradley, MD, Chair, Commission
Danny R. Hatfield, MD, CSC

References

1. Galibert P, Deramond H, Rosat P, et al. Preliminary note on the treatment of vertebral angioma by percutaneous acrylic vertebroplasty. Neurochirurgie 1987; 33(2):166–168.
2. Deramond H, Darrason R, Galibert P. Percutaneous vertebroplasty with acrylic cement in the treatment of aggressive spinal angiomas. Rachis 1989; 1:143–153.
3. Weill A, Chiras J, Simon JM, et al. Spinal metastases: indications for and results of percutaneous injection of acrylic surgical cement. Radiology 1996; 199:241–247.
4. Cotten A, Dewatre F, Cortet B, et al. Percutaneous vertebroplasty for osteolytic metastases and myeloma: effects of the percentage of lesion filling and the leakage of methyl methacrylate at clinical follow-up. Radiology 1996; 200:525–530.
5. Deramond H, Galibert P, Debussche-Depriester C. Vertebroplasty. Neuroradiology 1991; 33(Suppl):S177–S178.
6. Debussche-Depriester C, Deramond H, Fardellone P, et al. Percutaneous vertebroplasty with acrylic cement in the treatment of osteoporotic vertebral crush fracture syndrome. Neuroradiology 1991; 33(Suppl):S149–S152.
7. Gangi A, Kastler BA, Dietemann JL. Percutaneous vertebroplasty guided by a combination of CT and fluoroscopy. Am J Neuroradiol 1994; 15:83–86.
8. Cardon T, Hachulla E, Flipo RM, et al. Percutaneous vertebroplasty with acrylic cement in the treatment of Langerhans cell vertebral histiocytosis. Clin Rheumatol 1994; 13(3):518–521.
9. Chiras J, Deramond H. Complications des vertebroplasties. In Echecs et Complications de la Chirurgie du Rachis: Chirurgie de Reprise. G Saillant, C Laville (eds). Paris: Sauramps Medical, 1995:149–153.
10. Dousset V, Mousselard H, de Monck d'User L, et al. Asymptomatic cervical hemangioma treated by percutaneous vertebroplasty. Neuroradiology 1996; 38(4):392–394.
11. Jensen ME, Evans AJ, Mathis JM, et al. Percutaneous polymethylmethacrylate vertebroplasty in the treatment of osteoporotic vertebral

body compression fractures: technical aspects. Am J Neuroradiol 1997; 18:1897–1904.
12. Deramond H, Depriester C, Toussaint P, et al. Percutaneous vertebral surgery: techniques and indications. Semin Musculoskel Radiol 1997; 1(2).
13. Chiras J, Depriester C, Weill A, et al. Percutaneous vertebroplasty. J Neuroradiol 1997; 24:45–59.
14. Lemley TJ, Barr MS, Barr JD, et al. Percutaneous vertebroplasty: a new technique for treatment of benign and malignant vertebral body compression fractures. Surgical Physician Assistant 1997; 3(3):24–27.
15. Mathis JM, Petri M, Naff N. Percutaneous vertebroplasty treatment of steroid-induced osteoporotic compression fractures. Arthritis Rheum 1998; 41(1):171–175.
16. Cotten A, Boutry N, Cortet B, et al. Percutaneous vertebroplasty: state of the art. RadioGraphics 1998; 18:311–320.
17. Barr MS, Barr JD. Invited commentary. Vertebroplasty: state of the art. RadioGraphics 1998; 18:320–322.
18. Do HM, Jensen ME, Cloft HJ. Percutaneous vertebroplasty in the treatment of patients with vertebral osteonecrosis (Kummell's disease). Neurosurgical Focus 1999; 7(1):article 2.
19. Barr JD, Barr MS, Lemley TJ, et al. Percutaneous vertebroplasty for pain relief and spinal stabilization. Spine 2000; 25:923–928.
20. Padovani B, Kasriel O, Brunner P, et al. Pulmonary embolism caused by acrylic cement: a rare complication of percutaneous vertebroplasty. Am J Neuroradiol 1999; 20:375–377.
21. Cooper C. The epidemiology of fragility fractures: is there a role for bone quality? Calcif Tissue Int 1993; 53(Suppl 1):S23–S26.
22. Cooper C, Atkinson EJ, Jacobsen SJ, et al. Population-based study of survival after osteoporotic fractures. Am J Epidemiol 1993; 137(9):1001–1005.
23. Riggs BL, Melton LJ, 3d. Involutional osteoporosis. N Engl J Med 1986; 314:1676–1686.
24. Riggs BL, Melton LJ, III. The worldwide problem of osteoporosis: insights afforded by epidemiology. Bone 1995; 17(Suppl):S505–S511.
25. Wasnich RD. Vertebral fracture epidemiology. Bone 1996; 18:S179–S183.
26. Silverman SL. The clinical consequences of vertebral compression fracture. Bone 1992; 13(Suppl):S27–S31.
27. Heaney RP. The natural history of vertebral osteoporosis. Is low bone mass an epiphenomenon? Bone 1992; 13(Suppl):S23–S26.

Part II QUALITY IMPROVEMENT GUIDELINES FOR PERCUTANEOUS VERTEBROPLASTY[*,†]

Preamble

The membership of the Society of Interventional Radiology (SIR) Standards of Practice Committee represents experts in a broad spectrum of interventional procedures from the private and academic sectors of medicine. Generally, Standards of Practice Committee members dedicate the vast majority of their professional time to performing interventional procedures; as such, they represent a valid, broad expert constituency of the subject matter under consideration for standards production.

Technical documents specifying the exact consensus and literature review methodologies as well as the institutional affiliations and professional credentials of the authors of this document are available on request from the Society of Interventional Radiology, 10201 Lee Highway, Suite 500, Fairfax, VA 22030.

Methodology

SIR produces its Standards of Practice documents with use of the following process: Standards documents of relevance and timeliness are conceptualized by the Standards of Practice Committee members. A recognized expert is identified to serve as the principal author for the standard. Additional authors may be assigned depending on the magnitude of the project.

An in-depth literature search is performed with use of electronic medical literature databases. Then, a critical review of peer-reviewed articles is performed with regard to the study methodology, results, and conclusions. The qualitative weight of these articles is assembled into an evidence table, which is used to write the document so it contains evidence-based data with respect to contents, rates, and thresholds.

When the evidence of literature is weak, conflicting, or contradictory, consensus for the parameter is reached by a minimum of 12 Standards of Practice Committee members with use of a Modified Delphi Consensus Method (1,2). For the purposes of these documents, consensus is defined as 80% Delphi participant agreement on a value or parameter.

The draft document is critically reviewed by the Standards of Practice Committee members by telephone conference call or face-to-face

---

[*] J. Kevin McGraw, John Cardella, John Dean Barr, John M. Mathis, Orestes Sanchez, Marc S. Schwartzberg, Timothy L. Swan, and David Sacks for the Society of Interventional Radiology Standards of Practice Committee.
[†] Reprinted with permission from *J Vasc Intervent Radiol* 2003; 14:S311–S315.

meeting. The finalized draft from the Committee is sent to the SIR membership for further input/criticism during a 30-day comment period. These comments are discussed by the Standards of Practice Committee and appropriate revisions are made to create the finished standards document. Before its publication, the document is endorsed by the SIR Executive Council.

Vertebral Fractures

Each year, more than 700,000 vertebral fractures secondary to osteoporosis are diagnosed in the United States population, resulting in 115,000 hospital admissions (3). The lifetime risk of a vertebral body compression fracture is 16% for women and 5% for men, and the incidence of osteoporotic fractures is anticipated to increase fourfold worldwide in the next 50 years (3). Other causes of painful compression fracture include malignant involvement of the spinal column (metastasis, myeloma, and lymphoma), hemangioma, and vertebral osteonecrosis. In addition to pain, spinal column instability may also be present. Regardless of etiology, treatment for compression fractures has been largely conservative and directed toward pain control, usually consisting of narcotic analgesia, bedrest, and back bracing. For osteoporosis, current preventive drug regimens, including hormonal replacement therapy, biphosphates, and calcitonin, often are not prescribed until the disease has been diagnosed by the presence of a fracture.

Percutaneous vertebroplasty is a therapeutic alternative for the treatment of pain associated with vertebral body compression fractures (4–22). The procedure entails placement of a large-caliber needle into the involved vertebral body and injection of radiopaque bone cement (e.g., polymethyl methacrylate). The injected bone cement does not reexpand the collapsed vertebra, but acts as an internal splint to reinforce and stabilize the fracture for pain alleviation.

These guidelines are written to be used in quality improvement programs to assess percutaneous vertebroplasty procedures. The most important processes of care are (1) selecting the patients, (2) performing the procedure, and (3) monitoring the patients. The outcome measures or indicators for these processes are indications, success rates, and complication rates. Outcome measures are assigned threshold levels.

Definitions

Percutaneous vertebroplasty is defined as the injection of radiopaque bone cement (e.g., polymethyl methacrylate) into a painful osteoporotic compression fracture (9,10,12–14,16,18,20–28) or painful pathologic vertebral body (e.g., multiple myeloma [7,8,29–32], metastatic disease [5–7,33], and hemangioma [4,33–38]) with use of imaging guidance. Radiologic imaging has been a critical part of percutaneous vertebroplasty from its inception. Most procedures are performed with use of fluoroscopic guidance for needle placement and to monitor bone cement injection. The use of computed tomography has also been described (39).

Although practicing physicians should strive to achieve perfect outcomes (e.g., 100% success, 0% complications), in practice, all physicians will fall short of this ideal to a variable extent. Therefore, indicator thresholds may be used to assess the efficacy of ongoing quality-improvement programs. For the purposes of these guidelines, a threshold is a specific level of an indicator that should prompt a review. *Procedure thresholds* or *overall thresholds* reference a group of indicators for a procedure, e.g., major complications. Individual complications may also be associated with complication-specific thresholds. When measures such as indications or success rates fall below a (minimum) threshold, or when complication rates exceed a (maximum) threshold, a review should be performed to determine causes and to implement changes if necessary. For example, if the incidence of fracture of rib or other bone is one measure of the quality of percutaneous vertebroplasty, values in excess of the defined threshold (in this case <1%) should trigger a review of policies and procedures within the department to determine the causes and to implement changes to lower the incidence of the complication. Thresholds may vary from those listed herein; e.g., patient referral patterns and selection factors may dictate a different threshold value for a particular indicator at a particular institution. Therefore, setting universal thresholds is very difficult, and each department is urged to alter the thresholds as needed to higher or lower values to meet its own quality-improvement program needs.

Complications can be stratified on the basis of outcome. Major complications result in admission to a hospital for therapy (for outpatient procedures), an unplanned increase in the level of care, prolonged hospitalization, permanent adverse sequelae, or death. Minor complications result in no sequelae; they may require nominal therapy or a short hospital stay for observation (generally overnight; see Appendix 1). The complication rates and thresholds described herein refer to major complications.

Indications

The major indication for percutaneous vertebroplasty is the treatment of symptomatic osteoporotic or neoplastic vertebral body compression fracture(s) refractory to medical therapy. Failure of medical therapy is defined by minimal or no pain relief with the administration of prescribed analgesics or adequate pain relief with narcotic dosages that produce undesirable side effects (excessive and intolerable sedation, confusion, or constipation). Other, less common indications, are outlined in Table 14.1. Absolute and relative contraindications are outlined in Table 14.2. The indications and contraindications for percutaneous

Table 14.1. Indications for Percutaneous Vertebroplasty: Threshold 95%.

1. Painful primary and secondary osteoporotic vertebral compression fracture(s) refractory to medical therapy
2. Painful vertebrae with extensive osteolysis or invasion secondary to benign or malignant tumor (i.e., hemangioma, multiple myeloma, or metastatic disease)
3. Painful vertebral fracture associated with osteonecrosis (Kummell's disease)

Note: When fewer than 95% of percutaneous vertebroplasty in an institution are performed for one or more of the above indications, it should prompt a review of practices related to selection of patients for percutaneous vertebroplasty.

vertebroplasty may change in the future as more research and information become available.

Success Rates

When percutaneous vertebroplasty is performed for osteoporosis, success is defined as achievement of significant pain relief and/or improved mobility as measured by validated measurement tools with a threshold of 80%.

When percutaneous vertebroplasty is performed for neoplastic involvement, success is defined as achievement of significant pain relief and/or improved mobility as measured by validated measurement tools with a threshold of 50 to 60%.

Complications

Major complications occur in less than 1% of patients treated for compression fractures secondary to osteoporosis and in less than 5% of

Table 14.2. Absolute and Relative Contraindications for Percutaneous Vertebroplasty.

Absolute contraindications
1. Asymptomatic vertebral body compression fractures
2. Patient improving on medical therapy
3. Prophylaxis in osteoporotic patients
4. Ongoing local or systemic infection
5. Retropulsed bone fragment resulting in myelopathy
6. Spinal canal compromise secondary to tumor resulting in myelopathy
7. Uncorrectable coagulopathy
8. Allergy to bone cement or opacification agent

Relative contraindications
1. Radiculopathy in excess of vertebral pain, caused by a compressive syndrome unrelated to vertebral collapse. Occasionally, preoperative percutaneous vertebroplasty can be performed before a spinal decompressive procedure
2. Asymptomatic retropulsion of a fracture fragment causing significant spinal canal compromise
3. Asymptomatic tumor extension into the epidural space

treated patients with neoplastic involvement (5–9,13,14,16,19,22,23,28, 40–49). Published complication rates and suggested thresholds are included in Table 14.3.

Published rates for individual types of complications are highly dependent on patient selection and are based on series comprising several hundred patients, which is a volume larger than most individual practitioners are likely to treat. It is also recognized that a single complication can cause a rate to cross above a complication-specific threshold when the complication occurs in a small volume of patients, e.g., early in a quality-improvement program, than is the published rate.

Overall procedure threshold for all complications resulting from percutaneous vertebroplasty performed for osteoporosis is 2% and performed for neoplastic indications is 10% (32).

Acknowledgments

Dr. J. Kevin McGraw authored the first draft of this document and served as topic leader during the subsequent revisions of the draft. Dr. John F. Cardella is Chair of the SIR Standards of Practice Committee. Dr. David Sacks is Councilor of the SIR Standards Division. Other members of the Standards of Practice Committee and SIR who participated in the development of this clinical practice guideline are (listed alphabetically): John Aruny, MD, Daniel B. Brown, MD, Patricia Cole, PhD, MD, Peter Drescher, MD, MS, Neil Freeman, MD, Jeff Georgia, MD, Clement Grassi, MD, Ziv Haskal, MD, Michael Todd Jones, MD, Patrick Malloy, MD, Louis Martin, MD, Timothy McCowan, MD, Steven Meranze, MD, Theodore Mirra, MD, Kenneth D. Murphy, MD, Calvin Neithamer, MD, Steven Oglevie, MD, Reed Omary, MD, Nilesh Patel, MD, Pavati Ramchandani, MD, Anne C. Roberts,

Table 14.3. Specific Complications for Percutaneous Vertebroplasty.

Specific Complication	Published Rates (%)	Suggested Thresholds (%)
Transient neurological deficit(<30 days)		
Osteoporosis	1	1
Neoplastic	5	10
Permanent neurological deficit (>30 days or requiring surgery)		
Osteoporosis	0	<1
Neoplastic	2	5
Fracture of rib or vertebra	<1	<1
Allergic or idiosyncratic reaction	<1	<1
Infection	<1	<1
Symptomatic pulmonary cement embolus	<1	<1
Significant hemorrhage or vascular injury	0	0
Death	0	0

MD, Mark I. Silverstein, MD, H. Bob Smouse, MD, Patricia E. Thorpe, MD, Richard B. Towbin, MD, Anthony C. Venbrux, MD, Daniel J. Wunder, MD, Thomas M. Vesely, MD, Curtis W. Bakal, MD, Elizabeth A. Drucker, MD, JD, Curtis A. Lewis, MD, MBA, Albert A. Nemcek, Jr, MD, and Kenneth S. Rholl, MD.

Appendix 1. SIR Standards of Practice Committee Classification of Complications by Outcome

Minor Complications

a. No therapy, no consequence, or
b. Nominal therapy, no consequence, includes overnight admission for observation only.

Major Complications

a. Require therapy, minor hospitalization (<48h),
b. Require major therapy, unplanned hospitalization (>48h),
c. Have permanent adverse sequelae, or
d. Result in death.

Appendix 2. Methodology

Reported complication-specific rates in some cases reflect the aggregate of major and minor complications. Thresholds are derived from critical evaluation of the literature, evaluation of empirical data from Standards of Practice Committee member practices, and, when available, the SIR HI-IQ system national database.

Consensus on statements in this document was obtained utilizing a modified Delphi technique (1,2).

Technical documents specifying the exact consensus and literature review methodologies, as well as the institutional affiliations and professional credentials of the authors of this document, are available on request from SIR, 10201 Lee Highway, Suite 500, Fairfax, VA 22030.

Note: The clinical practice guidelines of the Society of Interventional Radiology attempt to define practice principles that generally should assist in producing high-quality medical care. These guidelines are voluntary and are not rules. A physician may deviate from these guidelines, as necessitated by the individual patient and available resources. These practice guidelines should not be deemed inclusive of all proper methods of care or exclusive of other methods of care that are reasonably directed toward the same result. Other sources of information may be used in conjunction with these principles to produce a process leading to high-quality medical care. The ultimate judgment regarding the conduct of any specific procedure or course of management must be made by the physician, who should consider all circumstances relevant to the individual clinical situation. Adherence to the SIR Quality Improvement Program will not ensure a successful outcome in every situation. It is prudent to document the rationale for any deviation from suggested practice guidelines in the department policies and procedure manual or in the patient's medical record.

References

1. Fink A, Kosefcoff J, Chassin M, et al. Consensus methods: characteristics and guidelines for use. Am J Public Health 1984; 74:979–983.
2. Leape LL, Hilborne LH, Park RE, et al. The appropriateness of use of coronary artery bypass graft surgery in New York state. JAMA 1993; 269: 753–760.
3. Riggs BL, Melton III LJ. The worldwide problem of osteoporosis: insights afforded by epidemiology. Bone 1995; 17(Suppl):505S–511S.
4. Galibert P, Deramond H, Rosat P, Le Gars D. Preliminary note on the treatment of vertebral angioma by percutaneous acrylic vertebroplasty. Neurochirurgie 1987; 33:166–168 [in French].
5. Kaemmerlen P, Thiesse P, Bouivard H, et al. Percutaneous vertebroplasty in the treatment of metastases: technique and results. J Radiol 1989; 70: 557–562 [in French].
6. Weill A, Chiras J, Simon JM, et al. Spinal metastases: indications for and results of percutaneous injection of acrylic surgical cement. Radiology 1996; 199:241–247.
7. Cotton A, Dewatre F, Cortet B, et al. Percutaneous vertebroplasty for osteolytic metastases and myeloma: effects of the percentage of lesion filling and the leakage of methylacrylate at clinical follow-up. Radiology 1996; 200:525–530.
8. Cortet B, Cotton A, Boutry N, et al. Percutaneous vertebroplasty in patients with osteolytic metastases or multiple myeloma. Rev Rheum Engl Ed 1997; 64:177–183.
9. Jensen ME, Evans AJ, Mathis JM, et al. Percutaneous polymethylmethacrylate vertebroplasty in the treatment of osteoporotic vertebral body compression fractures: technical aspects. Am J Neuroradiol 1997; 18: 1897–1904.
10. Mathis JM, Petri M, Naff N. Percutaneous vertebroplasty treatment of steroid-induced osteoporotic compression fractures. Arthritis Rheum 1998; 41:171–175.
11. Deramond H, Depriester C, Galibert P, et al. Percutaneous vertebroplasty with polymethylmethacrylate: technique, indications, and results. Radiol Clin North Am 1998; 36:533–546.
12. Cortet B, Cotton A, Boutry N, et al. Percutaneous vertebroplasty in the treatment of osteoporotic vertebral compression fractures: an open prospective study. J Rheumatol 1999; 26:2222–2228.
13. Martin JB, Jean B, Sugiu K, et al. Vertebroplasty: clinical experience and follow-up results. Bone 1999; 24(Suppl):11S–15S.
14. Cyteval C, Sarrabere MPB, Roux JO, et al. Acute osteoporotic vertebral collapse: open study of percutaneous injection of acrylic surgical cement in 20 patients. Am J Roentgenol 1999; 173:1685–1690.
15. Jensen ME, Dion JE. Percutaneous vertebroplasty in the treatment of osteoporotic compression fractures. Neuroimaging Clin North Am 2000; 10:547–568.
16. Barr JD, Barr MS, Lemely TJ, et al. Percutaneous vertebroplasty for pain relief and spine stabilization. Spine 2000; 25:923–928.

17. O'Brien JP, Sims JT, Evans AJ. Vertebroplasty in patients with severe vertebral compression fractures. A technical report. Am J Neuroradiol 2000; 21:1555–1558.
18. Grados F, Depriester C, Cayrolle G, et al. Long-term observations of vertebral osteoporotic fractures treated by percutaneous vertebroplasty. Rheumatology 2000; 39:1410–1414.
19. Mathis JM, Barr JD, Belkoff SM, et al. Percutaneous vertebroplasty: a developing standard of care for vertebral compression fractures. Am J Neuroradiol 2001; 22:373–381.
20. Zoarski GH, Snow P, Olan WJ, et al. Percutaneous vertebroplasty for osteoporotic compression fractures: quantitative prospective evaluation of long-term outcomes. J Vasc Intervent Radiol 2002; 13:139–148.
21. Peh WC, Gilula LA, Peck DD. Percutaneous vertebroplasty for severe osteoporotic vertebral body compression fractures. Radiology 2002; 223:121–126.
22. McGraw JK, Lippert JA, Minkus DK, et al. Prospective evaluation of pain relief in 100 patients undergoing percutaneous vertebroplasty. Results and follow-up. J Vasc Intervent Radiol 2002; 13:883–886.
23. Levine SA, Perin LA, Hayes D, et al. An evidence-based evaluation of percutaneous vertebroplasty. Managed Care 2000; 9:56–60, 63.
24. Heini PF, Walchli B, Berlemann U. Percutaneous transpedicular vertebroplasty with PMMA: operative technique and early results. Eur Spine J 2000; 9:445–450.
25. Kaufmann TJ, Jensen ME, Schweickert PA, et al. Age of fracture and clinical outcomes of percutaneous vertebroplasty. Am J Neuroradiol 2001; 22:1860–1863.
26. Garfin SR, Yuan HA, Reiley MA. Kyphoplasty and vertebroplasty for the treatment of painful osteoporotic compression fractures. Spine 2001; 26:1511–1515.
27. Hardouin P, Grados F, Cotton A, Cortet B. Should percutaneous vertebroplasty be used to treat osteoporotic fractures? An update. Joint Bone Spine 2001; 68:216–221.
28. Amar AP, Larsen DW, Esnaashari N, et al. Percutaneous transpedicular polymethylmethacrylate vertebroplasty for the treatment of spinal compression fractures. Neurosurgery 2001; 49:1105–1115.
29. Deramond H, Depriester C, Toussaint P, et al. Percutaneous vertebroplasty. Semin Musculoskel Radiol 1997; 1:285–296.
30. Cotton A, Boutry N, Cortet B, et al. Percutaneous vertebroplasty: state of the art. RadioGraphics 1998; 18:311–320.
31. Murphy KJ, Deramond H. Percutaneous vertebroplasty in benign and malignant disease. Neuroimaging Clin North Am 2000; 10:535–545.
32. Jensen ME, Kallmes DE. Percutaneous vertebroplasty in the treatment of malignant spine disease. Cancer J 2002; 8:194–206.
33. Galibert P, Deramond H. Percutaneous acrylic vertebroplasty as a treatment of vertebral angiomas as well as painful and debilitating diseases. Chirurgie 1990; 116:326–334. [French]
34. Cortet B, Cotton A, Deprez X, et al. Value of vertebroplasty combined with surgical decompression in the treatment of aggressive spinal angioma. Rev Rheum Ed Fr 1994; 61:16–22. [French]
35. Ide C, Gangi A, Rimmelin A, et al. Vertebral haemangiomas with spinal cord compression: the place of preoperative percutaneous vertebroplasty with methyl methacrylate. Neuroradiology 1996; 38:585–589.
36. Dousset V, Mousselard H, de Monck d'User L, et al. Asymptomatic cervical haemangioma treated by percutaneous vertebroplasty. Neuroradiology 1996; 38:392–394.

37. Feydy A, Cognard C, Miaux Y, et al. Acrylic vertebroplasty in symptomatic cervical vertebral haemangiomas: report of 2 cases. Neuroradiology 1996; 38:389–391.
38. Cotton A, Deramond H, Cortet B, et al. Preoperative percutaneous injection of methyl methacrylate and n-butyl cyanoacrylate in vertebral hemangiomas. Am J Neuroradiol 1996; 17:137–142.
39. Gangi A, Kastler BA, Dietemann JL. Percutaneous vertebroplasty guided by a combination of CT and fluoroscopy. Am J Neuroradiol 1994; 15:83–86.
40. Padovani B, Kasriel O, Brunner P, et al. Pulmonary embolism caused by acrylic cement: a rare complication of percutaneous vertebroplasty. Am J Neuroradiol 1999; 20:375–377.
41. Ratliff J, Nguyen T, Heiss J. Root and spinal cord compression from methylmethacrylate vertebroplasty. Spine 2001; 26:E300–E302.
42. Vasconcelos C, Gailloud P, Martin JB, et al. Transient arterial hypotension induced by polymethylmethacrylate injection during percutaneous vertebroplasty. J Vasc Intervent Radiol 2001; 12:1001–1002.
43. Harrington KD. Major neurological complications following percutaneous vertebroplasty with polymethylmethacrylate. J Bone Joint Surg Am 2001; 83A:1070–1073.
44. Ryu KS, Park CK, Kim MC, et al. Dose-dependent epidural leakage of polymethylmethacrylate after percutaneous vertebroplasty in patients with osteoporotic vertebral compression fractures. J Neurosurg 2002; 96(Suppl 1):56–61.
45. McGraw JK, Heatwole EV, Strand BT, et al. Predictive value of intraosseous venography before percutaneous vertebroplasty. J Vasc Intervent Radiol 2002; 13:149–153.
46. Gaughen JR, Jensen ME, Schweickert PA, et al. Relevance of antecedent venography in percutaneous vertebroplasty for the treatment of osteoporotic compression fractures. Am J Neuroradiol 2002; 23:594–600.
47. Kaufmann TJ, Jensen ME, Gord G, et al. Cardiovascular effects of polymethylmethacrylate use in percutaneous vertebroplasty. Am J Neuroradiol 2002; 23:601–604.
48. Scroop R, Eskridge J, Britz GW. Paradoxical cerebral arterial embolization of cement during intraoperative vertebroplasty: case report. Am J Neuroradiol 2002; 23:868–870.
49. Vasconcelos C, Gaulloud P, Beauchamp NJ, et al. Is percutaneous vertebroplasty without pretreatment venography safe? Evaluation of 205 consecutive procedures. Am J Neuroradiol 2002; 23:913–917.

Section II
Case Studies

Case 1

Single-Level Vertebroplasty and Biopsy

John M. Mathis

Clinical Presentation

The patient is an 80-year-old man who has had multiple compression fractures in the past. He has some chronic back pain that is suspected to be related to noncritical spinal stenosis. He has prostate cancer, but no signs of metastasis clinically or by laboratory analysis. He presents with 2 weeks of new back pain after minor trauma at the junction of the mid and low back. His pain is worse with standing and movement but partially relieved by lying down. Oral narcotic analgesics produce considerable nausea and constipation. He is referred by his local physician with little change in the initial level of presenting symptoms and after undergoing magnetic resonance imaging (MRI).

This elderly gentleman has local tenderness at the thoracolumbar junction region on palpation. He is afebrile, and laboratory tests are normal with no signs of infection and normal clotting function.

Imaging Findings

The patient's MRI reveals an acute fracture involving the L2 vertebra with marrow edema and mild compression (Case Figure 1.1). Multiple old fractures are noted but are chronic by MRI signal analysis. The MRI does show moderate spinal stenosis below the level of new fracture. The MRI did not show signs of tumor involvement, but because of the history of prostate cancer it was decided to perform a biopsy at the time of percutaneous vertebroplasty.

Procedure

The patient received 1 gram of Ancef (cefazolin) intravenously (IV) 30 minutes before the procedure. Procedural sedation was accomplished by titrating IV fentanyl and Versed.

Local anesthesia was administered to the skin, subcutaneous tissue, and periosteum over the L2 vertebra at the sites of intended needle

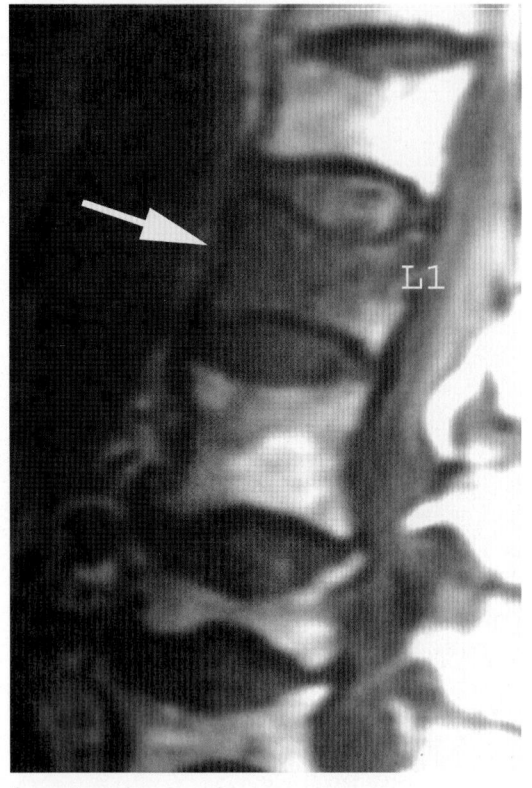

A

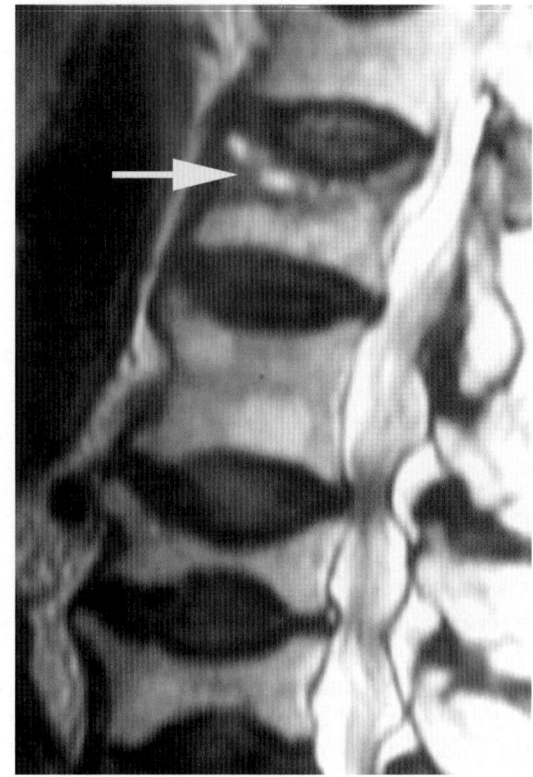

B

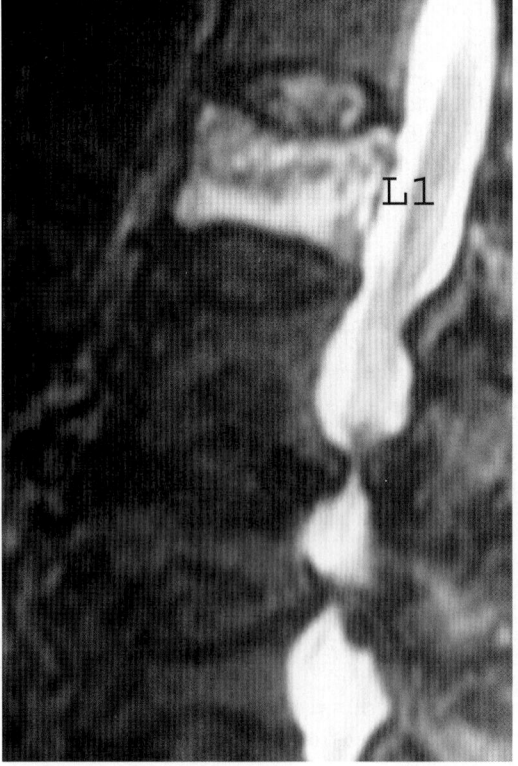

C

Case Figure 1.1. (A) T1-weighted MRI reveals acute marrow edema (low signal) in the L1 vertebra (white arrow). Chronic compressions of T12, L3, and L4 are noted. These have normal bright marrow signal. **(B)** T2-weighted MRI demonstrates some focal bright signal in the L1 vertebra below the upper endplate (white arrow). This indicates fluid in a small cleft or cavity created during the fracture. This will preferentially fill with cement. **(C)** Fat saturation, inversion recovery (STIR) image shows the acute fracture at L1 as bright. All other vertebrae are low signal, again consistent with no acute injury.

introduction. A 13-gauge trocar–cannula for cement delivery was inserted through the pedicle of L2 bilaterally using fluoroscopic guidance (Case Figure 1.2A).

The needle tip of the first needle was stopped just beyond the posterior wall and a biopsy device inserted (Case Figure 1.2B). A biopsy specimen was obtained and submitted for analysis (Case Figure 1.2C,D). (It subsequently was negative for cancer.) Both needles were ultimately advanced to the junction of the anterior and middle thirds of the vertebra (shown in the lateral projection) (Case Figure 1.2E).

Simplex P was mixed with sterile barium sulfate (the barium level was brought to 30% by weight). The cement was injected and an adequate fill achieved with no significant leak or clinical complication. The patient had a small cavity in the upper part of the vertebra that preferentially filled with cement during the cement injection (Case Figure 1.3A). The cement fill on this vertebroplasty was not homogenous (Case Figure 1.3B,C). This occurs commonly and does not indicate a problem with the ultimate outcome. One does not need to reinsert additional needles to try to fill the parts of the vertebra not filled with cement. A more homogenous fill is shown in Case Figure 1.4. This fill gives a better visual result but the clinical outcome should be the same.

Results

Postprocedure the patient was monitored for 2 hours total. He was maintained recumbent for 1 hour and then gradually ambulated. He experienced good pain relief by about 4 hours postprocedure and was able to discontinue narcotic analgesics. His chronic back pain remained.

Discussion

This patient demonstrates the common situation of coexistent spine problems accompanying new compression fracture and new, severe pain. The new pain is often superimposed on more chronic but less severe pain. In discussing this procedure with patients and their family, it is important to point out that the new pain related to the compression fracture should be relieved by the percutaneous vertebroplasty. The more chronic pain will likely remain. In this patient's case, the chronic pain was related to spinal stenosis, which was not critical and did not have radicular symptoms.

This patient had known prostate cancer but no evidence of systemic spread. Because vertebroplasty can be performed effectively in either benign or malignant disease, one does not have to wait for the result of the biopsy before continuing with the procedure. If malignant disease is ultimately found, appropriate therapy can be instituted at that time and will not be adversely affected by the

252   J.M. Mathis

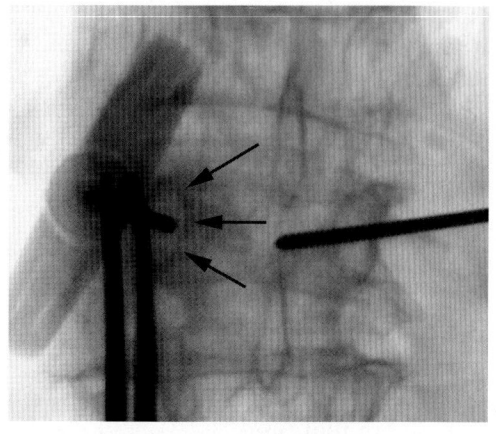

A

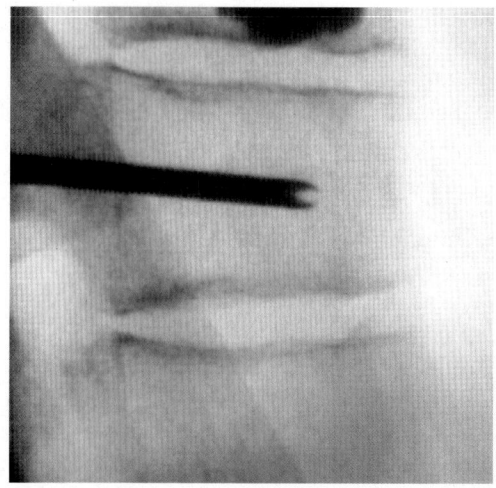

C

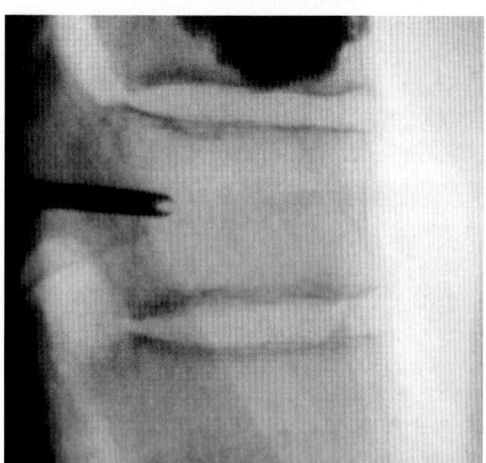

B

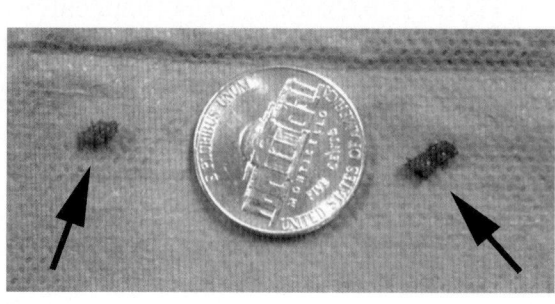

D

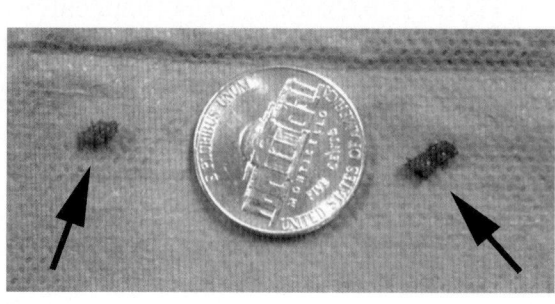

E

Case Figure 1.2. (A) Oblique radiograph shows the pedicle appearance (black arrows) as the needle is being directed through the pedicle into the vertebral body. (B) Lateral radiograph showing a biopsy device exiting the cannula, which was initially stopped at the posterior margin of the vertebra (this is a different case used for this demonstration). (C) The biopsy device is advanced into the vertebra to take a bone core. (D) The bone cores (black arrows) obtained with the biopsy device. (E) The lateral image shows the final position of the first needle, with the tip at the junction of the anterior and middle thirds of the vertebra.

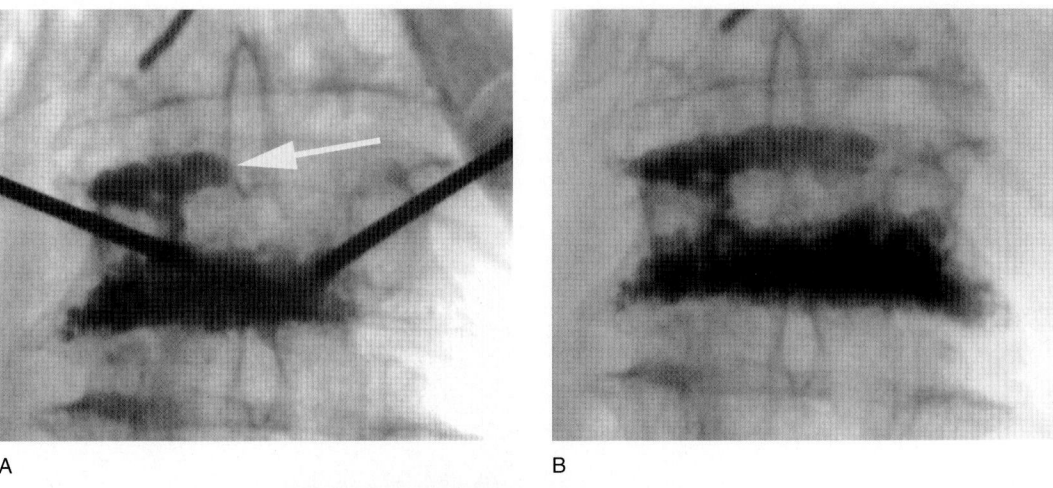
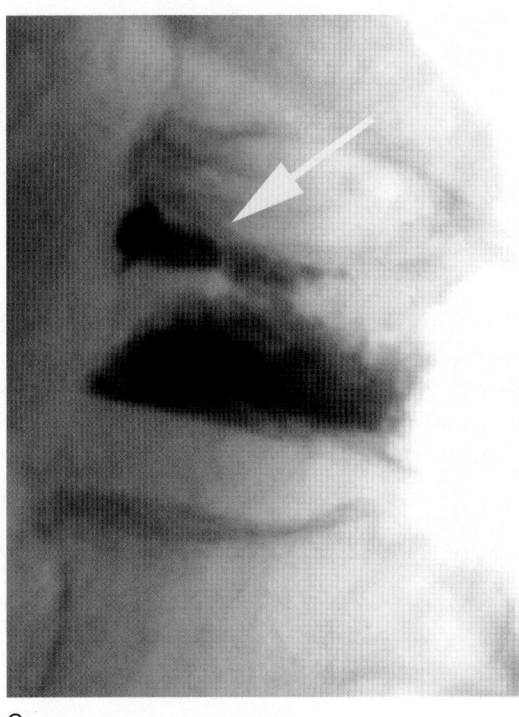

Case Figure 1.3. **(A)** Anteroposterior radiograph shows initial cement filling. Note that the small cleft below the superior endplate (white arrow) is preferentially filling even though the needle tip is not close to this area. **(B,C)** The final fill result. The cleft has filled (C, white arrow), but there is little cement in the center of the vertebra. This fill is not homogenous, but the outcome was good with expected pain relief.

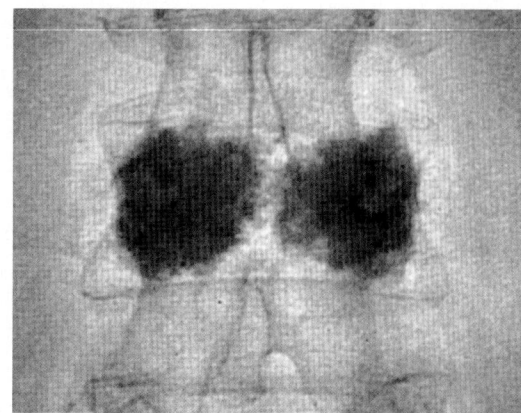
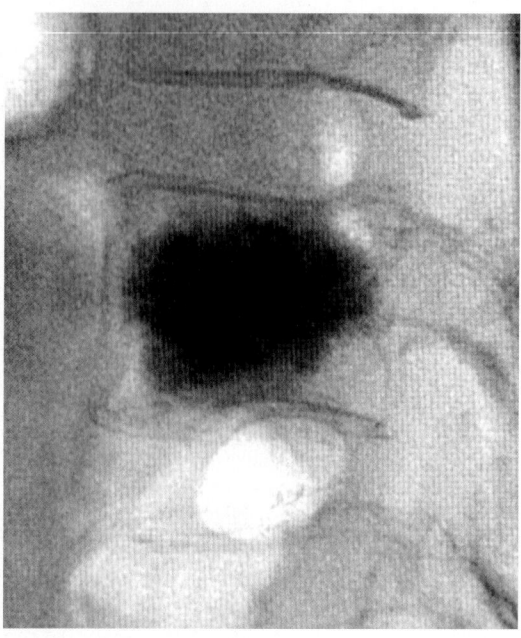

Case Figure 1.4. (A,B) Anteroposterior and lateral radiograph of a more homogenous cement fill produced by a bilateral transpedicular vertebroplasty. This is visually nicer than the fill shown in Case Figure 1.3. However, the clinical outcomes were the same.

vertebroplasty. Specifically, vertebroplasty will not interfere with radiation therapy.

Biopsy devices are available in multiple styles and can be placed through either 11- or 13-gauge guide needles. The biopsy is preformed during the procedure but before the injection of cement.

Case 2

Multilevel Vertebroplasty

James Ball and John M. Mathis

Clinical Presentation

A 78-year-old woman presented with new, severe back pain. This patient was a frail, thin person with chronic obstructive lung disease, congestive heart failure, atrial fibrillation, hyperlipidemia, hypertension, asthma, a 50 pack year smoking history osteoporosis, and she was taking oral steroids. The patient had undergone a prior L3 compression fracture and subsequent percutaneous vertebroplasty (PV). This resulted in good pain relief for the acute symptoms.

Imaging Findings and Procedures

A magnetic resonance image (MRI) (taken November 5, 2003) revealed a new compression fracture at L2 with chronic compressions of L3 (with prior PV) and L4 (Case Figure 2.1). Based on the finding of new compression fracture and a consistent pain location, PV at L2 was performed.

This patient again got good pain relief from the PV at L2. However, within days new fractures occurred, and by December 4, 2003, the patient had undergone PV at T11 and T12 and was complaining of new pain in the low lumbar area. A repeat MRI revealed marrow edema (low signal) in L4 and L5 consistent with additional compression fractures (Case Figure 2.2).

Over a period of approximately 1 year, the patient experienced nine vertebral compression fractures, sacral insufficiency fracture, and right hip fracture. The vertebral compression fractures and the sacral insufficiency fracture were all treated percutaneously with good pain relief and no clinical complication (Case Figure 2.3).

Discussion

This patient demonstrates the cascade of progressive compression fractures and other osteoporotic fractures that some individuals can experience. It is important for all patients experiencing a compression

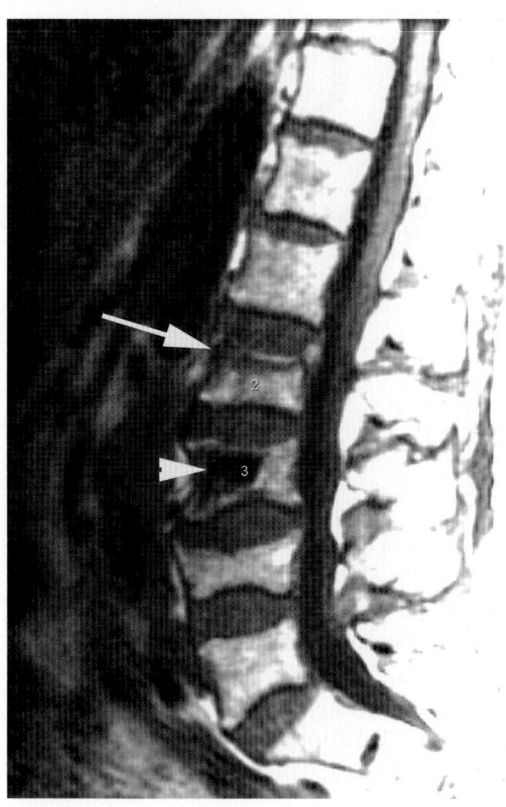

Case Figure 2.1. Lateral T1 MRI reveals a new compression fracture at L2 (white arrow). L3 shows central low signal consistent with a prior vertebroplasty (white arrowhead). The bone cement creates a signal void. L4 has experienced a prior compression. The bright signal indicates that this fracture is chronic.

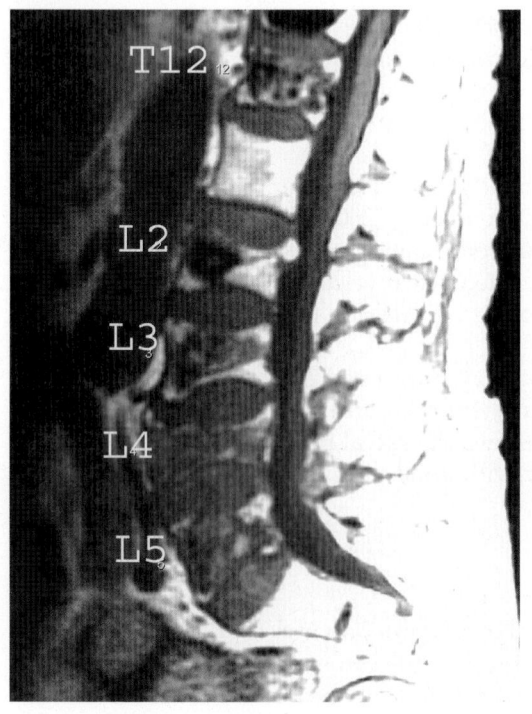

Case Figure 2.2. Lateral T1 MRI now showing vertebroplasties at T11, T12, L2, and L3. New compression fractures are present at L4 and L5.

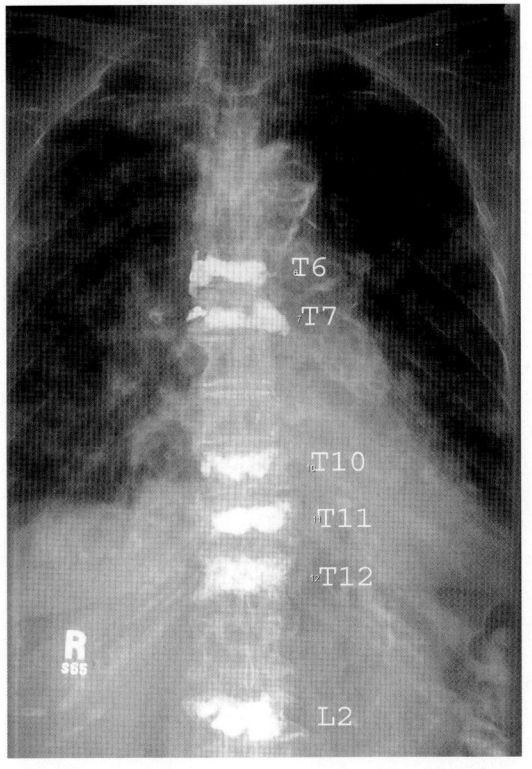
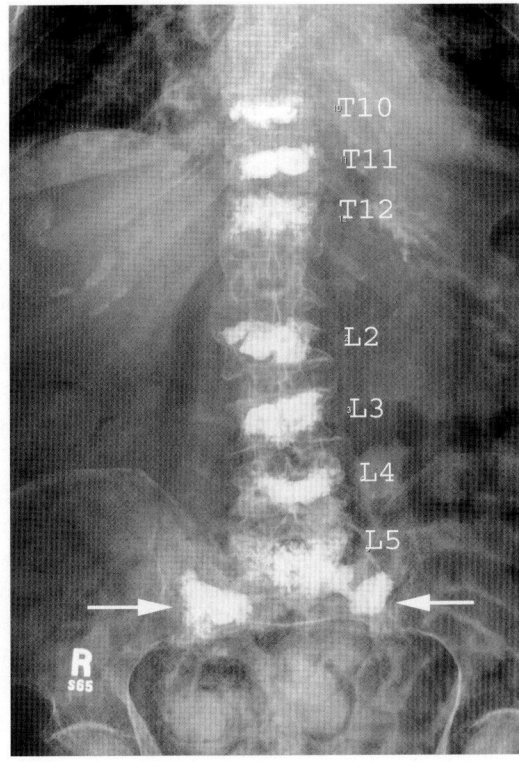

Case Figure 2.3. (A,B) Anteroposterior radiographs show nine vertebral levels that have been treated with percutaneous vertebroplasty as well as sacroplasty (white arrows). **(C)** Coronal CT images of the sacroplasty (white arrows).

fracture to undergo appropriate workup and pharmacologic therapy in an attempt to avoid future fractures. Even with this help, progressive debility due to additional fractures can occur. The additional fractures can usually be treated with PV or kyphoplasty. It is possible that, for such patients, prophylactic vertebral therapy would help avoid future compressions, but we presently have no way of detecting vertebrae that will actually fracture in the future. Also, reimbursement guidelines specifically exclude vertebrae that are not fractured.

Finally, we have no data about the physiologic outcomes following multilevel therapy. For example, older individuals make their blood products progressively in the central marrow space (largely the spine). Will filling these vertebrae result in chronic anemia or force the body to provide blood precursors through extramedullary hematopoiesis (also a pathologic condition)?

Multilevel therapy, although controversial for many reasons, is nonetheless indicated for patients who present with multiple fractures or experience repeated fractures over time. The risk of cardiopulmonary complications increases as the number of vertebrae treated increases (during a single session). This happens because every vertebroplasty (or kyphoplasty) pushes marrow fat and blood precursors out of the bone as cement is introduced. This material ultimately is filtered by the lungs, creating pulmonary emboli. Most patients tolerate these events well and have no clinical complications. However, these emboli can result in cardiopulmonary compromise and even death in patients with poor pulmonary or cardiac function. We recommend that patients be assessed for an underlying cardiopulmonary disease that would put them at increased risk from PV or kyphoplasty. Procedures should be minimized for these individuals (limiting the number of vertebrae and amount of cement injected).

Even for patients with normal cardiopulmonary function, the number of levels that can be performed safely is not known. For this reason, we recommend limiting the number of levels treated at one setting to three in patients with normal function. For high-risk patients, more stringent criteria should be considered. Remember, compression fractures do not constitute a medical emergency, and therefore treatment should be timed to maximize safety.

Presently, there are no scientific data to support prophylactic therapy with vertebroplasty or kyphoplasty, and reimbursement is only for compression fractures resulting from osteoporotic or malignant disease. Prophylactic treatment of noncompressed vertebrae should be undertaken only with internal review board approval and with specific discussions with and consent obtained from the patient.

Case 3
Vertebra with a Cleft or Cavity

John M. Mathis

Clinical Presentation

A 74-year-old woman presented with new, severe pain in the lower thoracic region. She was tender over the region of the thoracolumbar junction, and the pain was worse with standing. She had no particular additional risk factors besides age. Her primary physician ordered magnetic resonance imaging (MRI) after several weeks of analgesic therapy provided little overall improvement.

Imaging Findings

Standard radiographs demonstrated a compression fracture of T11 and a vacuum cleft in the superior aspect of the vertebra (Case Figure 3.1). The MRI again showed the compression fracture and established it as acute with marrow edema. T2 images disclosed a high-signal zone below the superior endplate where the vacuum cleft had been seen on x-ray (Case Figure 3.2). No other fractures were found.

Procedure

The patient underwent a single-level percutaneous vertebroplasty (PV) following the usual consent, intravenous (IV) antibiotics, and IV procedural sedation. Two needles were placed via the transpedicular route with fluoroscopic guidance. Needle tips were in the lower part of the vertebra, away from this vertebral cleft. This was not intentional, but did allow a good example of the fact that clefts and cavities will usually preferentially fill during cement injection (Case Figure 3.3). This occurred in this case as well. Cement migrated into the sub-endplate cleft, and there was poor filling of the inferior part of this vertebra (Case Figure 3.4). The procedure was tolerated well, and the fill pattern was accepted without attempts at additional needle placement or filling.

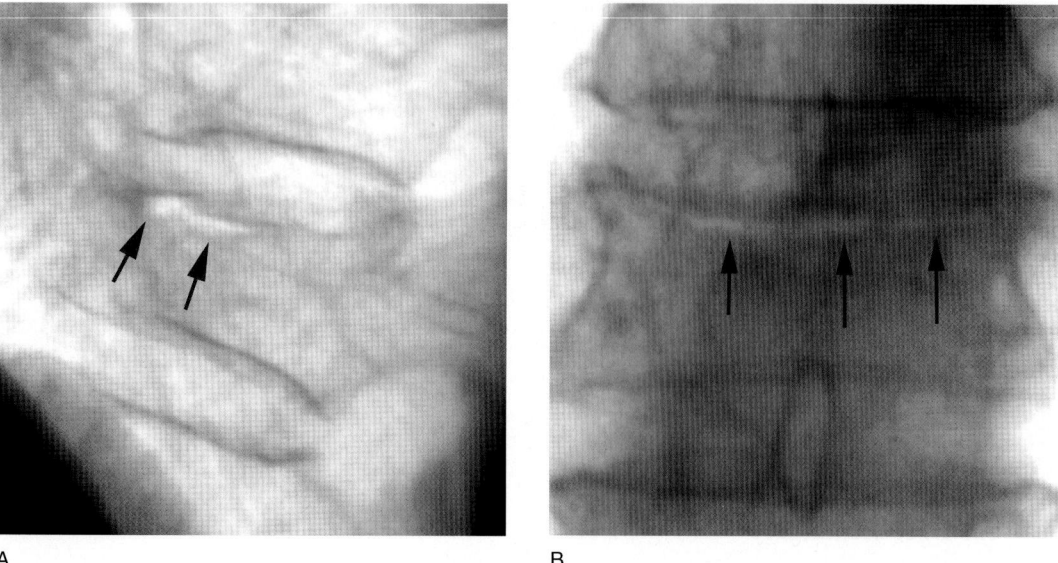

Case Figure 3.1. (A) Lateral radiograph showing compression fracture of T11 with an air-filled cavity below the superior endplate (black arrows). (B) The same cavity (black arrows) on an anteroposterior radiograph.

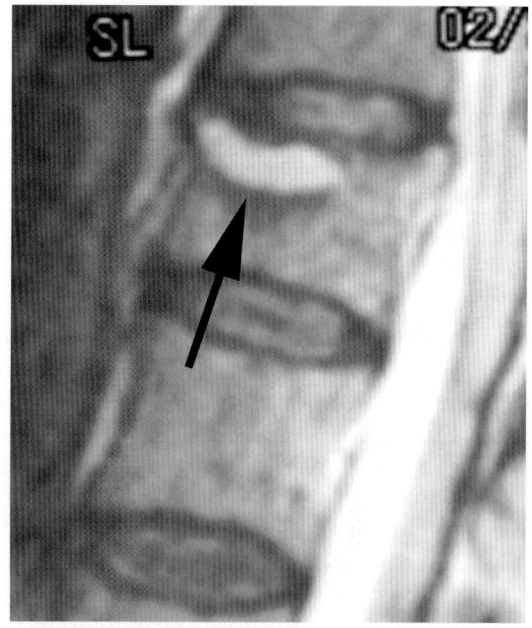

Case Figure 3.2. A T2-weighted sagittal MRI shows a sub-endplate cavity (black arrow) exhibiting high signal. This indicates that the cavity is fluid filled.

Case 3 Vertebra with a Cleft or Cavity 261

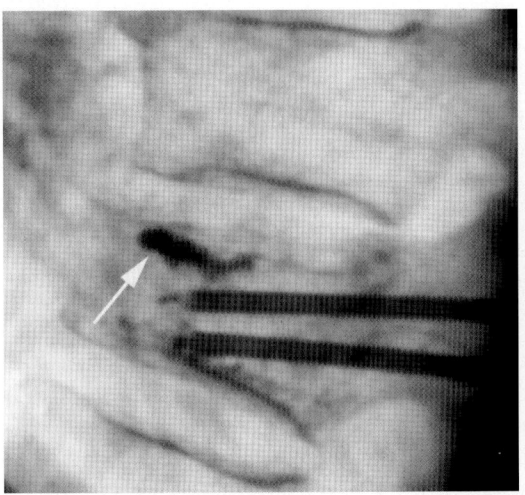 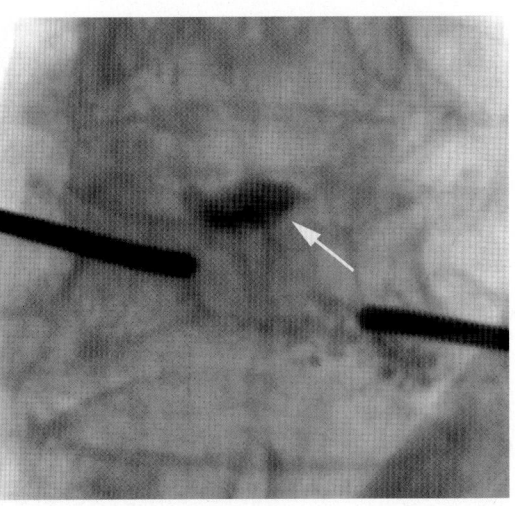

Case Figure 3.3. Lateral **(A)** and anteroposterior **(B)** views of the vertebra early in the process of cement injection. Note that the needle tips are remote to the cavity itself. These images show cement tracking to the cavity and preferentially filling the cavity (white arrow) rather than the more proximal vertebral body.

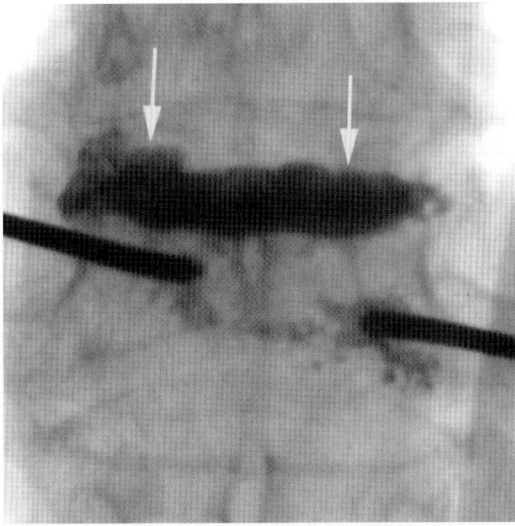

Case Figure 3.4. Anteroposterior radiograph taken near the end of the PV procedure demonstrates that cement has continued to fill the cavity (white arrows) rather than the rest of the vertebral body.

Results

This patient was monitored for 2 hours postprocedure and experienced almost complete resolution of pain during that period. She was discharged and resumed usual activity. Three years later, she remains well with no additional fracture or recurrence of pain.

Discussion

This case demonstrates the relatively common occurrence of a cleft or cavity in a vertebral body following a compression fracture. It is believed that natural distraction on the vertebra by the muscles and ligaments postfracture opens up the region of cavity. This can be associated with vertebral motion and allows height restoration when these patients are positioned prone for the PV or kyphoplasty procedure. The height gain is captured during cementation in either procedure. These patients seem to have an excellent pain response to PV or kyphoplasty. Pain relief is usually dramatic and rapid.

Filling of the cleft or cavity is usually easy to accomplish even if the needles are not placed into or near the cavity itself. The cavity provides a low resistance space, and cement usually tracks into the cavity easily, as it did in this case. Other portions of the vertebra may or may not fill as well (Case Figure 3.4). As with this patient, filling of the rest of the vertebra does not seem crucial for pain relief.

Case 4

The Mobile Vertebra: Height Restoration

John M. Mathis

Clinical Presentation

A 65-year-old man presented with new, severe back pain after a minor fall. The patient was known to have ankylosing spondylitis. The pain was so severe that the patient was confined to bed. The pain was focal at the thoracolumbar junction region, and there was no associated motor dysfunction. An initial trial of analgesics and bed rest was unsuccessful, and subsequently the primary care physician ordered magnetic resonance imaging (MRI).

Imaging Findings

Initial radiographs of the lumbar spine were obtained and revealed a compression fracture of L1 (Case Figure 4.1). The L1 vertebra was markedly compressed, with only 35% of its original height anteriorly. An MRI demonstrated the fracture with a central cavity (Case Figure 4.2A). Height was regained by simply placing the patient supine on the MRI table. Height restoration compared with initial radiographs was estimated at 35%. The MRI also demonstrated that the fracture extended into the posterior elements (Case Figure 4.2B). Based on the findings, a vertebroplasty was planned.

Procedure

The patient received 1 gram of Ancef and procedural sedation intravenously. He was placed prone on the procedure table and sterile preparation and local anesthesia were administered. The 13-gauge needles were placed transpedicularly with fluoroscopic guidance. It was noted that the vertebral height was almost complete in the prone position (Case Figure 4.3A) and markedly changed compared with the initial postfracture radiograph (Case Figure 4.1B). Cement was injected, and the cavity created within the vertebra filled preferentially.

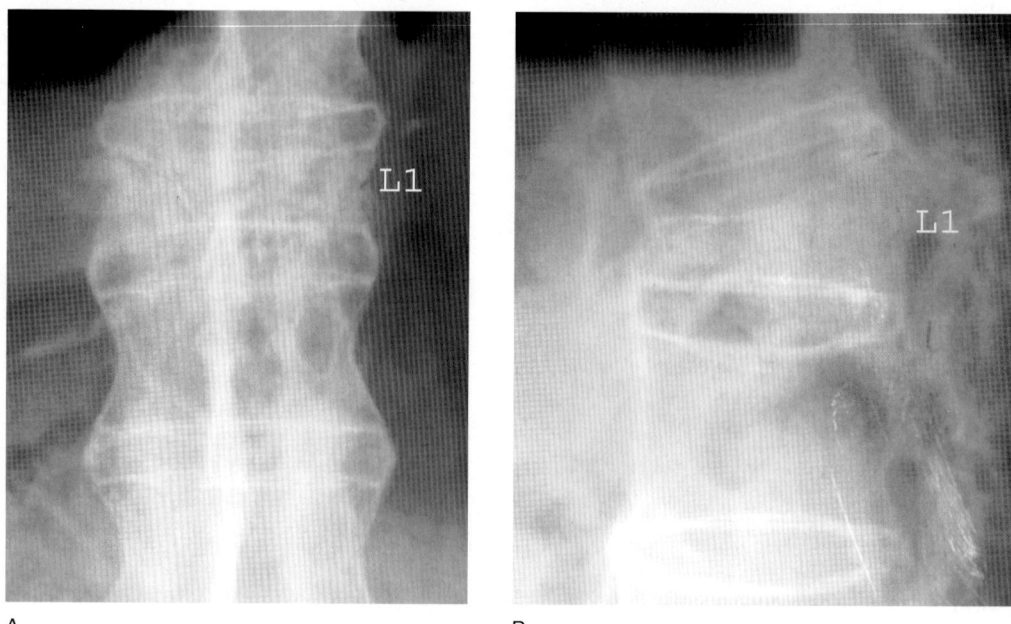

Case Figure 4.1. (A) An anteroposterior radiograph shows typical signs of ankylosing spondylitis. There is a compression fracture of L1. **(B)** A lateral radiograph demonstrates again the severe compression fracture of L1. The anterior height is 35% to 40% of the anterior height of the adjacent L2 vertebra.

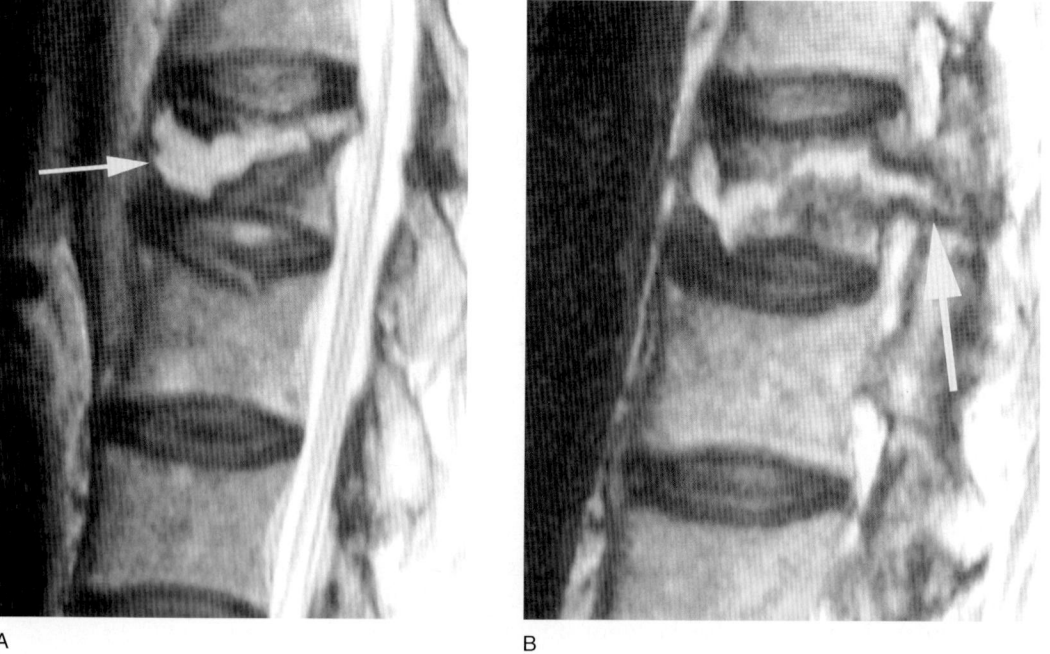

Case Figure 4.2. (A) A sagittal T2 MRI demonstrates a cavity within the L1 vertebra (white arrow). Note that the anterior height is now 75% to 80% of the anterior height of the adjacent L2 vertebra. With the patient supine for the MRI, the vertebra is distracted, producing partial height restoration and opening the central cavity. **(B)** A more lateral image for this MRI series shows the fracture line extending into the posterior elements (white arrow). This is a common occurance with fractures in ankylosing spondylitis.

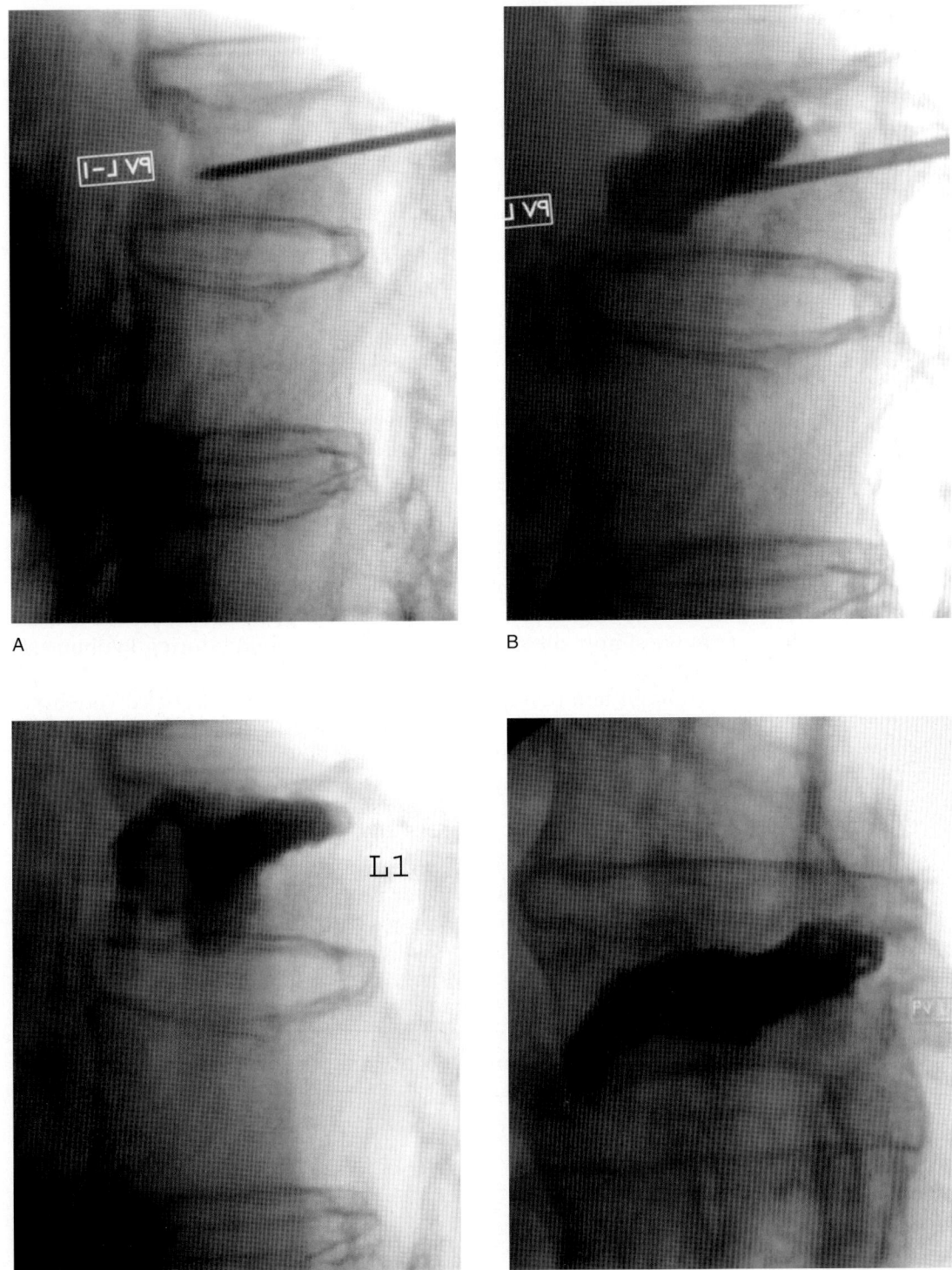

Case Figure 4.3. (A) A lateral radiograph after transpedicular needle introduction for percutaneous vertebroplasty. Again, height restoration is substantial compared with the initial postfracture radiograph shown in Case Figure 4.1B. (B) A lateral radiograph taken in the early phase of cement filling shows preferential filling of the central cavity. Lateral (C) and anteroposterior (D) radiographs show the final cement fill achieved in this percutaneous vertebroplasty. Filling is predominately of the cavity, with little cement extending into other parts of the vertebra.

Results

There were no clinical complications. The patient was observed for 2 hours postprocedure, and his pain was totally gone by the end of this observation period. The patient resumed routine activity and has had no additional problems over a 3-year period of follow-up.

Discussion

The postprocedure images reveal that essentially all of the original height of the vertebra was regained with positioning, and this height restoration was permanent following cement injection (Case Figures 4.2 and 4.3). The cement filled the cavity created by opening up of the vertebra during prone positioning. This height restoration was achieved without additional devices such as the balloon tamp used during kyphoplasty.

Many fractured vertebrae are mobile to some degree following fracture, and some height restoration is common with percutaneous vertebroplasty kyphoplasty. One of the big questions is whether this mobility is all that is attainable regardless of which procedure is used. (Are we simply measuring this inherent mobility during kyphoplasty rather than a primary effect of the balloon?)

An important point to note when mobility of a fractured vertebra is observed is that pain relief is usually very quick (sometimes within minutes after coming off the operative table) and dramatic.

Signs of a potentially mobile vertebra include a cleft or cavity seen on the radiographs or MRI images. Change in vertebral height when different images are compared also indicates mobility. This is most commonly observed when images made in different positions are compared (standing versus supine or prone).

The cavity seen in these fractures will often fill preferentially during cement injection. This will be sufficient to create pain relief and provide durable fracture fixation. More vertebral filling is not necessary for a good outcome. Filling of the posterior elements was not attempted, as this increases the risk of a serious leak. Even without posterior element filling, this patient enjoyed a very good outcome that was durable.

Case 5

Extreme Vertebral Collapse

John M. Mathis

Clinical Presentation

A 97-year-old woman presented with new, severe pain in her back around the T12 level. She had experienced compression fractures before but had never had vertebroplasty. She had mild age-related medical problems and was ambulatory with minimal assistance before this injury. Her pain was focal and without radicular symptoms. The pain was worse with standing and bending. She did not tolerate strong analgesics and therefore was made basically immobile by the new problem.

Imaging Findings

A magnetic resonance image (MRI) was obtained that revealed old compression fractures at L2 and L5. Acute compression fractures were present at T11 and L1 (Case Figure 5.1A). The T11 compression was about 25% and was typical. The L1 compression showed severe loss of height estimated at 75% to 80%. The central portion of the vertebra was almost completely collapsed, and the lateral aspects had some more residual space for needle and cement placement (Case Figure 5.1B). A small amount of central bright signal on T2 suggested that there was a small central cavity (Case Figure 5.1C).

Procedure

The patient received intravenous antibiotics and procedural sedation. The T11 vertebra was treated in the usual fashion with a bipedicular approach and cement reinforcement.

The L1 vertebra was approached in the same manner, but here it was technically harder to get adequate needle positioning. The lower edge of the pedicle was positioned over the residual vertebral body (Case Figure 5.2; see also Figure 2.17C). The needle entry site was through

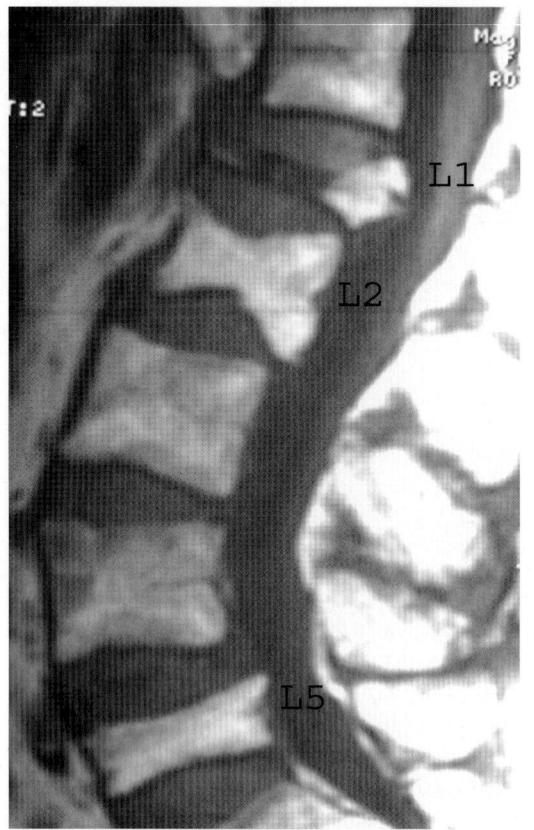
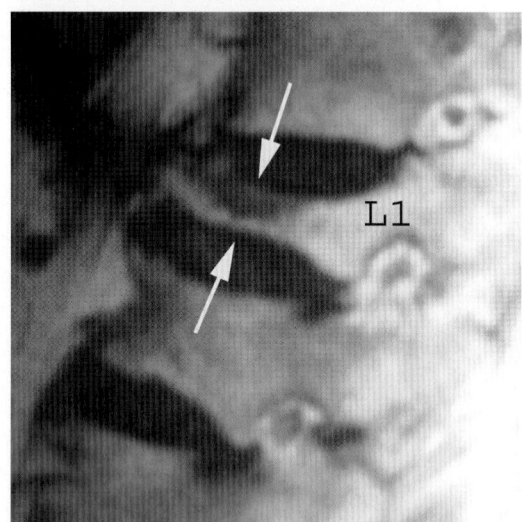
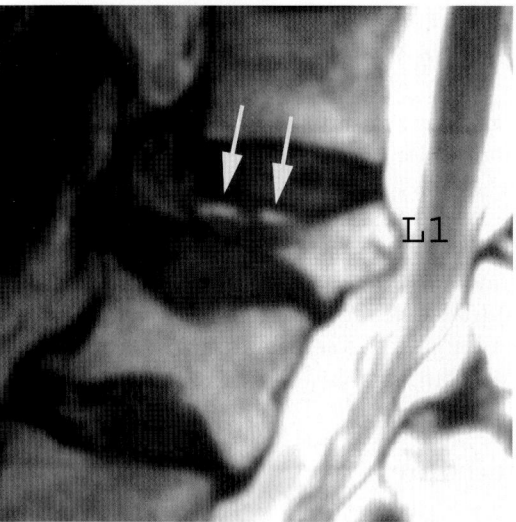

Case Figure 5.1 (A) A lateral T1-weighted MRI demonstrates old fractures of L2 and L5. The L1 vertebra is almost completely collapsed in the midline, with buckling of the posterior wall. **(B)** A more lateral MRI image demonstrates more residual height to the L1 vertebra (white arrows), which allows room for needle introduction. **(C)** A T2-weighted MRI image shows a small amount of bright signal in the central part of the vertebra (white arrows). This indicates a small cleft or cavity.

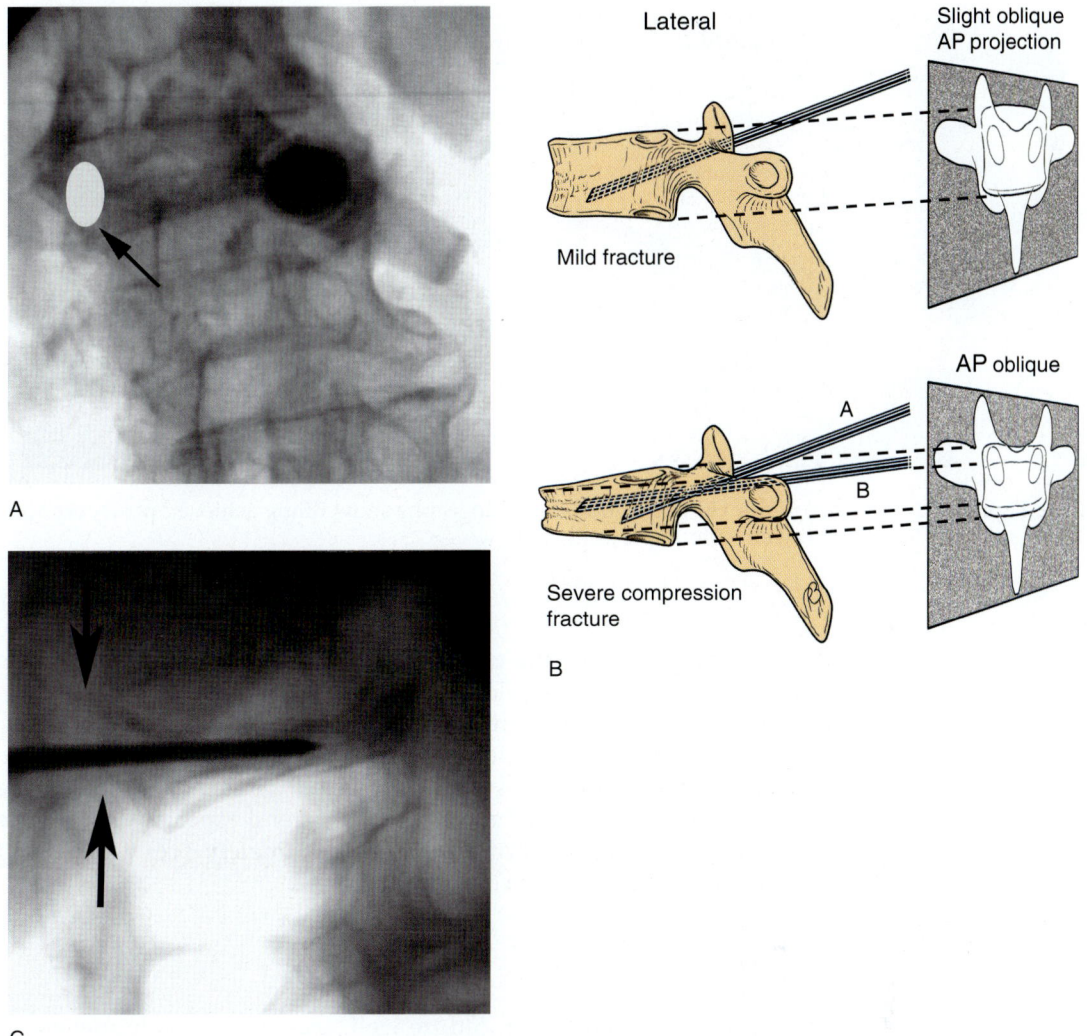

Case Figure 5.2. **(A)** An anteroposterior oblique image with the needle in place on the right. The left pedicle is highlighted (white oval). It is larger than the residual height of the vertebra. The inferior margin was positioned over the vertebra and the needle placed through the inferior pedicle (black arrow indicated the region of interest), but on the opposite side. **(B)** Artist's sketch of the angle that must be maintained for proper needle positioning in a very collapsed vertebra. A more cephalad-to-caudad angle works with minimal compression. As compression increases, a needle angle parallel to the vertebral endplates is necessary to gain access to the anterior part of the body. **(C)** Lateral radiograph showing the needles in place. The black arrows mark the inferior and superior pedicle margins. Note the flat or horizontal needle trajectory.

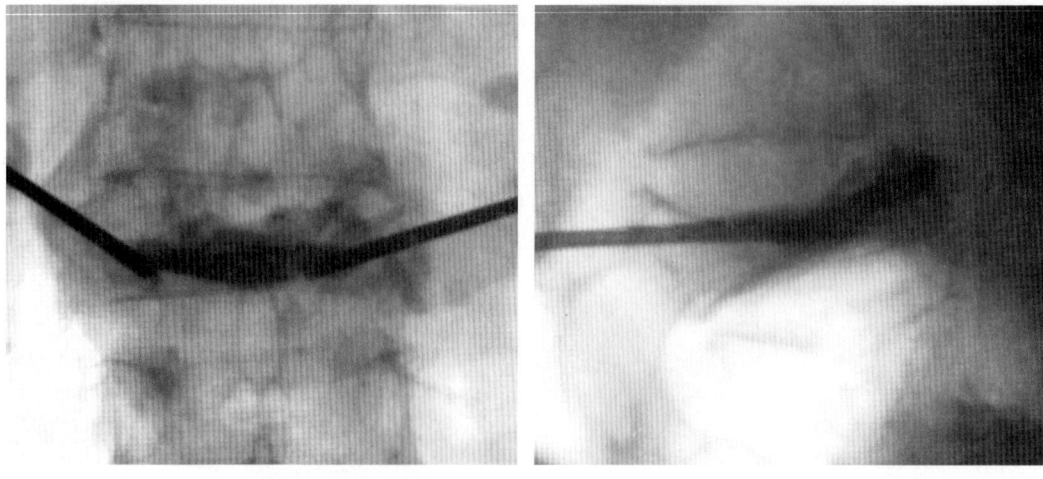

Case Figure 5.3. Anteroposterior **(A)** and lateral **(B)** radiographs show filling achieved postprocedure. The majority of the cement went into the central cleft.

this inferior portion of the pedicle, with care taken to ensure that the trajectory of the needle would allow access to the anterior vertebra once inserted. This usually dictates that the needle trajectory be horizontal or parallel to the residual vertebral endplates. Two needles were placed. Polymethylmethacrylate was injected, and a small cavity in the center of the vertebra filled more than the lateral aspects (Case Figure 5.3). A very small amount of cement (approximately 1 cc) was needed for this fill. There were no complications.

Results

The patient tolerated the procedure well, and there was an uneventful recovery. Pain relief was near total within 6 hours, and the patient was able to ambulate in her room with assistance on the day of the procedure. She returned to her usual daily routine within 48 hours.

Discussion

This case deals with the technical difficulties faced when a vertebra is almost completely collapsed. Because of the extreme loss of height, it is usually not possible to perform kyphoplasty on such a vertebra. Just placing 13-gauge needles can be technically challenging, as it was here.

It is common to find some sparing of vertebral height laterally even when there is extreme and near total collapse centrally. That was the case here. The pedicle height may be larger than the residual height of the vertebral body. A high position on the pedicle will usually make the entry angle too steep to allow the tip of the needle to reach the anterior part of the vertebral body (Case Figure 5.2B; see also Figure 2.17C). Cement would then have to be injected too far posterior in the vertebra to be safe (easy leak into the epidural space). Taking a low position through the pedicle (with this part of the pedicle first lined up over the residual portion of the vertebral body) provides the trajectory to allow the needle tip to reach the anterior vertebra, as it did in this case (Case Figure 5.2C). Two needles are usually needed because the extreme central collapse will often not allow cement to cross from side to side during filling. Only a small volume of cement is needed to adequately reinforce this type of fracture.

These cases are technically difficult, and the results from percutaneous vertebroplasty may not be as good as for less compressed vertebra. However, very compressed vertebra can respond to percutaneous vertebroplasty, and they should be treated when possible.

Case 6

Anterior Cervical Approach

John D. Barr and John M. Mathis

Clinical Presentation

A 43-year-old man was referred with severe neck pain and imaging findings consistent with diffuse metastatic disease to bone. The onset of pain had been gradual over several months, and there were no other neurologic symptoms at the time of presentation. The patient had no known primary cancer. An image-guided biopsy was requested.

Imaging Findings

Magnetic resonance imaging (MRI) demonstrated diffusely abnormal signal in the cervical spine with the largest lesion in C4 (Case Figure 6.1A,B). A computed tomography (CT) scan showed that the central portion of C4 was destroyed and the vertebra partially collapsed (Case Figure 6.1C,D). There was no extension of tumor into the spinal canal.

Procedure

A C4 biopsy was planned, which would be followed by vertebroplasty. There is no contraindication to percutaneous vertebroplasty (PV) in conjunction with biopsy before the cell type of a metastatic or primary tumor of bone is known. The approach to C4 used was anterior oblique with a small guide needle to first ensure that no critical structures (i.e., carotid artery) were punctured. A right side approach is always preferred to avoid the esophagus, found centrally or to the left behind the trachea.

The vascular structures on the right are manually pushed aside during the insertion of a 20-gauge guide needle (Case Figure 6.2A,B; see also Figure 2.3). After introduction, the guide needle position can be confirmed with CT scanning. As opposed to fluoroscopy, CT scanning can show the internal structures of the neck and help ensure that the guide needle adequately misses critical structures. Subsequently, a

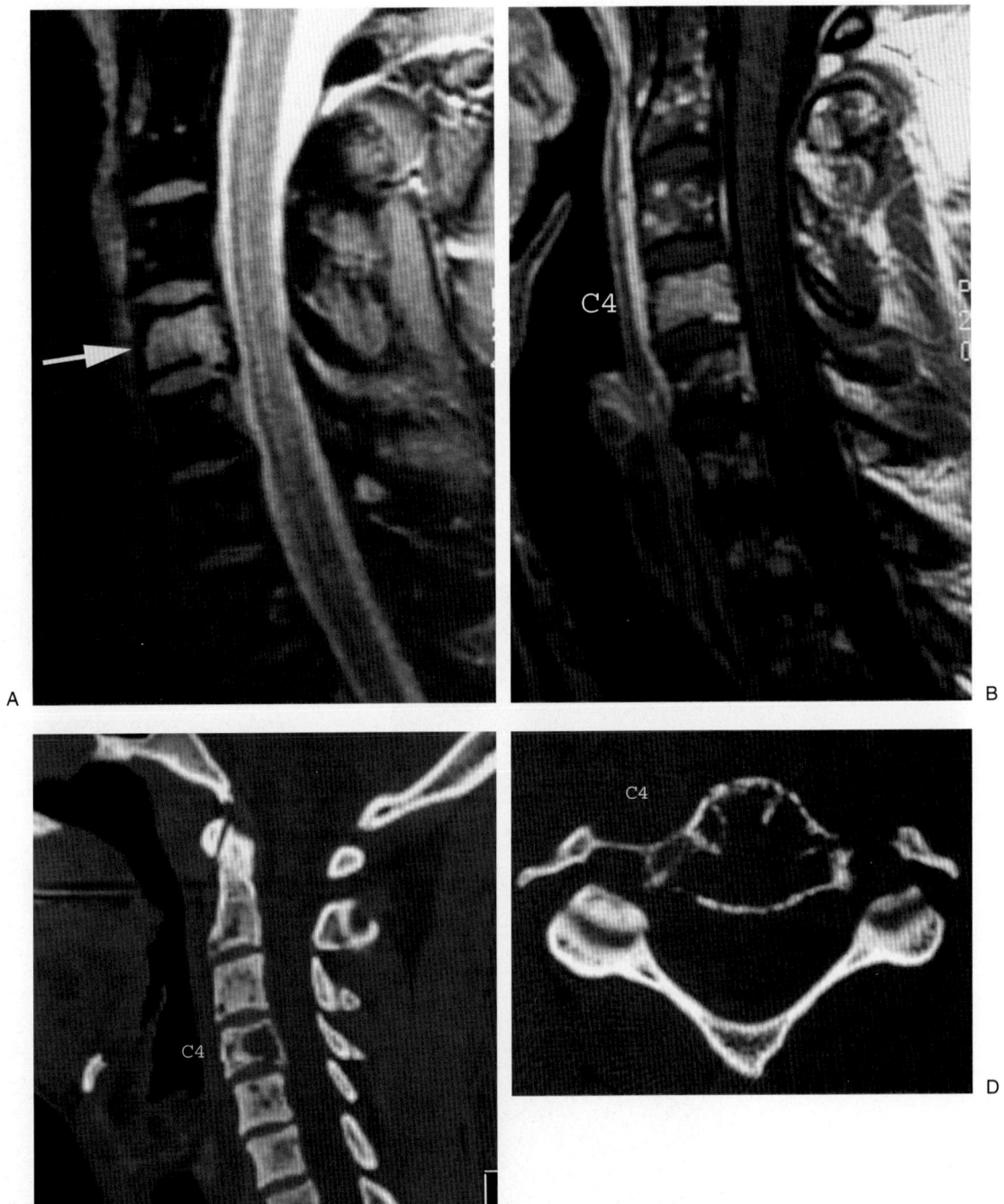

Case Figure 6.1. **(A)** Lateral T2 sagittal MRI shows diffuse abnormal signal in cervical vertebra with a large area of marrow replacement within C4 (white arrow). **(B)** A postcontrast T1 sagittal MRI demonstrates diffuse metastatic disease to bone, with the largest area of enhancement at C4. **(C)** A sagittal CT reconstruction reveals the loss of height at C4 consistent with a compression fracture. **(D)** The axial CT image of C4 also shows destruction and replacement of the osseous structure of this vertebral body.

Case Figure 6.2. (A) An artist's sketch of the cervical approach used for guide needle introduction to C4. Note that the approach is on the right, with the vascular structures manually pushed laterally during needle introduction. This technique is commonly used for cervical discography. **(B)** A lateral radiograph shows the guide needle (black arrow) in place, with the tip touching the anterior lateral margin of C4. **(C)** The cannula has been coaxially introduced over the guide needle. **(D)** A biopsy device has been inserted through the guide cannula to allow a core of tissue to be extracted. The cannula can remain in place for the subsequent PV.

larger cannula is placed coaxially over the 20-gauge guide needle to the surface of C4 (Case Figure 6.2C). The 20-gauge needle is removed and the trocar replaced into the cannula and advanced into the body of C4. The trocar can now be removed and a biopsy device placed through the cannula to obtain a bone core (Case Figure 6.2D).

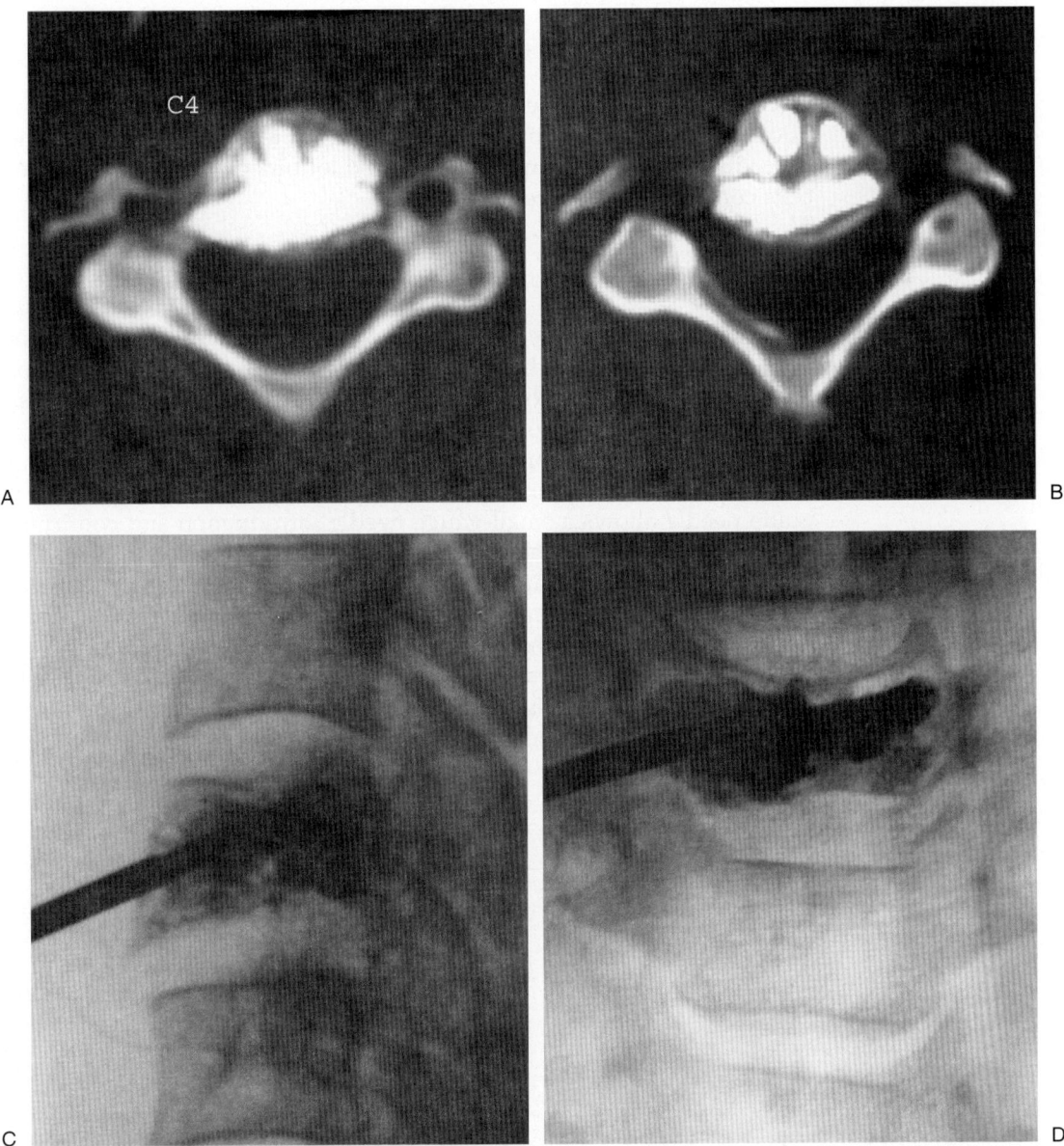

Case Figure 6.3. **(A,B)** Two adjacent level axial CT scans of C4 post-PV. Note good filling of the vertebra and no significant leak of cement. **(C,D)** Lateral and anteroposterior radiographs post-PV demonstrate the appearance of C4 following cement injection. The vertebral margins and exact location of the cement are harder to confirm than with CT.

After the biopsy material is obtained, bone cement (polymethylmethacrylate) is mixed and injected in small aliquots (i.e., 0.1–0.2 mL) with CT images obtained between injections. Computed tomography gives excellent visualization of the cement location, and small injections ensure that any potential leaks will be detected before becoming large enough to create clinical symptoms (Case Figure 6.3A,B). Radiographs of C4 give poorer definition of cement position by comparison (Case Figure 6.3C,D).

Results

The patient tolerated the procedure well. There were no clinical complications, and substantial pain relief was noted within hours of the procedure. The biopsy material revealed a homogenous infiltration of cells consistent with myeloma.

Discussion

This case illustrates an acceptable approach to cervical and high thoracic vertebrae for both biopsy and PV therapy. An alternate route for the clivus and C1–2 region is transoral. However, the needle must pass through oral mucosa for this approach, and seeding of bacteria is always a concern. Computed tomography offers good visualization and surpasses that obtained with fluoroscopy. Also, the placement of a guide needle allows a small-gauge needle introduction and confirmation of location before the large bone cannula is placed.

The cervical spine is rarely involved by a compression fracture unless there is underlying tumor invasion and vertebral destruction. Pure osteoporotic fractures are essentially never seen in this region.

The amount of bone cement needed is usually only 1–2 mL. There is no contraindication to PV before radiation or chemotherapy, so PV can follow immediately after the biopsy, as was done in this case.

Case 7

Vertebral Refracture After Percutaneous Vertebroplasty

Jon Kim and John M. Mathis

Clinical Presentation

The patient is an 81-year-old male who experienced good pain relief with percutaneous vertebroplasty (PV) of two lumbar vertebrae (L1–L2). Two weeks following the procedure, the patient experienced recurrence of pain after a mild traumatic event. He described severe pain in the upper lumbar region that worsened on standing and ambulation.

Imaging Findings

Initial post-PV radiographs demonstrated typical PV filling of L1 and L2 with no cement leak or apparent complication (Case Figure 7.1A). A repeat set of radiographs was obtained after the onset of new pain. Both vertebrae had lost additional height since the PV, with a fracture line extending through the superior-anterior aspect of L1 suggesting there may be a bone fragment (Case Figure 7.1B). Magnetic resonance images (MRI) were obtained to look for additional sites of injury not apparent on the radiographs. No other abnormalities were found, and the presumption was that the patient had refractured L1 and L2 and that this was the source of his recurrent pain.

Procedure

Prior to the procedure, 1 gram of cefazolin was administered intravenously to the patient for antibiotic prophylaxis. The patient was given intravenous procedural sedation with fentanyl and Versed, titrated for comfort.

Following sterile preparation and local anesthesia, 13-gauge needles were introduced into the vertebral bodies using a transpedicular route under fluoroscopic guidance (Case Figure 7.2B). Once the needles were in place, bone cement (polymethylmethacrylate with 30% barium

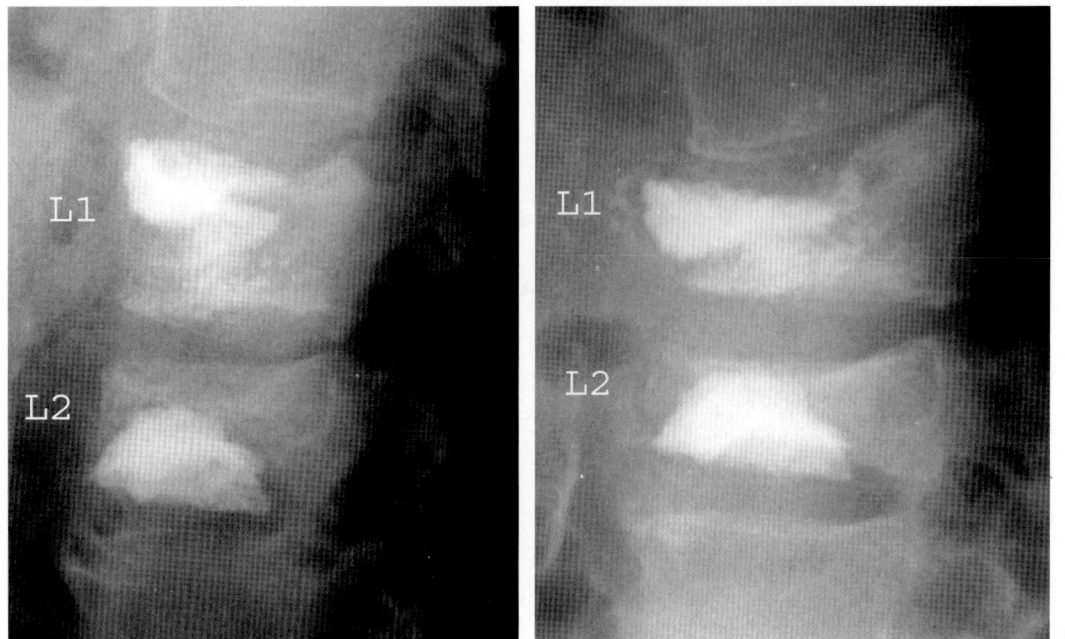

Case Figure 7.1. (A) Lateral radiograph post-PV at L1 and L2. (B) Lateral radiograph obtained following the onset of new pain. This examination shows loss of height of both L1 and L2 since PV was performed, consistent with the diagnosis of refracture of both of these vertebral levels. (From Mathis [1], with permission.)

sulfate) was prepared and injected into L1 and L2, again with fluoroscopic guidance. The previously nonfilled portions of the vertebrae were filled (Case Figure 7.2C). There were no leaks of cement, and the patient tolerated the procedure well.

Results

When the patient was placed prone on the operative table, sufficient pull on the spine was created to open up the previously recompressed vertebra (Case Figure 7.2A). The original post-treatment height of both vertebrae was recovered and maintained with retreatment (Case Figure 7.2B,C).

After a 2-hour observation period, the patient was released home with essentially total pain relief. The patient has been monitored for over 2 years postprocedure with no recurrence or additional fracture.

Discussion

The literature contains little discussion of vertebral refracture following PV (1). Fracture of other vertebrae after PV can occur and is the most common cause of recurrent fracture-related pain after PV.

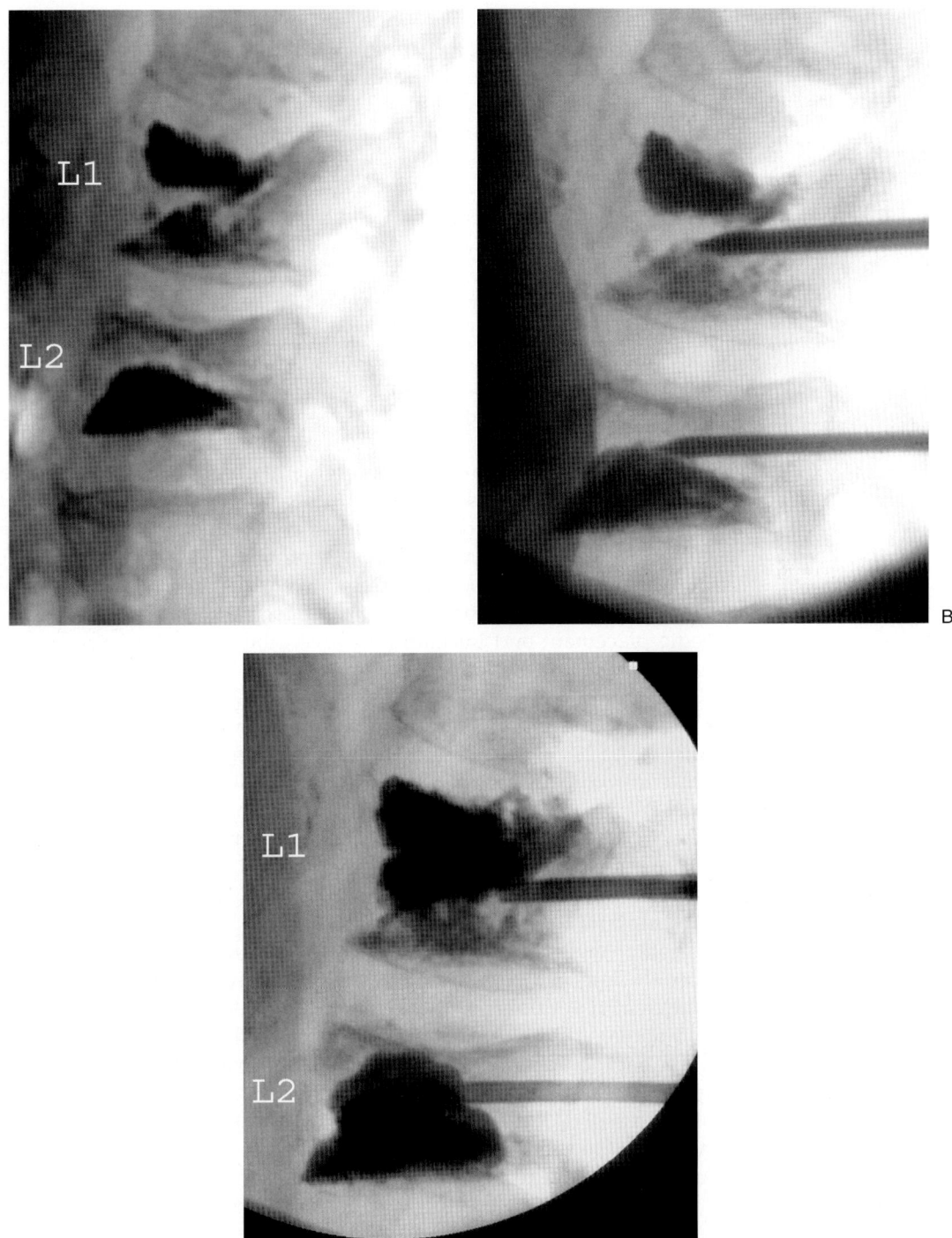

Case Figure 7.2. (A) With the patient prone on the operative table, there is natural distraction on the vertebral elements that has produced height restoration in both L1 and L2. This lateral radiograph shows vertebra height and configuration similar to that shown in Case Figure 7.1A (after the initial PV but before refracture). **(B)** Lateral image with needles in place prior to cement injection. **(C)** After cement injection in L1 and L2. Height gain is permanently recaptured. There is no cement leak or other complication. (From Mathis [1], with permission.)

However, as our treatment numbers have increased, we have seen an occasional refracture after treatment with PV. In our first 1,000 patients who underwent PV, we found 3 who experienced refracture in the treated vertebra (incidence of 0.3%). All were successfully retreated with PV with good secondary pain relief.

The cause of refracture is not known. Refracture may occur when insufficient amounts of cement are injected, resulting in suboptimal biomechanical reinforcement of the vertebra. Belkoff et al. (2) performed an ex vivo study on osteoporotic cadaver vertebrae, randomized to various injection volumes, to determine the quantity of cement needed to restore the original vertebral strength after fracture. These amounts were 2.3–3.0 mL in the upper thoracic spine, 3.0–4.0 mL at the thoracolumbar junction, and 6.0–8.0 mL in the lower lumbar spine. We know that pain relief has been poorly correlated (if at all) with the quantity of cement injected. This is not the case with biomechanical reinforcement. Additionally, some vertebrae prove to be so fragile that, even with reasonable amounts of cement injected to produce pain relief, there is still a risk of refracture. Repeat imaging and physical examination are required to exclude a new fracture that would better explain the patient's recurrence of symptoms. When a recurrent fracture is diagnosed, it should be retreated with PV. This can be challenging, because the initial cement can pose a substantial problem for needle placement and injection; however, these vertebrae can be successfully retreated with good pain relief.

The greatest difficulty associated with treatment of refracture is loss of visualization of the anatomic landmarks and the extremely hard cement that is now in place. The first problem can be overcome by needle introduction through the original needle tract, a remnant of the initial PV treatment. The needle tract can usually be seen as a circular defect in the cement in anteroposterior or anteroposterior oblique projection, effectively "looking down the original needle tract." By using the initial tract for needle placement, the operator is not dependent on anatomic landmarks.

Another method to overcome the lack of landmark visualization is to use the interpedicular line. We can approximate the pedicle location of the treated vertebra as it lies on a line between the pedicle of the vertebra above and below. After assessing pedicle location we can then take a parapedicular or transpedicular approach to enter the refractured vertebra. The second method for needle placement is less acceptable, as it will usually place the needle outside the original needle tract. This may result in the needle encountering bone cement, which is very hard and difficult to penetrate.

References

1. Mathis JM. Percutaneous vertebroplasty: complication avoidance and technique optimization. Am J Neuroradiol 2004; 24:1697–1706.
2. Belkoff SM, Mathis JM, Jasper LE, et al. The biomechanics of vertebroplasty: the effect of cement volume on mechanical behavior. Spine 2001; 26: 1537–1541.

Case 8

Percutaneous Sacroplasty

John M. Mathis

Clinical Presentation

This patient is a 96-year-old man who had been very active for age and sustained a relatively minor fall that resulted in severe back and pelvic region pain. He had been confined to bed and a wheelchair for 2 months with analgesic therapy. He had one bout of pneumonia from which he had recovered. A nuclear medicine scan was obtained, and the diagnosis was made of a sacral insufficiency fracture with a coexistent lumbar vertebral compression fracture. He was referred for percutaneous therapy of these lesions.

Imaging Findings

The radionuclide scan was very revealing and showed the typical H configuration of a sacral insufficiency fracture (Case Figure 8.1). A fracture of L1 was also present. A computed tomography (CT) scan at the time of treatment demonstrated bilateral fractures of the sacral wings (Case Figure 8.2).

Procedure

The L1 vertebroplasty was performed in the typical fashion using fluoroscopic guidance. This was successful and was performed the day before the percutaneous sacroplasty (PS). For the PS, the patient was given intravenous antibiotics (1 gram Ancef) and intravenous procedural sedation (fentanyl, midazolam). He was positioned prone on the CT table and initial localization scans were obtained. Two needles were inserted at a time (ultimately four needles were used). The two needles were inserted in a single CT scan plane so that the tips could each be visualized (Case Figure 8.3). This allows cement to be injected into two needles and the cement monitored with each CT evaluation. On each CT check, five slices are made (with a fast multislice machine) at

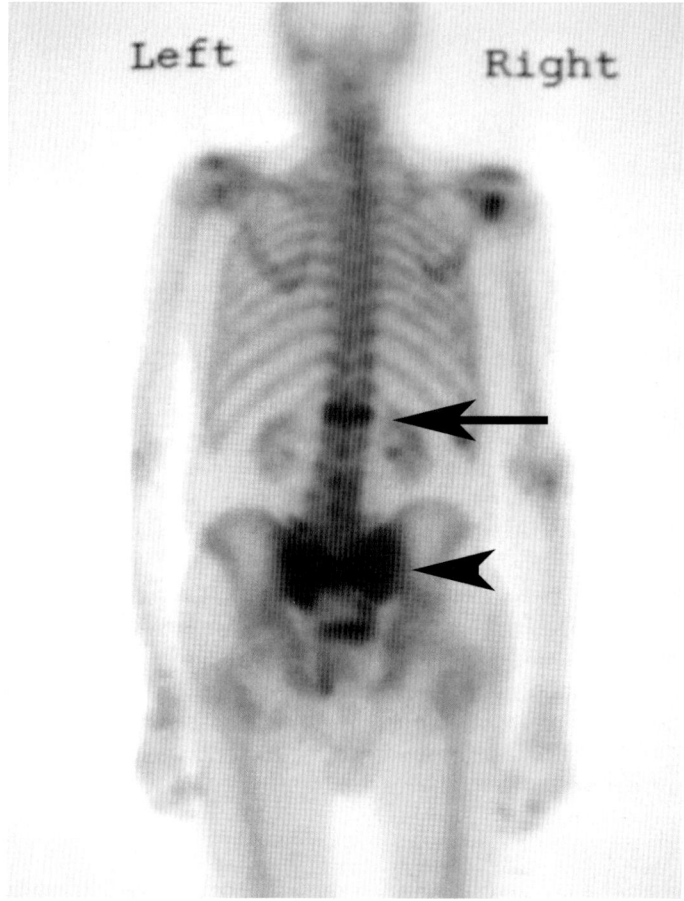

Case Figure 8.1. This bone scan image shows the typical H-shaped sacral insufficiency fracture (black arrowhead) and a coexistent L1 vertebral compression fracture (black arrow).

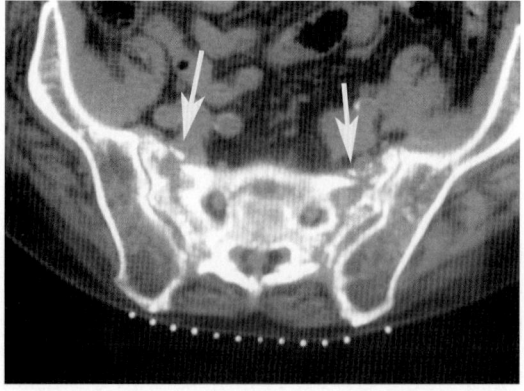

Case Figure 8.2. Pretreatment axial CT demonstrates the fractures in both sacral ala (white arrows). Note that the fractures are parallel to the sacroiliac joints.

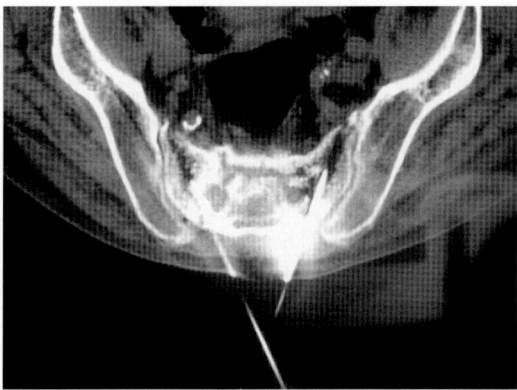

Case Figure 8.3. Axial CT showing two needles placed into the sacral fractures. Note that the needles extend along the fracture plane and that both needle tips are in the same CT plane for ease of monitoring.

0.5-cm intervals. This visualizes the needle tips and the surrounding area to look for adjacent leaks. Small aliquots of cement (0.5 mL) are injected through each needle at a time and CT images are obtained to look for leaks and filling patterns (Case Figure 8.4). As four needle locations were injected, approximately 2.5 mL of cement was injected at each site.

Results

The patient experienced almost complete pain relief over the 2 days of therapy. Analgesics were discontinued, and he underwent rehabilitation and ultimately resumed living alone.

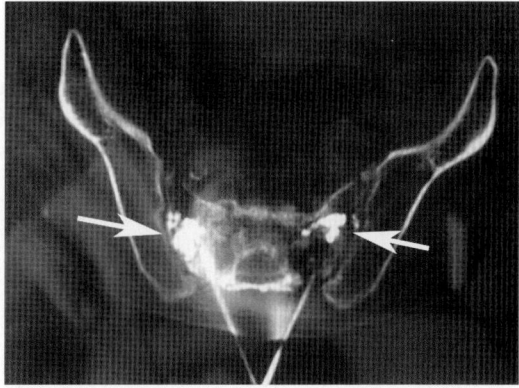

Case Figure 8.4. Cement is injected in small aliquots (typically 0.5 mL) and repeat CT images are obtained to evaluate the cement distribution (white arrows) and look for leaks.

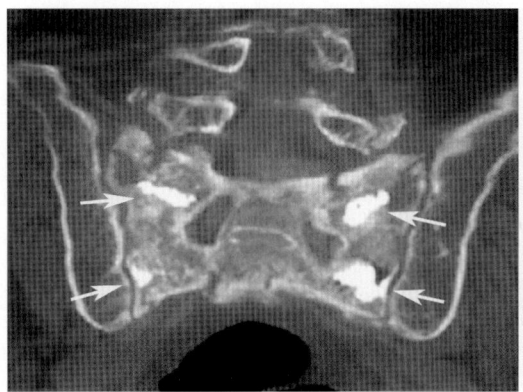 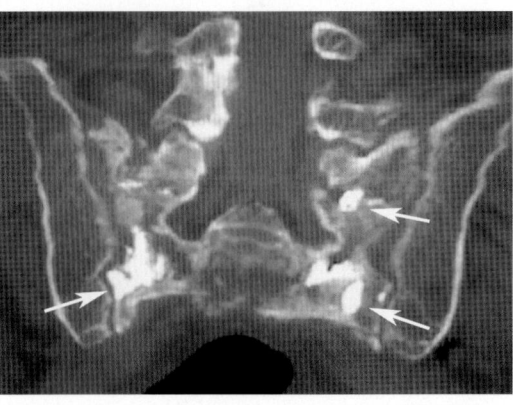

Case Figure 8.5. (A,B) These coronal reconstructions were obtained post-treatment and show the four cement injection sites (white arrows). By using four (or even six) injection sites, the total amount of cement that is needed at each site is reduced.

Discussion

This case is a classic example of a patient who sustained a sacral insufficiency fracture and did not recover with conservative therapy. Without percutaneous therapy, 50% of these patients will not regain their prefracture level of activity (see Chapter 12 further details). The case also shows the common finding of a coexistent vertebral compression fracture.

Computed tomography guidance was used, but others have described fluoroscopy. Computed tomography seems to better visualize the areas of potential complication (neural foramina and spinal canal) so that small cement leaks can be identified early and injections stopped.

Four needle injections were used in this patient to provide cement in several locations within the fracture (Case Figure 8.5). Two injections could be used, but more cement at each site would be recommended to ensure good bonding of the fracture fragments. Larger quantities at a single location present the increased risk of ultimate leak into an unwanted site. Even though this fracture involved the central portion of the sacrum, only the lateral fractures were treated. The patient recovered well, indicating that the central portion of the fracture does not necessarily need to be addressed to adequately achieve stabilization.

By placing two needles in a single scan plane and working both needles at one time, the procedure can be shortened and the total number of CT scans required is reduced. The needles are placed along the fracture line, which is usually parallel to the sacroiliac joints. The needle tip location should be sufficiently away from the foramina to allow filling without easy leak into these locations.

Case 9

Percutaneous Pelvic Augmentation: Supra-Acetabular Region

John M. Mathis

Clinical Presentation

A 57-year-old man, with known metastatic carcinoma to bone, presented with severe pain in the region of the right hip. The patient was unable to walk and was basically confined to bed, as even transfers to a wheelchair created severe pain. The patient had an indwelling pain pump, but this did not manage the acute pain caused by hip motion and weight bearing.

Imaging Findings

A computed tomography (CT) scan of the pelvis revealed bone destruction of the pelvis in the region above the right acetabulum by tumor (Case Figure 9.1A,B). Local radiographs of this area also confirmed the lytic process (Case Figure 9.1C). The adjacent femur was not involved.

Procedure

Percutaneous bone augmentation with cement was chosen because of the minimally invasive nature of the procedure with essentially no postprocedure recovery. The surgical procedure that was an alternative was discussed with the patient and declined because of the protracted recovery that would be necessary.

The patient received intravenous Ancef (1 gram) and intravenous procedural sedation with fentanyl and Versed. An 11-gauge trocar–cannula system was introduced along the pelvic axis into the supra-acetabular area (Case Figure 9.2A). Fluoroscopy along the tract of the needle and perpendicular to the needle axis allow needle positioning.

Simplex P was mixed with 30% sterile barium sulfate and then injected into the tumor mass above the acetabulum (Case Figure 9.2B). The needle was withdrawn as local filling was achieved (Case Figure

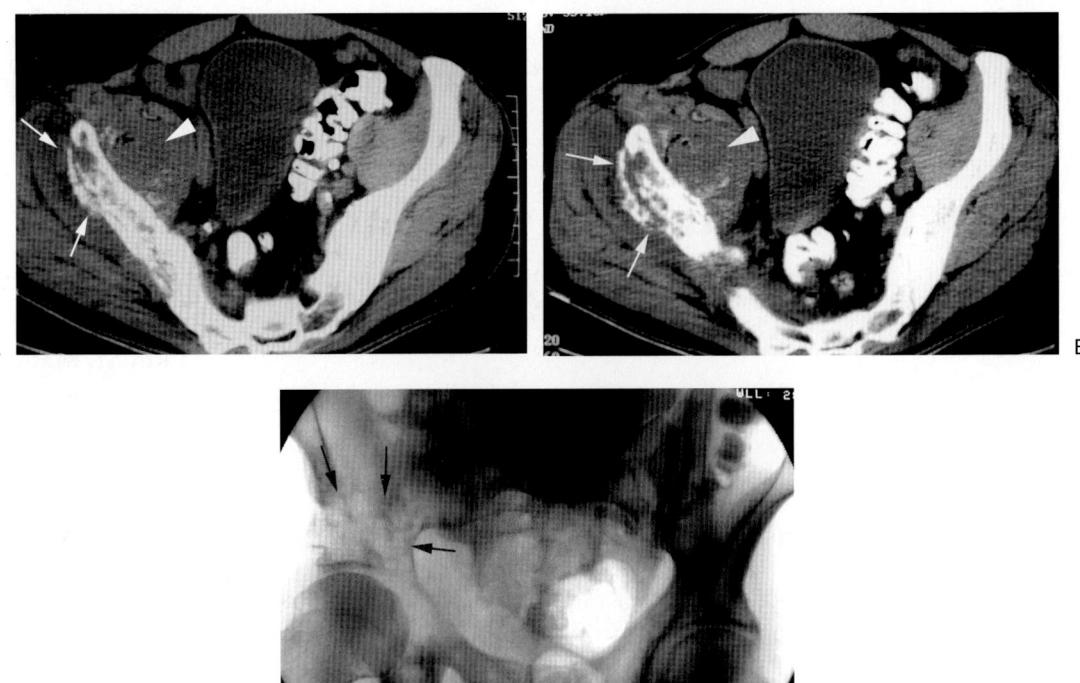

Case Figure 9.1. (A,B) Axial CT scans of the pelvis show destruction of the pelvis above the acetabulum on the right (white arrows). A soft tissue mass of tumor is seen adjacent to the affected bone (white arrowheads). **(C)** A pelvic radiograph demonstrates the lytic destruction of bone (black arrows) in the supra-acetabular region on the right.

9.2C,D). After the immediate region above the acetabulum was filled, a new needle was introduced above the original fill zone (Case Figure 9.3A). This allowed an additional layer of cement to be added to increase the augmentation of bone in this region (Case Figure 9.3B,C). This can be done several times as needed to eventually have the cement bridge areas of normal bone. The procedure was tolerated well by the patient, and there were no clinical side effects.

Results

The patient had substantial pain relief within 24 hours of the procedure. He was able to transfer from bed to wheelchair with assistance and with minimal pain. Also, he was able to walk with a walker with only mild pain. This was a tremendous improvement and allowed him to resume care at home by his family.

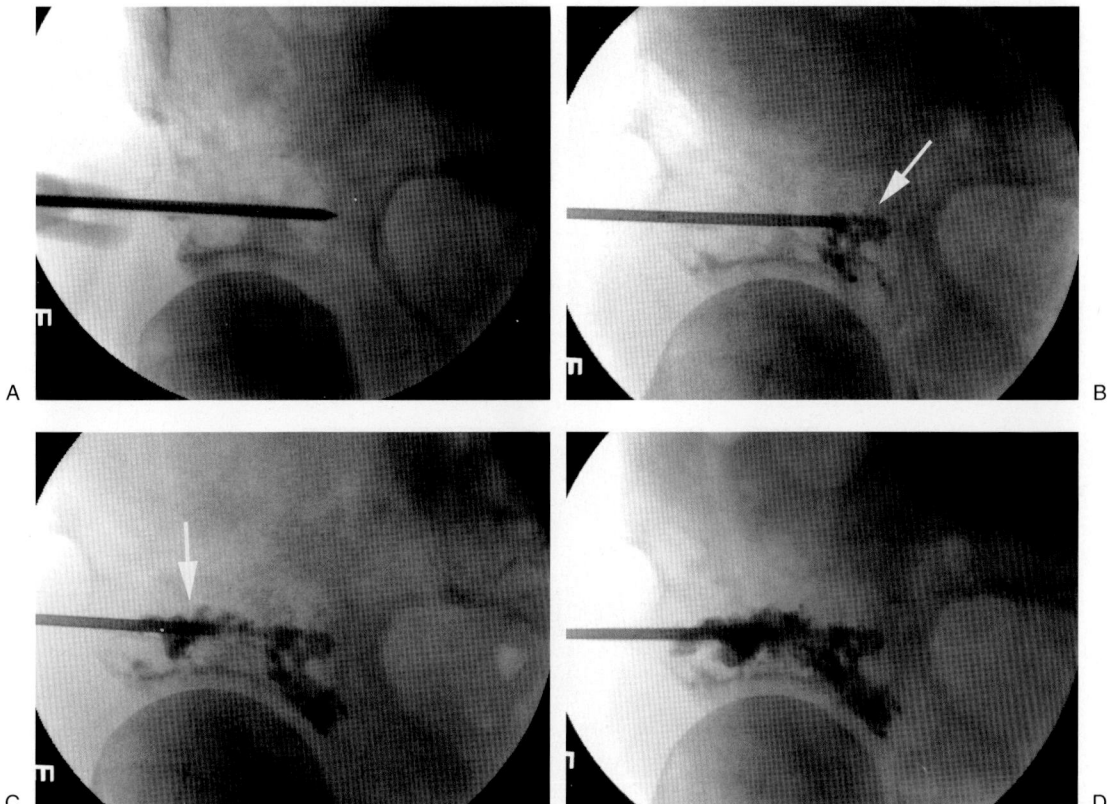

Case Figure 9.2. (A) Fluoroscopic image showing the cement injection needle in place above the acetabulum. **(B,C)** Cement (white arrows) is being injected at various locations along the needle track. **(D)** The final cement deposition in this first needle location.

Discussion

This case demonstrates the opportunity for percutaneous, image-guided bone augmentation in areas other than the spine. This patient's longevity was not affected by this treatment, but he did achieve an improved quality of life that allowed him to be at home with his family. The recovery from minimally invasive procedures is usually markedly shorter than for comparable open surgical procedures.

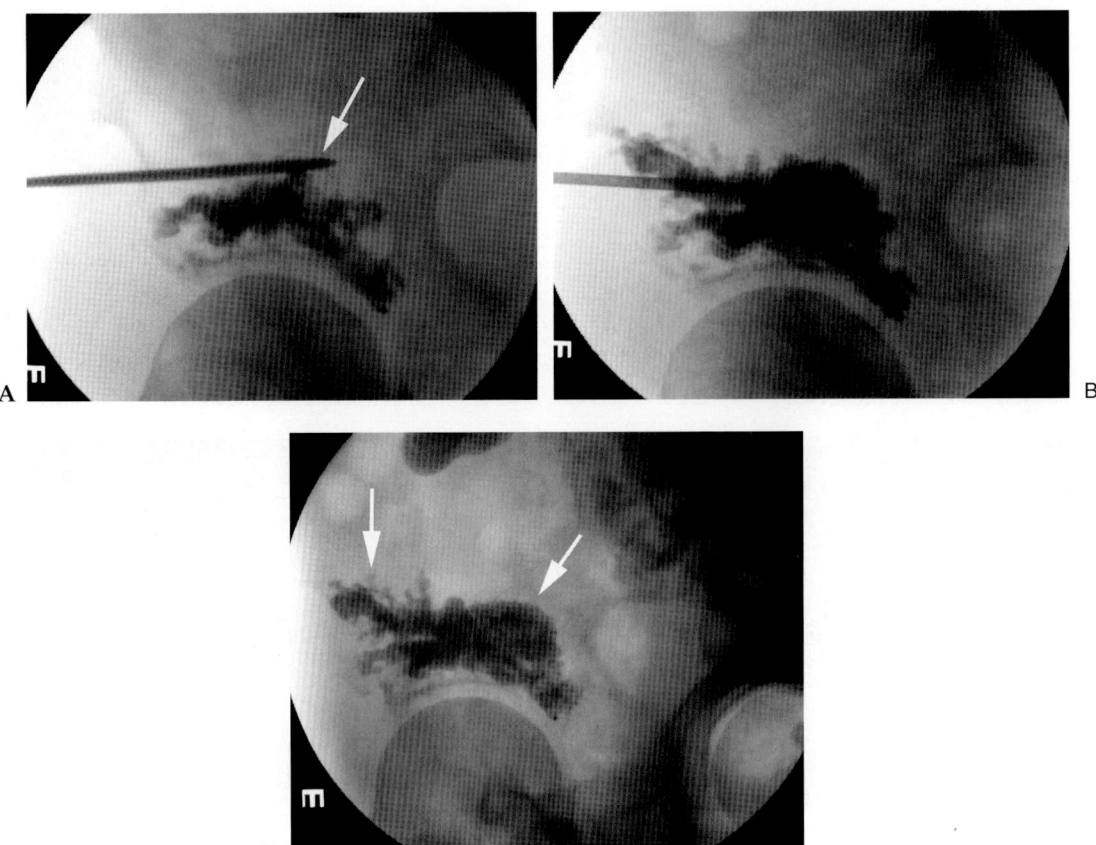

Case Figure 9.3. (A) Fluoroscopic image showing the second needle position (white arrow) but before more cement is injected here. (B) Additional cement has been injected through the second needle. (C) Final image shows the total cement (white arrows) volume placed in the supra-acetabular region, augmenting this portion of previously destroyed bone.

Case 10

Kyphoplasty in Osteoporotic Compression Fractures

A. Orlando Ortiz and John M. Mathis

Clinical Presentation

An 84-year-old man presented with severe back pain in the midthoracic spine. The patient had been experiencing pain for 6 weeks. There were no significant comorbidities in this individual. The pain was very limiting of his usual life style, and he had failed conservative therapy.

Imaging Findings

The patient was found to have moderate compression of the T8 and T9 vertebra (Case Figure 10.1), and there was associated kyphosis. These were subacute by bone scan. The level of pain correlated with the site of the fracture. Because there were two adjacent fractures, percutaneous kyphoplasty (KP) was chosen as the therapeutic option to try to restore as much height as possible to these vertebrae.

Procedure

The patient was given intravenous antibiotics prior to the procedure, which was performed in an angiography suite with intravenous procedural sedation (fentanyl and Versed). Sterile preparation of the back was followed by local anesthesia to the skin and periosteum of the bone.

Trocar and cannula systems were introduced using biplane fluoroscopic guidance via a transpedicular approach (bilaterally). When the cannula reached the posterior aspect of the vertebral body (Case Figure 10.2A), the trocar was removed and a drill inserted to develop a channel in the vertebral body for subsequent balloon insertion (Case Figure 10.2B). This was accomplished on both sides, and a balloon was inserted through each guide cannula (Case Figure 10.2D). The balloons were inflated, again using fluoroscopy for monitoring (Case Figure 10.2E). Balloon inflation was irregular in T9 (Case Figure 10.2F) and

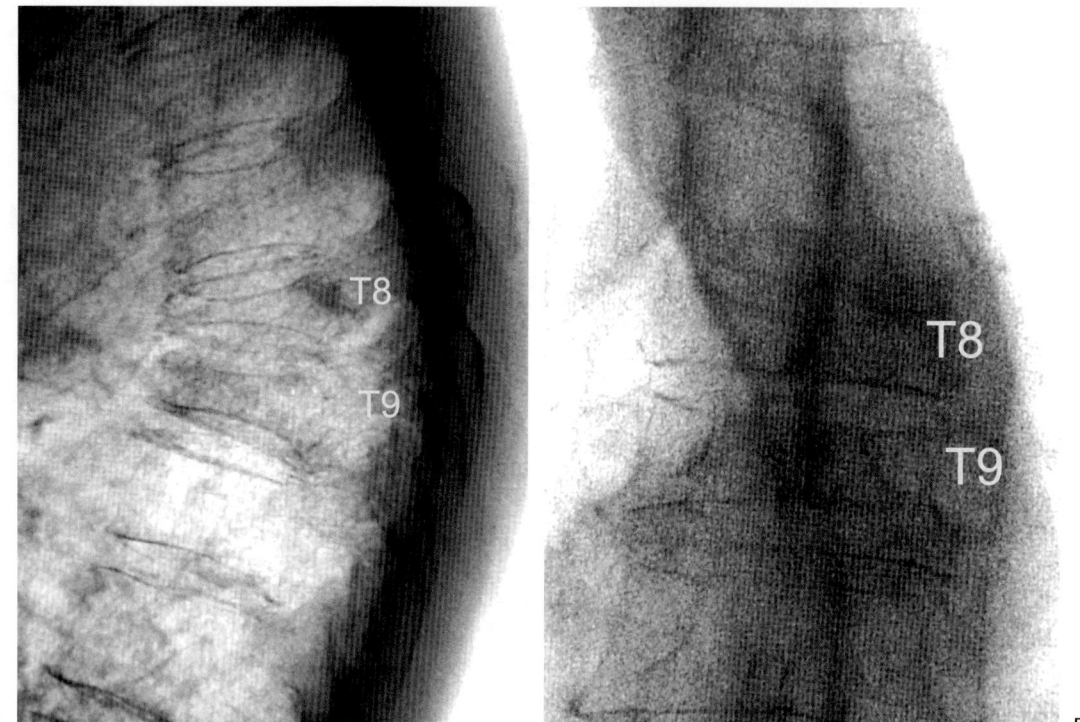

Case Figure 10.1. Lateral (A) and anteroposterior (B) radiographs showing moderately severe compression of T8 and T9.

reached maximum pressure (300 mm Hg). When a portion of one balloon reached the vertebral margin, additional inflation attempts were terminated and the balloons were removed from T9 for cement introduction. No appreciable height restoration was achieved in this vertebra. Cement leaked along the cannula track (Case Figure 10.2H).

Balloons were inserted into T8 (following the same procedure as for T9) (Case Figure 10.3A–C). Inflation was more uniform (Case Figure 10.3D) and progressed until maximal pressure (300 mm Hg) was achieved. The balloons were deflated and removed. Cement was introduced into the vertebral body of T8 (Case Figure 10.3E). This vertebra did gain height, and this was estimated to be 3–4 mm (Case Figure 10.3F). No cement leaks were experienced at this level.

Results

This patient experienced complete pain relief and had no clinical complications associated with the cement leak noted at T9. He returned to his daily routine and was able to discontinue analgesics.

Discussion

This case demonstrates the use of KP for the treatment of osteoporotic compression fractures. It resulted in good pain relief, but only gave minimal height restoration to the two levels treated. There was a cement leak, but, as with most leaks encountered in vertebroplasty, it was of no clinical significance. Overall, the result is clinically similar to that expected if vertebroplasty had been the method of treatment.

Pain relief seems to be similar for both KP and PV, as one would expect because both methods rely on final stabilization of the fracture with bone cement. Direct comparisons of biomechanical strength have been made that found similar resultant strengths.

Height restoration is variable from case to case. As of yet, there are no good data to help determine which patients are more appropriate for KP or for PV. Height restoration is seen with both procedures and is relatively meager generally. Very mobile vertebrae can achieve complete height restoration with either technique, and such cases are sometimes used as anecdotal examples. However, these are unrealistic outcomes for most cases. Until a direct prospective study comparing KP and PV is obtained, we will not be able to predict which procedure is more appropriate in a particular situation. We do know that there is a huge difference in the costs of KP and PV. Kyphoplasty tends to cost 10 times more than PV because of the materials used. The cost can be even greater if KP is performed in an operating room with general anesthesia (the technique used by most spine surgeons). The cost difference might be acceptable if there was demonstrative evidence of better outcomes, substantial height restoration, or improved safety with KP. However, this is not the case, and the actual reason for using KP generally is more driven by marketing to the public and to physicians than medical need. (See additional information in Chapters 8, 9, and 13.)

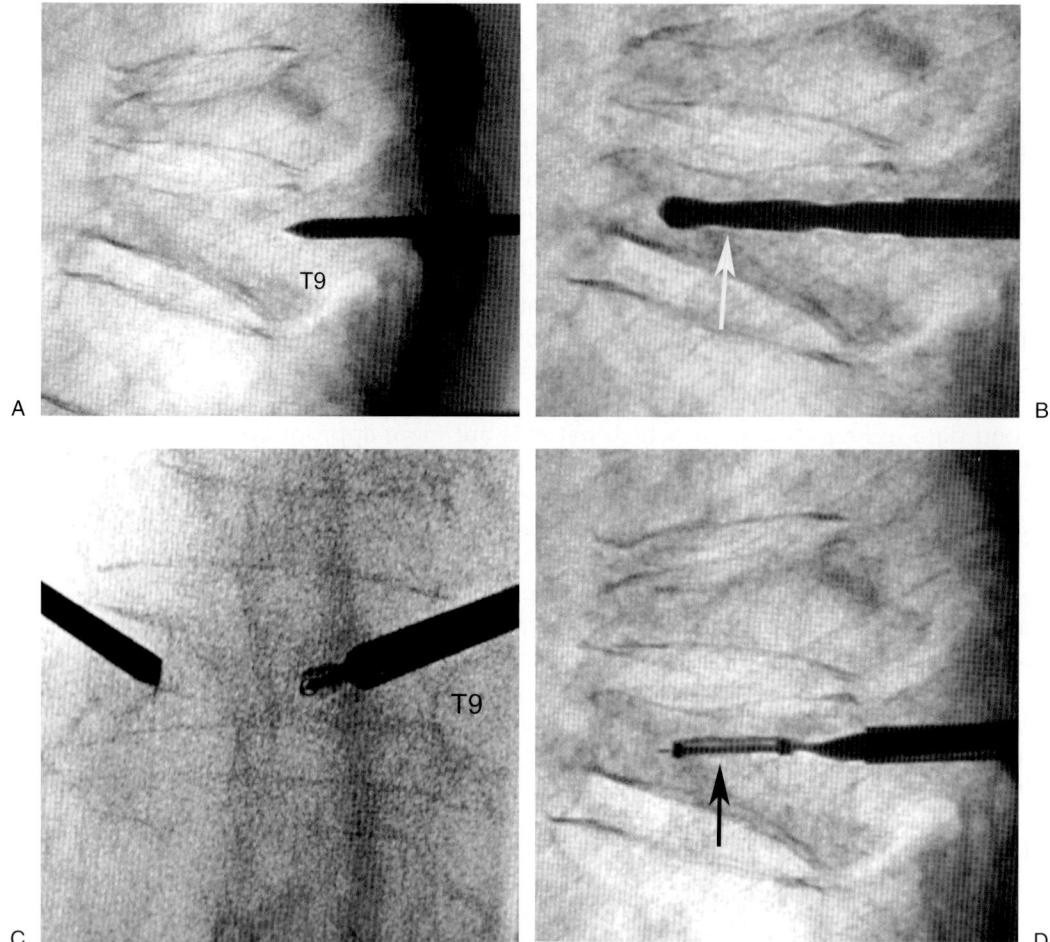

Case Figure 10.2. (A) Lateral image showing the guide cannula and trocar positioned at the posterior vertebral margin of T9. (B) Lateral image with the drill (white arrow) inserted through the cannula to produce a track for the balloon. (C) Anteroposterior image demonstrates both cannulas in place via a transpedicular approach. (D) Lateral image shows the balloon (black arrow) in place before inflation.

Case 10 Osteoporotic Compression Fractures 293

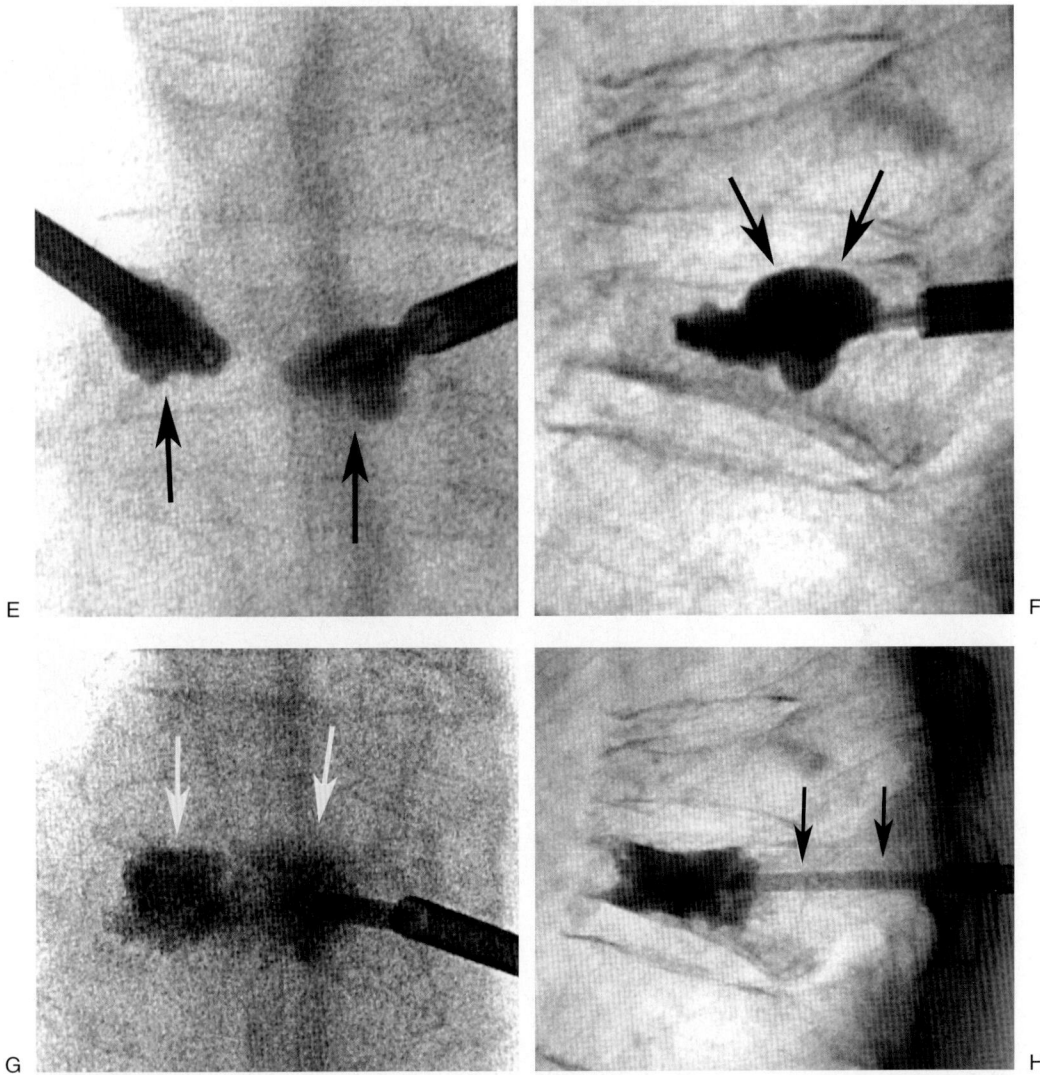

Case Figure 10.2. *Continued* **(E)** Anteroposterior image showing inflation of both balloons (black arrows). **(F)** The lateral radiograph shows the eccentric balloon configuration extending to the margin of the upper endplate (black arrows). **(G)** Anteroposterior image showing cement (white arrows) injection. **(H)** Lateral image after removal of the cement-introduction cannula. Note that cement has leaked along the cannula track into the soft tissues (black arrows).

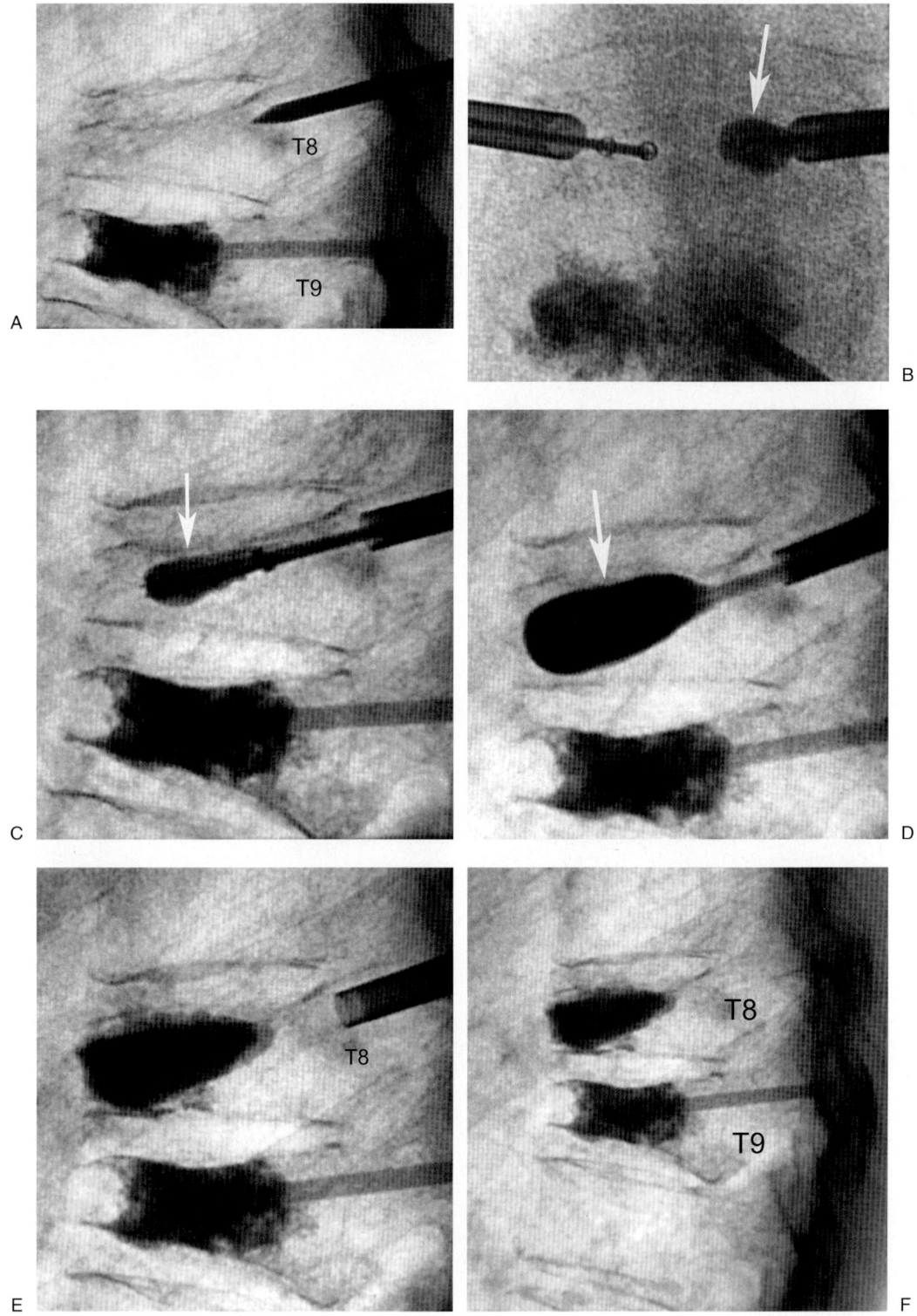

Case Figure 10.3. (A) Lateral fluoroscopic image showing the introductory trocar and cannula at the posterior aspect of T8. Note there is some height gain compared to Figure 10.1 even before the cannula is inserted. **(B)** Anteroposterior image demonstrates bilateral cannula with balloons in place. One shows early inflation (white arrow). **(C)** The corresponding lateral radiograph shows early inflation (white arrow) from this projection. **(D)** Lateral image with progressive inflation (white arrow). Note that the inflation of this balloon is more uniform than found at T9. Modest height recovery has been achieved at this level. **(E)** The lateral image following introduction of cement at T8. **(F)** A final lateral radiograph showing the result after treatment of both T8 and T9.

Case 11

Femoral Neck Augmentation

Paul F. Heini and Torsten Franz

Overview

The incidence of hip fractures worldwide is expected to almost quadruple in the next 60 years (1). In addition to the acute limitations associated with a hip fracture, most patients continue to suffer from difficulties in performing activities of daily living (2), and their related mortality is high. One third of patients do not survive beyond the first year after fracturing their hip. The risk of dying from a hip fracture equals that of dying of breast cancer (3). Osteoporotic fractures are associated with pain, limitation of mobility, and social dependency.

Osteoporotic fracture patients occupy 1% to 1.5 % of all hospital beds in Europe at any one time. This figure is expected to more than double during the next 50 years (4). Frailty of any population increases with longevity. Consequently, the present projections of fracture occurrence appear to be too conservative. The annual hip fracture incidence in Asia in 2050 might pass 10 million rather than the hitherto forecasted 3.2 million (5). Therefore, hip fracture prevention is of major importance. Protective devices have been developed in order to prevent fractures from a simple fall. Their effectiveness has been demonstrated in several studies; however, there is poor long-term compliance with their use (6–9). Energy-absorbing flooring, designed to prevent hip fractures, has been evaluated and shown to be cost effective (10). These measures and more will undoubtedly be increasingly employed in an attempt to stem the tide of increasing numbers of hip fractures.

Results

Based on the experience of reinforcement of osteoporotic vertebra (11–14), the potential of reinforcing the proximal femur was evaluated in an in vitro study. The technical feasibility was demonstrated, and the mechanical effect turned out to be significant (15) (Case Figure 11.1 and Case Table 11.1). However, the amount of polymethylmethacrylate (PMMA) needed to achieve a sufficient filling was on the order of

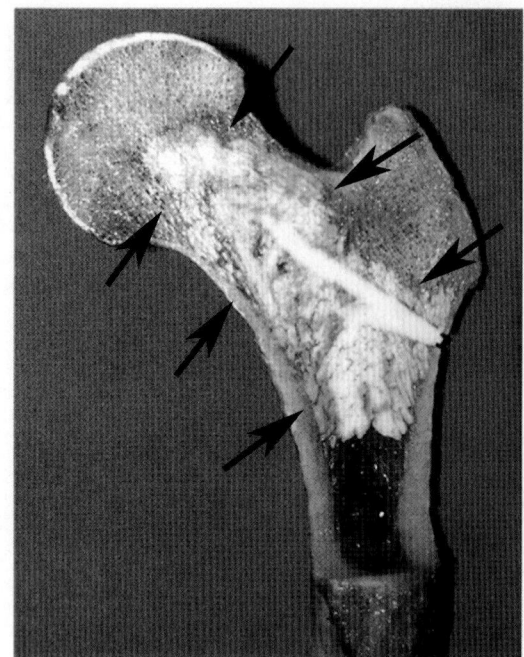 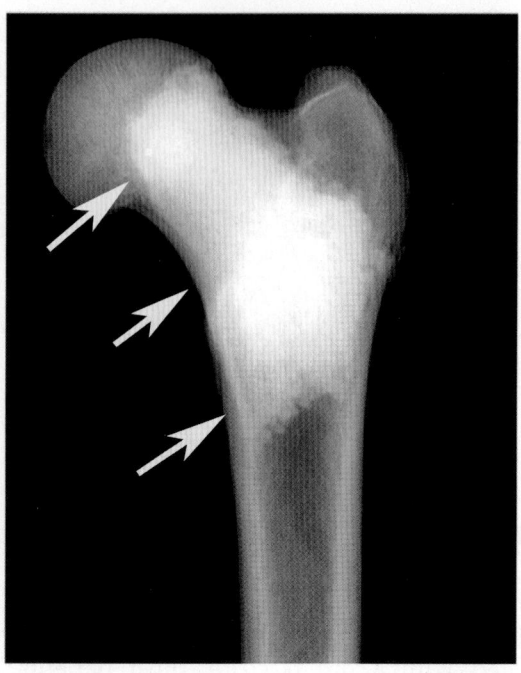

Case Figure 11.1. **(A)** Specimen photograph following percutaneous femoral neck augmentation with PMMA (black arrows). **(B)** Specimen radiograph shows the distribution of the PMMA within the femoral neck (white arrows).

36 mL (range, 28–41). This produced a substantial amount of heat, with the surface temperature of the femoral neck increased an average of 22°C (range, 18°–30°C). This increase endangers the blood supply of the femoral head. Therefore, the use of PMMA in clinical applications should be limited until less exothermic materials are available.

Discussion

Because of the problems mentioned, percutaneous augmentation of the femoral neck has been performed only in selected cases. In our series, this procedure was performed as prophylactic protection for patients with metastatic disease.

The demonstration case used prophylactic reinforcement in a nonfractured hip that had obvious metastatic involvement. This patient presented with a right hip fracture secondary to myeloma (Case Figure

Case Table 11.1. Average Failure Load of Native and Reinforced Femurs.

Load Application Type	Failure Load (Newtons)		Difference %, Statistics
	Control (N = 5 for each type)	Reinforced (N = 5 for each type)	
Single leg stance	5,764	6,986	21% $p < 0.002$
Simulated fall	2,499	4,548	82% $p < 0.002$

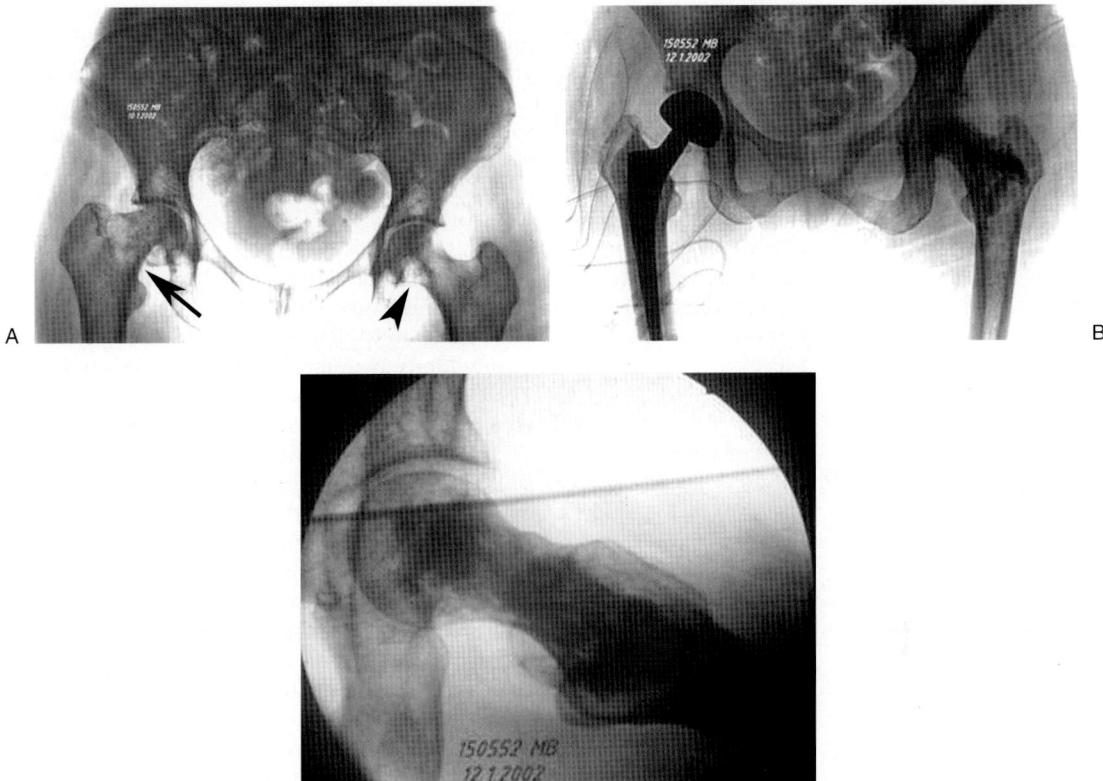

Case Figure 11.2. (A) Radiograph of the pelvis in a patient with myeloma. There is fracture of the right femoral neck (black arrow). Pathologic erosion of a portion of the left femoral neck is seen as well (black arrowhead). (B) A hemiarthroplasty was performed on the right. Percutaneous augmentation with PMMA was accomplished on the left. (C) An additional radiographic projection of the left femoral neck again shows the intramedullary PMMA.

11.2A). A hemiarthroplasty was performed on the right hip (Case Figure 11.2B). Percutaneous augmentation of the left hip was accomplished with PMMA and subsequently followed with radiation therapy (Case Figure 11.2D). This patient tolerated the procedures well and was able to resume ambulation after a period of rehabilitation.

New, low exothermic bone cements are in use (Cortoss, Orthovita, Malvern, PA) that have strength characteristics exceeding those of PMMA. These advances may allow this technique to be used in the prophylactic treatment of hips at risk because of osteoporosis.

References

1. Dubey A, Koval KJ, Zuckerman JD. Hip fracture prevention: a review. Am J Orthop 1998; 27(6):407–412.
2. Hochberg MC, Williamson J, Skinner EA, Guralnik J, Kasper JD, Fried LP. The prevalence and impact of self-reported hip fracture in elderly

community-dwelling women: the Women's Health and Aging Study. Osteoporos Int 1998; 8(4):385–389.
3. Keene GS, Parker MJ, Pryor GA. Mortality and morbidity after hip fractures. BMJ 1993; 307(6914):1248–1250.
4. Cooper C, Campion G, Melton LJ, 3rd. Hip fractures in the elderly: a worldwide projection. Osteoporos Int 1992; 2(6):285–289.
5. Elffors L. Are osteoporotic fractures due to osteoporosis? Impacts of a frailty pandemic in an aging world. Aging (Milano) 1998; 10(3):191–204.
6. Kannus P, Parkkari J, Poutala J. Comparison of force attenuation properties of four different hip protectors under simulated falling conditions in the elderly: an in vitro biomechanical study. Bone 1999; 25(2):229–235.
7. Kannus P, Parkkari J, Niemi S, Pasanen M, Palvanen M, Jarvinen M, Vuori I. Prevention of hip fracture in elderly people with use of a hip protector. N Engl J Med 2000; 343(21):1506–1513.
8. Kumar BA, Parker MJ. Are hip protectors cost effective? Injury 2000; 31(9):693–695.
9. Parker MJ, Gillespie LD, Gillespie WJ. Hip protectors for preventing hip fractures in the elderly. Cochrane Database Syst Rev 2000; 2.
10. Zacker C, Shea D. An economic evaluation of energy-absorbing flooring to prevent hip fractures. Int J Technol Assess Health Care 1998; 14(3):446–457.
11. Heini PF. The current treatment—a survey of osteoporotic fracture treatment. Osteoporotic spine fractures: the spine surgeon's perspective. Osteoporos Int 2004. 2004, March; 16 Suppl. 2:S85–92.
12. Heini PF, Orler R. [Vertebroplasty in severe osteoporosis. Technique and experience with multi-segment injection]. Orthopade 2004; 33(1):22–30.
13. Heini PF, Berlemann U, Kaufmann M, Lippuner K, Fankhauser C, van Landuyt P. Augmentation of mechanical properties in osteoporotic vertebral bones—a biomechanical investigation of vertebroplasty efficacy with different bone cements. Eur Spine J 2001; 10(2):164–171.
14. Heini PF, Walchli B, Berlemann U. Percutaneous transpedicular vertebroplasty with PMMA: operative technique and early results. A prospective study for the treatment of osteoporotic compression fractures. Eur Spine J 2000; 9(5):445–450.
15. Heini PF, Franz T, Fankhauser C, Gasser B, Ganz R. Femoroplasty-augmentation of mechanical properties in the osteoporotic proximal femur: a biomechanical investigation of PMMA reinforcement in cadaver bones. Clin Biomech (Bristol, Avon) 2004; 19(5):506–512.

Index

A
ACR. *See* American College of Radiology
Aging, bone metabolism changes with, 34–35
Ala. *See* Sacral wings
Alendronate therapies, 43–44
Allergies, 132, 221, 226
American College of Radiology (ACR)
 PV guidelines by, 223–243
 standards set by, 223–224
Anabolic agents, 46
Anatomy
 of cervical spine, 9–13, 10–13, CPII
 of coccyx, 9, 18, CPV
 of fractures, 23–31
 of lumbar spine, 9, 16–17, CPIV
 of sacrum, 9, 16–19, CPV
 of spine, 8–31, CPI
 of thoracic spine, 9, 13–16, CPIII–CPIV
 of vascular system in spine, 19–23, CPVII
Androgen deprivation therapy, 61
Anesthesia
 for KP, 136–137
 for lordoplasty, 137, 140–141
 modified solutions of, 117
 for PS, 205
 for PV, 117–118, 136–137
Ankylosing spondylitis, 263–264

Annual physical examination, 39–40
Anterior cervical approach, 272–276, CPII
Anterior column
 compressive stresses on, 93–94
 structural reconstruction of, 55–56
Anterior endplate, 24
Anterior lever arm, 54
Antibiotics
 for cement, 101, 117, 215–216
 for PS, 203
 for PV, 116–117, 215
Anticoagulants, 81
Antiresorptive therapies, 43–45
Aortic arterial branch, 20, CPVII
Arterial supply, for vertebrae, 19–20, 220, CPVII. *See also* Aortic arterial branch; Vertebral artery
Assessment
 of bone health, 37–41
  diagnostic tools for, 37–39
  medical evaluation for, 39–41
  recommendations for, 37
 of VCFs, 53–54
Axial loads, 51–53, 93

B
Back pain. *See* Pain
Balloon, for KP

 inflation of, 139–140, 150–151, 289–290, 293–294
 Kyphx inflatable, 146
 positioning of, 139–140
 size of, 139
Balloon kyphoplasty. *See* Kyphoplasty
Biomechanics. *See also* Anterior lever arm; Axial loads; Force vectors
 of loading on spine, 54, 93–94
 of PV, 89–106
 of stabilization, 93–98
 of VCFs, 51–53
Biopsy, with PV, 118, 249–254, 252, 272, 274–275
Bisphosphonates, 43–45
Body weight, for bone health, 43
Bone matrix proteins, 36
Bone mineral density, 37, 44, 75, 94
Bone needle. *See* Needle
Bones
 assessment of, 37–41
 augmentation of
  in femoral neck, 295–297
  in pelvis, 285–288
 biopsy of, 118
 formation and resorption coupling of, 36–37
 genetics of, 33–35
 health of, 33–46
 loss of, 34, 42

Bones (*cont.*)
  metabolism changes in, 33–37
  peak mass of, 33–35
  physiology of, 33–35
  resorption of, 44, 166–167
  retropulsion of, 63, 77, 226
  of spine, 8
  strength and fracture of, 36–37
  weakened, 53
Bone scintigraphy
  of malignant VCFs, 70
  of osteoporotic VCFs, 63–69
  of sacral insufficiency fractures, 198, 282
Burst fractures, 28–29, 51, 75, 104

C

Caffeine, 42
Calcitonin, 46
Calcium, 34–36, 40–44
Cancer
  bone metastases in, 157–158
  in patients undergoing PV, 162–164
Cannula, in lordoplasty, 141–142
Carbonated beverages, 35, 42
Cardiopulmonary compromise, 221, 258
Carotid-jugular complex, 120–122, CPII
Case study
  of anterior cervical approach, 272–276
  of extreme vertebral collapse, 267–271
  of femoral neck augmentation, 295–297
  of KP in osteoporotic VCF, 289–294
  of mobile vertebra, 263–266
  of multilevel vertebroplasty, 255–258
  of percutaneous pelvic augmentation in supra-acetabular region, 285–288
  of PS, 281–284
  of single-level vertebroplasty and biopsy, 249–254
  of vertebral refracture after PV, 277–280
  of vertebra with cleft or cavity, 259–262
Cauda equina, compression of, 55, 177
Cauda equina syndrome, 174
Cavity
  in KP, 139–140
  in vertebra, 24, 26, 259–262, 264
  filling of, 259, 261–263, 265–266
Celiac disease, 36, 40
Cement. *See also* Polymethylmethacrylate (PMMA) cement
  allergic reaction to, 132
  alterations of, 99–101
  antibiotic addition for, 101, 117, 215–216
  bioresorbable, 104
  calcium-phosphate, 104
  compressive strengths of, 100
  Conformitè Europèene approval of, 99
  cytotoxicity of, 92, 104
  distribution of, 167–168
  embolization of, 213, 219
  fatigue of, 101–102
  FDA approval of, 99, 112
  fill of, 251, 253–254, 259, 261–262
  for hips, 297
  injection of, 100, 113–115, 124–128, 137
    in extreme vertebroplasty, 189–190
    in PS, 200–202, 205
    in PV, 163–164
  leakage of, 10, 21, 29, 75, 77, 80, 95, 97–98, 100, 112, 124–128, 131, 177, 216–218
    in disc space, 213–214
    in extreme vertebroplasty, 185–186, 189, 190–191
    imaging of, 115–116, 212, 217–218
    in KP, 134, 146, 211, 290, 293
    in KP v. PV, 148–149, 152
    in PS, 200, 205, 207, 284
    in PV, 163–165, 167, 180, 211
    in thoracic vertebra, 15
    in treatment of metastatic lesions, 158–159
  mixing devices for, 126
  monomer-to-polymer ratio of, 99
  necrosis around, 89–90, 104
  pain relief v. dose of, 94–95, 127–128
  pedicle screw augmentation with, 57
  PMMA alternatives of, 3, 104
  preparation of, 124
  for PS, 205
  radio-opacification of, 4, 99–100
  tests of, 101–102
  thickness of, 127, 211, 213
  viscosity of, 97
  visualization of, 80
  volume of, 94–96, 127–128, 186–187, 205, 280
Center of gravity, 93–94
Cervical spine, 273
  anatomy of, 9, 10–13, CPII–CPIII
  CT visualization of PV for, 115
  extreme vertebroplasty for, 185–189
  fracture biomechanics in, 51–53
  metastases in, 77, 159, 161, 272–276
  needle approaches for, 11–13, 120–121, 272–276, CPII–CPIII
  PV in, 10–11, 272–276
  vertebral lesions in, 77
Chance fractures, 28–29
Channels, in KP, 139–140
Chemical mechanisms, in PV, 92
Chemotherapy, with PV, 157, 166, 169–170
Chronic obstructive pulmonary disease (COPD), 113, 213, 221
Classification, of VCFs, 51–52
Cleft, in vertebra, 24, 26, 150, 250, 253, 259–262, 264

Coagulopathy, 161, 203, 219–220, 226
Coaxial needle exchange, 189, 191
Coaxial needle placement, 191
Coccyx, anatomy of, 9, 18, CPV
Complications
   definition of, 239
   of extreme vertebroplasty, 185–186, 189
   in KP, 146–147, 210–221
   in KP v. PV, 152–153
   minimizing of, 210
   in PV, 78–80, 100, 131–132, 146, 164–165, 179–180, 210–221, 240–241
   rate of, 214–215, 233–234, 241
   SIR Standards of Practice Committee classification of, 242
Compression. See also Vertebral compression fracture
   of cauda equina, 55, 177
   for cement tests, 101–102
   severe, 24, 26–27, 76–77, 194, 267–270, CPVIII
   of spinal cord, 55, 71, 78, 159, 161, 166, 169, 177–178, 216–218
   of spine, 93–94
   of vertebrae, 23–30
   for vertebral body tests, 102–104
Compressive modulus, 101–102
Compressive yield strength, 101–102
Computed tomography (CT)
   of aggressive VHs, 171–173
   for anterior cervical approach, 272–273, 275–276
   of asymptomatic VHs, 170–171
   for bone health assessment, 39
   of cement leak, 212, 217–218
   continuous, 191
   with fluoroscopy, for extreme vertebroplasty, 185–191
   for KP and PV, CPX
   of malignant compression fractures, 70
   of osteoporotic VCFs, 63–65
   of pelvic augmentation, 286
   of posterior wall destruction, 162, 186, 188
   for PS, 200–206, 257
   with PV for VHs, 179
   of sacral insufficiency fractures, 198–199, 282–284
   with thecal sac marked by myelographic contrast, 188
   of tumor infiltration, 187
   of VHs, 73–74
   visualization with, 11–13, 100, 113–116, 137
Conformitè Europèene, cements approved by, 99
Contraindications, for PV, 71, 76–78, 116, 158–161, 225–226, 239–240
COPD. See Chronic obstructive pulmonary disease
Corticosteroids, 61
Cost, for KP v. PV, 147, 153, 291
CT. See Computed tomography
CT fluoroscopy, 206
Cytotoxicity, of cement, 92, 104

D
Death
   from KP, 220–221
   in KP v. PV, 152
   from PV, 132, 220–221
Decompression
   anterior, 55–56
   indirect, 56
   neural, 55–57
   before PV, 71
Deformity, progressive, 54–55, 55
Denis classification, of VCFs, 51–52
Deramond, Hervé, 145
DEXA. See Dual energy x-ray absorptiometry
Diagnostic tools, for assessing bone health, 37–39
Discharge, following PV, 128–130
Discitis, 76
Disc space leaks, 213–214
Discs, pressure on, 98

Disease states
   bone metabolism changes with, 35–36
   in causes of VCFs, 60–73
Documentation, in PV, 232–234
Dual energy x-ray absorptiometry (DEXA), 37–39, 40
   International Society for Clinical Densitometry Criteria for Diagnosis by, 38

E
Emboli
   cement, 213, 219
   pulmonary, 131, 211–213, 219, 221, 258
Emergency support, for PV, 230
Environmental factors, bone metabolism changes with, 35
Epidural abscess, 76
Estrogen, 43–45
Ethanol
   glue v., 179
   injection of, 166, 175–177, 179–180
Evaluation, of patient, 60–81
Exercise. See Physical activity
Extravasation. See Cement
Extreme vertebral collapse, 192–195, 226, 267–271

F
Facility, for PV, 230
Family history, for bone health assessment and osteoporosis screening, 39
Family, PV expectations of, 80–81
FDA. See Food and drug administration
Femoral neck augmentation, 295–297
Femurs, failure and load of, 296
Fever, following PV, 216
Fluoroscopy
   biplane equipment for, 113–114
   of cement leak, 212

Fluoroscopy (cont.)
  with CT, for extreme
      vertebroplasty,
      185–191
  examination under, 81
  of KP, 294
  of pelvic augmentation,
      287–288
  for PS, 200, 206–207
  single-plane equipment for,
      113–114
  for visualization during
      cement injection, 100,
      113–115, 137
Folate, 42
Food and Drug Administration
    (FDA)
  cements approved by, 99, 112
  PMMA warning by, 148
Foramina, 29, 200, 204–207,
    CPVI
Force vectors, of fracture, 51–52
Fractures. See also Extreme
    vertebral collapse;
    Malignant
    compression fractures;
    Sacral insufficiency
    fractures; Vertebral
    compression fracture
  acute v. chronic, 62–69
  adjacent, 98
  anatomy of, 23–31
  biomechanics of, 51–53
  blow-out, from KP, 211–212
  bone strength and, 36–37
  burst, 28–29, 51, 75, 104
  chance, 28–29
  classification of, 51–52
  compression, 23–30
  following PV, 130–131
  of hip, 295–297
  ipsilateral pubic, 207
  ischial ramus, 207
  multiple adjacent, 53–54
  of pedicles, 28
  in posterior elements of
      vertebra, 29, 263–264
  of ribs, 216
  sheer, 29–31
  simple, 23–29
  successive, 54–55
  traumatic, 226
  vertical, 28
  in weakened bone, 53

FSU. See Functional spine unit
Functional spine unit (FSU),
    augmented v.
    unaugmented, 98
Fusion, of spinal levels, 98

G
Genetics, of bones, 33–35
Glue
  ethanol v., 179
  injection of, 177–179
Guide wire, insertion of,
    138–141, CPXI

H
Height
  loss of, 24, 192–195, 267–271
  restoration of, 76, 97,
      192–193, 262, 264–265
    by KP, 134–136, 146–147,
      291
    KP v. PV, 148–153
    by lordoplasty, 135, 141
    in mobile vertebra,
      263–266
    in vertebral refracture,
      278–279
Hemiarthroplasty, 297
Hemorrhage, 219–220
Hemostasis, following PV,
    128
Hip fracture, 295–297
History
  of KP, 145–147
  of PV, 3–5, 145–147
H-shaped fracture, 198–201,
    203, 281–284
Hyperextension, 134, 136–137,
    192, CPX

I
Image guidance
  during KP, 137–138
  during PV, 113–116, 137–138
Incidents, in PV and KP,
    211–214
Indications
  for KP, 134–135
  for PV, 73–76, 158–161,
      225–226, 239–240
  for PV, KP, and lordoplasty,
      134–136
  for surgery, 55
  of VHs, 173–174

Infection, 76, 116, 131, 161, 203,
    234
  PV risk of, 101, 117
  spinal, 215–216
Inferior endplate, 24
Informed consent, 112–113, 203,
    233
Injection. See also Cement
  of absolute ethanol, 166,
      175–177, 179–180
  of glue, 177–179
  pressure of, 97, 148
  unipedicular, 96–97, 128, 129
Instability
  of fracture, 192
  of spine, 53–54
Instant vertebral assessment,
    38
International Society for
    Clinical Densitometry,
    DEXA diagnosis
    criteria of, 38
Intraarterial embolization,
    166
Intravenous procedural
    sedation, 117–118
Ischemia, 92, 164

J
Jargon. See Marketing

K
Kinematics, of spine, 98
KP. See Kyphoplasty
Kummell's disease, 63, 68
Kyphoplasty (KP), 8, 24, 76, 97,
    134–143, 150, 292–294.
    See also Balloon, for
    KP
  adjacent disc pressure
      changes by, 98
  blow-out fractures from,
      211–212
  cement leaks in, 134, 146,
      148–149, 152, 211, 290,
      293
  complications in, 132,
      146–147, 152–153,
      210–221, 214–215
  costs of, 147, 153, 291
  fluoroscopic image of, 294
  height restoration by,
      134–136, 146–153, 291
  history of, 145–147

image guidance for, 137–138
incidents in, 211–214
indications for, 134–136
injection pressure in, 148
kyphosis reduction by, 151–152
lordoplasty v., 135
marketing jargon for, 147–148
mechanical stabilization by, 147–148
monitoring for, 136–137
for osteoporotic VCF, 289–294
oxygen administration during, 136
pain relief by, 146–147
patient positioning in, 136–137
PV v., 145–154, 216–217
research needed in, 152–153
safety of, 152–153
side effects of, 112
surgical technique for, 136–140, CPXI
    percutaneous extrapedicular, 140
    percutaneous transpedicular, 137–140
training for, 210
treatment timing in, 150–151
visualization during, 137–138, CPX
Kyphosis, 8–9, 40, 51–53, 75, 289, CPI
reduction of, 57, 97, 134–136, 142–143, 151–152, 192
Kyphx inflatable balloon. See Balloon, for KP

L
Laminectomy, with PV, 180
Lateral sparing, 24, 27, 192, 270, CPVIII
Lesions. See also Metastases; Vertebral hemangioma
    benign, PV for, 170–180
    extreme vertebroplasty for, 185–195
    sclerosis of, 175–176, 179
Ligamentotaxis, 142–143
Local anesthetics. See Anesthesia

Lordoplasty, 134–143, 137, 140–141
    differentiated indications for, 134–136
    height restoration by, 135, 141
    KP v., 135
    kyphosis reduction by, 135, 142–143
    reduction maneuver in, 142–143
    surgical technique for, 140–143, CPXII
Lordosis, 8–9, 51–53, CPI
Lumbar spine
    anatomy of, 9, 16, 17, CPIV
    fracture biomechanics in, 51–53
Lytic lesions, 163, 167, 285–286

M
MAC. See Monitored anesthesia care
Magnetic resonance imaging (MRI)
    of arterial system in vertebra, 220
    of cavity in vertebra, 260, 264
    of cervical spine, 273
    of extreme compression, 194, 268
    of height restoration, 264
    of Kummell's disease, 63
    of malignant compression fractures, 71
    of multilevel vertebroplasty, 255–256
    of multiple myeloma, 167
    of osteoporotic VCFs, 62–69
    of paravertebral vessels, 220
    of sacral insufficiency fractures, 199, 202
    of single-level vertebroplasty, 249–250
    of tumor infiltration, 187
    of venous system in vertebra, 213, 220
    of VHs, 73–74, 170–173
Malignant compression fractures, 69–71, 70, 71, 77, 78
Marketing, for KP, 147–148
Mechanical mechanisms, in PV, 92

Medical evaluation, for bone health assessment and osteoporosis screening, 39–41
Medical history, for bone health assessment and osteoporosis screening, 39
Medical physicist, qualifications and responsibilities of, 229
Medical therapy, failure of, 225, 239
Medication history, for bone health assessment and osteoporosis screening, 39
Menopause, 35, 43–44
Metastases, 157, 162
    in cervical spine, 77, 159, 161, 272–276
    ethanol injection for, 166
    intraarterial embolization for, 166
    needle approach for, 163
    osteolytic, 69–70
    pathology of, 157–158
    patient demographics for, 157–158
    posterior wall destruction by, 158–159
    PV treatment of, 75, 157–166
    radicular pain in PV of, 159
    RFA treatment of, 166
    spinal, 157–158
    surgery for, 166
    thermal ablation for, 166
    VCFs with, 158
Metastatic adenocarcinoma, 72
Metastatic carcinoma, 285
Metastatic disease, 296
Microfracture, 75, 164
Micromotion, 94–95
Monitored anesthesia care (MAC), 136–137
Monitoring
    for KP, 136–137
    for PV, 136–137
Monomer-to-polymer ratio, 99
Motor deficit, following PV, 131
Multiple myeloma, 69, 71
    imaging of, 167
    pathology of, 166–167

Multiple myeloma (cont.)
  patient demographics of, 166–167
  PV for, 166–170
  VCFs in, 167
Myelographic contrast, 186, 188, 217–218
Myeloma, 157, 276, 296–297
Myelopathy, 174

N
N-butyl cyanoacrylate glue, 177
Necrosis, 90–92, 164
  by cement, 89–90, 104
Needle approach
  anterolateral, 11–12, 16, 23, 77, 118, 120–122
  in cervical spine, 11–13, 120–121, 272–276, CPII–CPIII
  considerations for, 21–23
  for extreme vertebral collapse, 192–195, 270–271
  lateral, 77, CPIII
  in lumbar spine, 16, CPIV
  for metastatic lesions, 163
  parapedicular, 16–17, 23, 77, 118–121, 219–220, 280, CPIV
  in pelvic augmentation, 287–288
  posterior-oblique, 19, CPVI
  posterolateral, 16, 118, 180, 204, CPVI
  for PS, 203–205, 283–284
  for refracture, 280
  in sacrum, 19, CPVI
  in severe compression, 24, 76–77, 267–270, CPVIII
  in thoracic spine, 14–16
  trans-oral, 11, 23, 77
  trans-SI, 19, 204, CPVI
Needles. See also Coaxial needle exchange; Coaxial needle placement
  Chiba, 191
  double v. single technique, 123–124
  for extreme vertebroplasty, 190
  introduction of, 118–124
  positioning of, 122–123, 137–138, 140, 189, 211–212
  size of, 118, 163–164
Neoplastic disease, 121, 225, 240
Neurologic compression, following PV, 131
Neurologic deficit, 55
Nonunion, of vertebral bodies, 24, 26
Nursing, qualifications and responsibilities of, 229
Nutrition assessment, for bone health assessment and osteoporosis screening, 39
Nutrition, for bone health, 41–42

O
Opacification, of PV cement, 4, 99–100
Osteomyelitis, 76, 226
Osteonecrosis, 24, 45, 176–177, 226
Osteopenia, 36, 40, 42–43, 63, 94
  DEXA definition of, 37–38
Osteoporosis, 94, 134, 225, 238, 255, 295
  bone scintigraphy of VCFs of, 63–69
  in cervical spine, 11
  CT of VCFs of, 63–65
  definition of, 33
  DEXA definition of, 37–38
  medical management of, 33–36
  MRI of VCFs of, 62–69
  pharmacologic therapy for, 44–46
  laboratory screening for, 40
  prevention of, 41–46
  primary, 23, 61, 64–65
  prophylactic treatment of, 75
  public health impact by, 33
  radiographs of VCFs of, 63–67
  screening for, 37–41
  secondary, 23, 39, 61, 75
  successive fracture and progressive deformity in, 54–55
  success rates for, 240
  traction for, 192–193
  treatment of, 41–46
  VCFs resulting from, 5, 55–57, 60–69, 78
Overfilling, 10
Oxygen administration, for PV and KP, 136

P
Pain, 24
  in back, 73, 161–162, 173–174
  cement dose v. relief of, 94–95, 127–128
  chronic v. new, 251
  differentiation of, 60, 78
  diffuse v. focal, 159, 161
  following PV, 128, 131, 216
  as indication for PV, 73
  as indication for surgery, 55
  from malignant compression fractures, 69
  mechanism for PV relief of, 89–92
  postvertebroplasty stiffness relief of, 95
  as PV complication, 79
  radicular, 159
  relief of
    by KP, 146–147
    by PV, 76–77, 80, 89, 130–131, 146, 164, 169–170, 179, 240, 262
  in PV v. KP, 291
  by radiation therapy, 170
  of sacral insufficiency fractures, 197–198
  sacroiliac, 207–208
  from VCF, 62
Palpitation, of painful vertebrae, 81
Paraplegia, 217–218
Paraspinous hematoma, 120
Parathyroid hormone derivatives, 46
Paravertebral vessels, 21–23, 220
Patient
  discharge of, 128–130
  education concerns for, 234
  evaluation of, 60–81, 174–175
  high v. low risk, 112–113
  with malignant compression fractures, 69

with metastases, 157–158,
    161–162
with multiple myeloma,
    166–167
physician-referred, 78
positioning of, 134–137, 192,
    203, 263, 266, 279, CPX
postprocedural care of,
    231–232
preprocedural care of, 231
procedural care of, 231
PV expectations of, 80–81
PV instructions for, 81
selection of, 60–81, 161–162,
    202–203
self-referred, 78
with VCF, presentation of,
    62
with VHs, 170–175
Pedicles, 13–14, 16, 28, 70, 163
Pedicle screw instrumentation,
    56–67
Pedicle subtraction osteotomy,
    57
Pelvis. *See* Percutaneous pelvic
    augmentation
Percutaneous pelvic
    augmentation, in
    supra-acetabular
    region, 285–288
Percutaneous sacroplasty (PS),
    8, 197–208, 281–284
    diagnosis for, 197–200
    incidence of, 197
    needle trajectories for, 204
    patient selection and
        evaluation for,
        202–203
    puncture sites for, 203–205
    technique for, 203–207
        with CT guidance, 200–206
        with fluoroscopic
            guidance, 206–207
Percutaneous vertebroplasty
    (PV), 8, 60, 116–118,
    136–137, 215–216,
    238
    antitumoral effect of, 163–164
    for benign lesions, 170–180
    biomechanical considerations
        of, 89–106
    with biopsy, 272, 274–275
    for burst fractures, 75
    in cancer patients, 162–164

cement leaks in, 148–149,
    152, 163–165, 167, 180,
    211
of cervical vertebrae, 10–11,
    272–276
chemical mechanisms of, 92
with chemotherapy, 157, 166,
    169–170
clinical outcomes for, 234
complications in, 78–80, 100,
    131–132, 146, 152–153,
    164–165, 179–180,
    210–221, 240–241
    rates and thresholds for,
    214–215, 233–234, 241
contraindications for, 71,
    76–78, 116, 158–161,
    225–226
costs of, 147, 153, 291
definition of, 238–239
early development of, 3–5
evaluation of VH patients
    for, 174–175
external traction for, 192–193
extreme, 185–195
    for cervical spine, 185–189
    complications of, 185–186,
        189
    CT for, 185–191
    fluoroscopy for, 185–191
    for thoracic spine, 185–189
    for extreme vertebral
        collapse, 192–195
first case of, 3–4
fluoroscopic visualization of,
    100
height restoration by,
    148–153
hemostasis following, 128
history of, 3–5, 145–147
image guidance for, 113–116,
    137–138
incidents in, 211–214
increased fracture risk with,
    130–131
indications for, 73–76,
    158–161, 225–226
infection risk of, 101, 117
informed consent for,
    112–113, 233
injection pressure in, 148
KP v., 145–154, 216–217
kyphosis reduction by,
    151–152

materials for, 99–104
    mechanical tests of,
        101–104
mechanical mechanisms of,
    92
mechanical stabilization by,
    147–148
for metastatic lesions,
    157–166
    cement injection in,
        163–164
    patient selection and
        evaluation in, 161–162
    results of, 164
    side effects of, 164–165
    technique for, 162–164
monitoring for, 136–137
of multiple levels, 80–81
for multiple myeloma,
    166–170
    cement distribution in,
        167–168
    results of, 169
    technique for, 167–169
needle introduction during,
    118–124
needles for, 118–119
oxygen administration
    during, 136
pain following, 128, 131, 216
pain relief by, 76–77, 80, 89,
    130–131, 146, 164,
    169–170, 179, 240, 262,
    291
patient and family
    expectations for, 80–81
patient care in, 231–232
patient discharge after,
    128–130
patient instructions for, 81
patient positioning in,
    134–137, 192
postprocedure care for,
    128–130
postvertebroplasty stiffness
    by, 95
preprocedure consultation
    for, 79–81
preprocedure laboratory
    studies for, 81
for preventing secondary
    osteonecrosis with
    ethanol injection,
    176–177

Percutaneous vertebroplasty (PV) (cont.)
  procedure technique for, 112–132
  for prophylactic treatment, 75–76
  quality improvement guidelines for, 237–243
  with radiation therapy, 75, 157, 165–166, 169–170, 251–254
  refracture after, 277–280
  research needed in, 152–153
  results of, 130–131
  risks in, 233
  for sacrum, 200
  safe performance of, 80, 225
    knowledge and skills required for, 228–229
  safety of, 152–153
  for secondary osteoporosis, 75
  side effects of, 112
  standards for performance of, 223–243
  surgical and emergency support for, 230
  surgical technique for, 136–137
  above T5 or T6 level, 77
  technical points of, 3–4
  technical requirements for, 230
  thermal mechanisms of, 90–92
  timing of, 73–75
  training for, 210
  for traumatic VCFs in young patients, 75, 77
  treatment timing in, 150–151
  for tumor infiltration, 75
  for VCF treatment, 4–5, 55
  for VH treatment, 71–73
    with complementary ethanol injection, 175–177, 179, 180
    with complementary glue injection, 177–179
    CT with, 179
    with laminectomy, 180
    with radiation therapy, 180
    results of, 179
    side effects and complications of, 179–180
    with surgical excision, 180
    technique for, 175–179
    with transarterial embolization, 180
    visualization and imaging during, 137–138, CPX
    volume fill in, 94–96
Pharmacologic therapies, for osteoporosis, 44–46
Physical activity, for bone health, 42–43
Physician
  certification of, 227
  knowledge and skills of, 228–229
  maintenance of competency by, 229
  qualifications and responsibilities of, 226–229
  residency or fellowship of, 227–228
Physician-referral, of patients, 78
Physiology, of bones, 33–35
Plain film imaging, 70, 73
PMMA cement. See Polymethylmethacrylate cement
Pneumothorax, 23, 77, 80, 120
Polymerization, of PMMA cement, 90–92
Polymethylmethacrylate (PMMA) cement, 3, 80–81, 89, 90–92, 104, 148, 295–296
Postprocedure care, for PV, 128–130
Postvertebroplasty stiffness, 95
Preprocedure consultation, for PV, 79–81
Presentation
  for anterior cervical approach, 272
  of extreme vertebral collapse, 267
  for KP, 289
  of malignant compression fracture, 69
  of multilevel vertebroplasty, 255
  for percutaneous pelvic augmentation, 285–288
  of PS patient, 281
  of single-level VCF, 249
  of VCF patients, 62
  of vertebral refracture after PV, 277
  of vertebra with cleft or cavity, 259
Prevention, of osteoporosis, 41–46
Prophylaxis, 75–76, 258, 296
PS. See Percutaneous sacroplasty
Public health, osteoporosis impact on, 33
Pulmonary compromise, 75, 112–113, 132, 226
Pulmonary disease, 219
Pulmonary emboli, 131, 211–213, 219, 221, 258
Pulmonary infarct, 219
Puncture sites, for PS, 203–205
PV. See Percutaneous vertebroplasty

Q

Quality control, 234
  of PV equipment, 232
Quality improvement, 234
  for PV, 232–234, 237–243
    complications in, 240–241
    contraindications in, 239–240
    definitions in, 238–239
    deviation from SIR guidelines for, 242–243
    indications in, 239–240
    preamble of, 237
    SIR methodology for development of guidelines in, 237–238
    success rates for, 240

R

Radiation therapy, 75, 157, 165–166, 169–170, 180, 251–254
Radiculopathy, 71, 77, 164–165, 208, 216, 226
Radiofrequency ablation (RFA), 166

Radiographs
  of ankylosing spondylosis, 264
  of asymptomatic VHs, 170–171
  of biopsy, 252
  of cavity in vertebra, 260–261
  of cement filling, 253–254
  of cervical spine, 275
  of extreme vertebral collapse, 269–270
  of femoral neck, 296–297
  of height restoration, 265
  of KP, 292–294
  of multilevel vertebroplasty, 257
  of multiple myeloma, 167
  of osteoporotic VCFs, 63–67
  of pelvic augmentation, 286
  of sacral insufficiency fractures, 198
  of severe VCF, 264
  with thecal sac marked by myelographic contrast, 188
  of VCF, 290
  of vertebral refracture, 278–279
  of VH, 74
Radiological technologist, qualifications and responsibilities of, 229
Radio-opacification. See Opacification
Raloxifene, 43–45
Recommended dietary allowances
  for calcium, 41
  for vitamins, 41–42
Reduction maneuver, in lordoplasty, 142–143
Refracture, following PV, 277–280
Reiley, Mark, 146
Reproductive function assessment, for bone health assessment and osteoporosis screening, 39
Retroperitoneal hematoma, 219
RFA. See Radiofrequency ablation
Ribs, fractures in, 216
Risks, in PV, 233

S

Sacral insufficiency fractures, 19, 29–31, 255, CPIX, CPV–CPVI
  conventional treatment of, 200
  CT visualization of PV for, 115
  diagnosis of, 197–200
  fractures concurrent with, 207
  incidence of, 197
  morbidity and mortality of, 197
  patterns of, 198–201, 203, 281–284
  PS for, 281–284
Sacral wings, 18, 30–31
Sacroiliac (SI) joints, 16–19, CPV
Sacroplasty. See Percutaneous sacroplasty
Sacrum, 30, CPIX. See also Percutaneous sacroplasty; Sacral insufficiency fractures; Sacral wings
  anatomy of, 9, 16–19, CPV
Safety, 234
  in KP v. PV, 152–153
Sclerosis, of lesion, 175–176, 179
Sedation, 203. See also Intravenous procedural sedation
  conscious, 158–159
Selection, of patient, 60–81, 161–162, 202–203
Selective estrogen receptor modulators, 43–45
Self-referral, of patients, 78
Sheer fractures, 29–31
Side effects, of PV and KP, 112, 164–165, 179–180
SI joints. See Sacroiliac joints
Simple fracture, 23–29
Single x-ray absorptiometry, 38
SIR. See Society of Interventional Radiology
Social history, for bone health assessment and osteoporosis screening, 39
Society of Interventional Radiology (SIR)
  PV guidelines by, 223–243
  Standards of Practice Committee of, 237
  complications classification by, 242
Soda. See Carbonated beverages
Solitary bone plasmacytoma, 167, 169
Spinal cord, compression of, 55, 71, 78, 159, 161, 166, 169, 177–178, 216–218
Spine
  altered kinematics of, 98
  anatomy of, 8–31, CPI
  asymptomatic lesions of, 159–160
  biomechanical loading of, 54, 93–94
  bones of, 8
  columns of, 93
  compressive stresses on, 93–94
  curvature of, 8
  fusion in, 98
  infection in, 215–216
  multiple lesions of, 159–160
  segments of, 8–9
  stability of, 147–148
  stress concentration in, 98
Spineplex, 124, 126
Stability, of spine, 147–148
Stabilization, biomechanical, 93–98
Standards, for PV performance, 223–243
  development of, 224
  documentation in, 232–234
  equipment quality control in, 232
  indications and contraindications for PV in, 225–226
  patient care in, 231–232
  personnel qualifications and responsibilities in, 226–230
  procedure specifications in, 230–232
  quality improvement in, 232–234

Standards, for PV performance (*cont.*)
  surgical and emergency support for, 230
  technical requirements for, 230
Statins, 46
Stenosis, 77, 249, 251
Stress, on spine, 93–94, 98
Strontium, 46
Supplements, vitamin, 41–42
Supra-acetabular region, percutaneous pelvic augmentation in, 285–288
Surgery
  for metastatic lesions, 166
  with PV, 180
  for VCFs, 51–58
    indications for, 55
    open anterior approach for, 55–56
    open combined approach for, 57
    open posterior approach for, 56–57
    primary considerations of, 51–54
Surgical support, for PV, 230
Surgical technique
  for KP, 136–140, CPXI
  for lordoplasty, 140–143, CPXII
  for PV, 136–137
Systems review, for bone health assessment and osteoporosis screening, 39–40

T
Tai Chi, for bone health, 43
Temperature. *See* Thermal mechanisms
Testosterone replacement therapy, 45
Thecal sac, 186, 188, 217–218
Thermal ablation, 166
Thermal mechanisms, in PV, 90–92
Thoracic spine
  anatomy of, 9, 13–16, CPIII–CPIV
  CT visualization of PV for, 115
  extreme vertebroplasty for, 185–189
  fracture biomechanics in, 51–53
Thoracolumbar junction
  compression fracture of, 67
  osteoporotic VCFs at, 61–62
  pain in, 259, 263
Thresholds
  definition of, 239
  for PV complications, 233–234, 241
Topping off/bottoming off syndrome, 56–57
Traction, for vertebral height restoration, 192–193
Transarterial embolization, with PV, 180
Treatment
  of osteoporosis, 41–46
  timing of, 73–75, 150–151
Tumors, 157–180
  displacement of, 77, 115
  extrusion of, 186, 188, 226
  growth of, 91–92
  infiltration by, 75, 187
  PV impact on, 163–164
  as PV indication, 225

U
Ultimate compressive stress, 101–102
Ultrasound, 38–39

V
Vascular anatomy, 19–23, CPVII
VCF. *See* Vertebral compression fracture
Venogram, for PV injection, 125
Venography, 124
Venous supply, 19–23, 213, 220, CPVII
Vertebrae, CPI
  anterior body of, 24
    posterior body separation from, 28
  anterior collapse of, 53
  anterior margin of, 13–15, 211–212
  body of
    bilateral transpedicular injection in, 129
    mechanical tests of, 102–104
    unipedicular injection in, 129
  in cervical spine, 10–11, CPII–CPIII
  cleft or cavity in, 24, 26, 150, 250, 253, 259–262, 264
  compression of, 23–30
  fluoroscopy examination of, 81
  in lumbar spine, 16, 17, CPIV
  mechanical property restoration of, 94–95
  mobile, 263–266
  palpitation of, 81
  posterior body of
    anterior body separation from, 28
    malignant compression fracture involvement of, 70, 77
    spinal instability caused by weakness in, 53–54
  posterior margin of, 13–14
  posterior wall of, 24, 25
    destruction of, 185–186, 188, 217–218
    CT detection of, 162
    by metastatic lesions, 158–159
    fracture extended in, 263–264
  PV volume fill of, 94–96
  size of, 8–10
  in thoracic spine, 13, CPIII–CPIV
  vascular supply to, 19–23, CPVII
  volume of, 10
Vertebral artery, 11–13, CPIII
Vertebral compression fracture (VCF), 4, 23–30, 145, 225, 238
  with anterior cleft, 150
  asymptomatic, 76
  biomechanics of, 51–53, 89–106
  bone scintigraphy of, 63–69
  causes of, 60
  classification of, 51–52
  complications in PV treatment of, 78

CT of, 63–65
diagnosis of, 94
disease demographics of, 5
disease processes resulting in, 60–73
force vectors contributing to, 51–52
health consequences of, 61
instability of, 192
kyphotic deformity of, 124
with metastatic lesion, 158
MRI of, 62–69
multiple, 255–258
in multiple myeloma, 167
osteoporotic, 4–5, 60–69
presentation of patients with, 62
as PV indication, 225–226
PV relief of pain from, 130–131
quick assessment of, 53–54
radiographs of, 63–67
stabilization of, 94
surgical options for, 51–58
  indications for, 55
  open anterior approach in, 55–56
  open combined approach in, 57
  open posterior approach in, 56–57
  primary considerations of, 51–54
  treatment in, 55–57
traumatic, 75, 77
Vertebral hemangioma (VH), 3, 71–73, 225
aggressive, 170–174, 177, 180
  ethanol injection for, 176
asymptomatic, 170–171, 173–174
in cervical spine, 77
classification of, 173–174
CT of, 73–74
evaluation of patients with, 174–175
imagining of, 74
indications of, 173–174
pathology of, 170–173
patient demographics of, 170–173
plain film imaging of, 73
PV for, 71–73
  results of, 179
  side effects and complications of, 179–180
PV technique for, 175–179
  with complementary ethanol injection, 175–177, 179–180
  with complementary glue injection, 177–179
Vertebrectomy, 169
Vertebroplasty, 3. *See also* Percutaneous vertebroplasty
adjacent disc pressure changes by, 98
differentiated indications for, 134–136
increased fracture risk with, 98
multilevel, 255–258
with PS, 281–284
single-level with biopsy, 249–254
Visualization, during PV and KP, 137–138, CPX
Vitamin A, 42
Vitamin B complex, 42
Vitamin D, 34–35, 39–43
Vitamin K, 42
Volume
of cement fill, 94–96, 127–128, 186–187, 205, 280
of vertebrae, 10